The Selective Mutism Resource Manual – Access your online resources

The Selective Mutism Resource Manual is accompanied by a number of printable online materials, designed to ensure this resource best supports your needs.

Activate your accompanying online resources:

- Go to www.routledge.com/cw/speechmark then click on the cover of this book

- Click the 'Sign in or Request Access' button and follow the instructions, in order to access your accompanying online resources

T0132707

AUTHOR BIO

Maggie Johnson FRCSLT is a speech and language therapist specialising in childhood communication disorders and selective mutism. Her experience in education and community settings spans over thirty years in mainstream and special schools, language units, clinics and multi-agency centres. Maggie works for Kent Community Health NHS Foundation Trust.

Alison Wintgens is a speech and language therapist. Having worked for many years as a consultant SLT in the Department of Child and Adolescent Mental Health at St. George's Hospital, London, she has extensive experience of children and adolescents with a range of communication disorders and additional behavioural or mental health problems.

THE
SELECTIVE MUTISM
RESOURCE MANUAL

SECOND EDITION

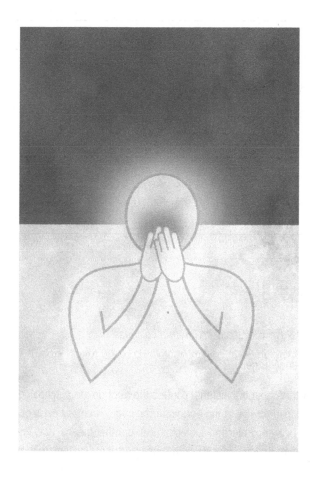

MAGGIE JOHNSON
AND ALISON WINTGENS

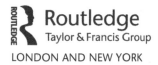

Routledge
Taylor & Francis Group

LONDON AND NEW YORK

Courage is resistance to fear, mastery of fear – not absence of fear.

Mark Twain (1835–1910)

Notes on the text

- Please note that, throughout this manual, the abbreviation 'SM' is used to refer to 'selective mutism'.

- We often specify which age group we are talking about (early years, younger children, adolescents or teenagers) but 'child' or 'children' is used where it is intended to be fairly general.

- 'Parent' refers to parent or guardian.

- 'Practitioner' refers to any therapist, psychologist or clinician working with the child and their family.

Dedications

To my Little Wurrit, who turned out to be the bravest of us all.

To Peter for his support, encouragement and patience.

First published in 2016 by Speechmark Publishing Ltd

Published 2017 by Routledge
2 Park Square, Milton Park, Abingdon, Oxon OX14 4RN
711 Third Avenue, New York, NY 10017, USA

Routledge is an imprint of the Taylor & Francis Group, an informa business

British Library Cataloguing in Publication Data

A catalogue record for this book is available from the British Library

ISBN 978 1 90930 133 7 (pbk)

CONTENTS

Part 1 Understanding Selective Mutism

Part 2 Guidelines for Identification and Assessment

Part 3 Management

Part 4 Reflective Practice: Learning from Experience

Part 5 Online Resource Library

References (research references – see Appendix E;
resource references – see Appendix F)

FOREWORD

Twenty years ago, I met the first child with selective mutism (SM) in my clinical practice. I still remember the unpleasant feeling of incompetence and the literature gave few answers. This triggered me to start researching SM for the next two decades.

In 2016, the literature and knowledge about SM have improved considerably, and there is greater agreement among clinicians on how to understand and treat the condition. Maybe the most important progress has been to categorise SM as an anxiety disorder. Nevertheless, it is still a challenge to offer adequate help for these children.

This excellent resource manual presents updated information on important aspects of SM and – above all – practical and detailed information on how to deal with the problem that is relevant for clinicians, teachers, children and adolescents with SM and their family members. It also provides lots of useful handouts. The case stories are representative, illustrate the variation of symptoms in SM and emphasise the importance of tailoring interventions for each child.

The two authors have an extensive and unique experience with children and adolescents who have SM, and their deep respect for each individual is reflected in all of the chapters. They also address muteness in all relevant arenas and the impact on important people in each child's life. This is essential for treatment success and is a clear message to our colleagues not to restrict their intervention to clinical settings.

This book contains a wealth of knowledge!

Hanne Kristensen, MD, PhD
Centre for Child and Adolescent Mental Health
Southern and Eastern Norway
(March 2016)

PREFACE

Despite more parent organisations, training, books, research and media coverage in the last 15 years, selective mutism (SM) continues to be a misunderstood condition. However, its importance is as great as ever for several reasons. Children who have SM are at a significant disadvantage both personally and socially. SM is a great barrier to learning and, if neglected or mismanaged, it may continue into adulthood with devastating effects. Yet SM is hidden and easily overlooked – 'the quiet child is the forgotten child' – and more attention and resources are directed towards children who are disruptive. Different disciplines may not agree on who should take responsibility for it; and many professionals do not have adequate training or see enough children who have SM to build up much experience.

SM has a significant and powerful effect on other people around the child, especially parents and teachers. The very nature of SM disrupts the normal process of interaction; and it is unnerving and even threatening when attempts to draw out a child are apparently rejected. It is our experience that people encountering SM for the first time rarely have sufficient information to feel confident about how to manage the child or put a treatment programme into practice, even when they are familiar with the principles involved. Furthermore, parents and professionals are sometimes afraid to intervene, in case they make the situation worse.

The earlier the situation can be addressed, the better for everyone involved.

When we met, both speaking about SM at an international conference in York in 1999, we decided to pool our experiences and perspectives as two speech and language therapists working in two different services: child and adolescent mental health and community health. We wanted to set out practical assessment and treatment, advice and information on how to identify and manage SM that was accessible for parents and a range of professionals. The result was the first edition of *The Selective Mutism Resource Manual*, published in 2001. Now, 15 years later, we have a total of over 60 years of working alongside several hundred children and young people with SM, directly and through supervision, acting as advisers, running parent groups, and teaching both in the UK and overseas.

Our ideas have inevitably developed but our approach has not changed fundamentally. This second edition of the manual is again based on the importance of having a good understanding of the nature of SM to create the right environment to manage it wisely; and the behavioural principles for building graded exposure programmes within a broader model of confident talking.

Part 1 starts with an expanded 'frequently asked questions' chapter which signposts you to other sections in the manual; the second chapter explains the rationale and framework for our methods in the light of research findings and our clinical experience. Parts 2 and 3 again give detailed ideas on assessment and management, respectively. You will see more emphasis on how parents can help their children; informal approaches for round-the-clock support; a fuller look at understanding and managing anxiety; new handouts, forms and checklists for you to access and print; and additional materials for older children and young people. We focus on home, community and educational settings, rather than clinical settings. This is because we believe that these are the environments where clinicians need to focus their involvement, either through direct work with the child or by supporting the child's family and school.

Part 4 begins with troubleshooting – practices that prevent or hinder progress. There is a chapter on identifying and managing coexisting conditions alongside SM; and a chapter with examples of interventions with various children and young people. The manual ends with insights and reflections from adults who have experienced SM in the past. We recognise that attention now needs to turn to adults who still have SM.

Please don't be put off by the size of this manual – you don't have to read it all! It remains a *resource* manual, written for a wide range of people, including teachers, clinical and educational psychologists, speech and language therapists, child psychiatrists and importantly parents, and young people and adults who have SM. It contains a lot of material which you can dip into, whichever part suits and helps you best. For example, you might start with Chapter 1 'Frequently asked questions' or head for Part 2 on assessment. The parental interview forms are more suitable for clinicians, whereas the advice in 'Ensuring an anxiety-free environment' and 'Facing fears at home and in the community' has a much wider application.

We recommend that you access and print any online resources that are relevant to your situation and the age of your child or young person. Schools or teams managing a caseload may prefer to print out all of the resources and keep them in an accompanying file for ease of access. With different readers in mind, we have aimed for a style that is appropriate for everyone. Whoever you are, we hope that this manual gives you a better understanding of SM and the confidence and tools to help alleviate it.

Maggie Johnson and Alison Wintgens
(March 2016)

AUTHORS' ACKNOWLEDGEMENTS

This book could not have been written without all the children, young people and parents with whom we have had the privilege to work. We have learned so much through them and are sure they will recognise their contributions throughout this manual. We are also most grateful to the adults who have shared their experience of SM with us and generously provided feedback as we wrote the manual or allowed their stories to be published here.

We have also benefited from the shared knowledge and practice of good colleagues and professionals we have worked alongside or been fortunate to meet. Although there are too many to name individually, after so many years in the field, we would like to especially mention Una Freeston and Peter Hill, to whom we dedicated the first edition, 'for their wisdom and the ability to communicate it'. Their inspiration lives on!

Last but not least, we would also like to thank our immediate and wider families and close friends for encouraging, supporting and bearing with us while we were writing this second edition.

LIST OF TABLES

LIST OF FIGURES

LIST OF BOXES

LIST OF ONLINE RESOURCES

Progress charts

PART 1
UNDERSTANDING SELECTIVE MUTISM

CONTENTS

FREQUENTLY ASKED QUESTIONS ABOUT SELECTIVE MUTISM

Introduction

Despite a significant increase in awareness and professional interest since the first edition of this manual, there is still much misunderstanding and disagreement about the nature of selective mutism (SM). In order to treat any condition effectively, it is important to know what we are dealing with and to dispel some of the myths. This chapter begins by listing the frequently asked questions about SM. The answers that follow will direct you to various sections of the manual or the online resource library for further reading.

Frequently asked questions

1   Does my child have SM?

2   Some children are just shy. How can I tell the difference?

3   Can't speak or won't speak?

4   Won't they just grow out of it?

5   What causes SM?

6   No child of mine would behave like that – why do parents put up with it?

7   Isn't this child just being stubborn?

8   The child was smirking at me – what's that about?

9   Is SM about having control?

10   Have children who have SM been traumatised or abused?

11   My child can talk at school so I was told it can't be SM. Is that right?

12   My child has stopped talking at playgroup. Is it SM?

13   My child does not talk at all. Does that rule out SM?

14   Why has my child stopped talking to the family too?

15   My child is getting increasingly resistant to *everything*, not just talking. What can I do?

16   Is it advisable to separate twins so that the one who has SM can't lean on the other?

17   My child found school much too stressful. Am I right to consider home-schooling?

18   Why does my child talk to strangers but not people he knows well?

19   My child is making progress but doesn't talk if I'm around, Why is that?

20   Should we be more protective of children who have SM?

21   How common is it?

22   At what age does it start?

1   Does my child have SM?

The essential feature of SM is that, in certain situations, the child speaks little or not at all while, in other situations, they are uninhibited and talk freely. The pattern is predictable and has persisted for at least a month (two months in a new setting such as school). Beyond this, no two children who have SM are exactly alike.

After many years of misunderstanding, SM is now recognised as an anxiety disorder. This does not mean that your child is anxious all the time; it's at specific times when they sense an expectation to speak that their anxiety levels shoot up. For example, it may be easy to talk to parents in a large, noisy, impersonal supermarket but impossible in the corner shop where every word can be heard. Suddenly their body and face stiffen and their communication becomes non-existent or reduced to whispers, single words, short phrases or simple gestures. Similarly, a child may talk happily to their friends in the playground but clam up as soon as a teacher approaches. Everyone involved becomes expert at predicting what will happen in each situation the child is exposed to. This is very different from the 'mood-dependent' communication of emotionally disturbed children and typical teenagers which can vary on a daily basis.

Nothing characterises SM more than the sudden swings from relaxed and chatty, to wary and reticent as the child becomes aware of another person's presence. But only people in the child's comfort zone will see these swings; others only see a quiet child and may not even realise that the child speaks at all. If your child does not present these marked changes, or talks on some days but not others *in identical circumstances*, they are unlikely to have SM.

Below are a few final points to consider.

★   SM may exist alongside other diagnoses or considerations.

★   SM may be confused with other diagnoses.

★ The presentation of SM changes over time, and a child may also stop talking at home.

★ Short-lived or isolated episodes of silence do not satisfy the criteria for SM.

★ SM does not only affect speech. Children can become so anxious about talking that extreme muscular tension can interfere with their ability to point, handle objects, walk or run.

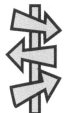

Chapter 1 'Why has my child stopped talking to the family too? (page 15)

Chapter 1 'Do I need an official diagnosis?' (page 21)

Chapter 2 A holistic view of selective mutism

Chapter 3 'Making a diagnosis' (page 53)

Chapter 13 When it is more than selective mutism

Online: Handout 2 'What is selective mutism?'

2 Some children are just shy. How can I tell the difference?

Children who have SM appear to be shy in many situations but are not necessarily shy by nature, as their families will confirm. They may appear very confident when there is no need to talk. But they become immediately tense and unresponsive when questioned by people outside their comfort zone, which does not abate until the pressure to talk has been removed.

> *Shy children may be worried about speaking; children who have SM are terrified.*

Shy children are generally unsure of themselves, slow to warm-up and slow to come forward, but they do not display the extreme aversion to speaking that characterises SM. Their facial expressions and body language convey uncertainty and hesitation rather than an unyielding stare and stiffness. With gentle support and encouragement, they gradually get used to new situations and new people, and talking comes as a natural part of gaining confidence and getting involved in activities. Having settled into school or nursery (this can take up to a month), shy children may still find it difficult to *initiate* interaction, but they are able and usually glad to respond if someone else makes the first move. Their expressive language will be no different from how they speak at home.

It is important to note that shy children may develop SM if they are subjected to ridicule or pushed into speaking before they are ready. Therefore all shy children and reluctant speakers need support and reassurance to settle in and participate at their own pace.

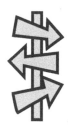

Chapter 1 'My child can talk at school so I was told it can't be SM' (page 13)

Online: Handout 3 'Quiet child or selective mutism?'

Handout 9 'Helping young children to speak at school'

3 Can't speak or won't speak?

Children who have SM speak happily to some people but clam up as soon as others enter the room. The stony look on their face can give the impression that their silence is deliberate, even defiant, and that the child is refusing to speak to certain people. This leads to remarks such as 'He'll speak when he wants to' and 'If she can't be bothered to talk to me, why should I talk to her?'

> *Understanding that selective mutism is a phobia is an important first step to providing sympathetic and appropriate support*

> Emma's teacher was frustrated: 'She's taking us all for a ride. She loves her daily session with the classroom assistant, but will only draw pictures or play. As soon as any speech is required, she digs in her heels and refuses.'

Everyone can withhold speech out of choice, but it is generally short-lived and feels nothing like being *unable* to speak. Children who have SM *want* to speak but have an irrational fear or dread – a phobia – of speaking aloud in certain situations: when expected to speak, they inwardly panic, become physically frozen and cannot utter a sound (similar to stage fright). The panic sensation is so distressing that they will go to great lengths to avoid it, including trying to prevent certain people finding out that they can speak.

It's not that they 'won't' speak; they simply can't face what happens to them when they try. Other forms of avoidance may include the use of alternative forms of communication such as gesturing, whispering, writing or using a modified voice – if these are accepted in the long term, they can become 'safe' habits which arouse no anxiety.

It is essential to regard and respond to SM as a phobia, rather than a choice to be silent.

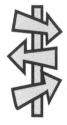

Chapter 2 A holistic view of selective mutism

Chapter 14 Examples of interventions (Daniel – whispering)

Online: Handout 5 'Selective mutism is a phobia'

4 Won't they just grow out of it?

Do children outgrow their fear of the dark? It may seem like this but, in fact, it is sympathetic handling and appropriate support that allows them to work through it. If they were repeatedly shut in a dark room despite their fear, they would grow up with a deep dread of darkness and losing control.

So it is with SM. Some children are lucky enough to get the right support and the SM is resolved. However, as SM is generally not well understood, many children are repeatedly put in situations where they are encouraged to talk, followed by disappointment or disapproval when they do not. Their dread of talking increases and their self-esteem, confidence, school work and friendships are all at risk. Left untreated for many years, some will become adults with SM. The disorder may progress until the young person no longer speaks to anyone, not even close friends or family. However, a good number work through their fears without formal intervention but inevitably experience much unhappiness along the way.

Since there is no way to identify which children will receive appropriate support or discover their own ways to face their fears, there is no guarantee that children will overcome SM. Therefore, all cases of SM should be taken seriously. Timely intervention will result in positive changes almost immediately.

> Chapter 1 'At what point should action be taken?' (page 22)
>
> Chapter 2 'The importance of early intervention' (page 44)
>
> Online: Booklet for teenagers and adults 'When the words won't come out'

> No one had heard of selective mutism when I was little. All I remember is feeling really afraid whenever someone came to our house and hiding behind the dressing table in my mother's room. I knew my behaviour was upsetting her but I didn't know how to change.
>
> 'Luckily, I had a really understanding teacher. She visited me at home and spent extra time with me at school. She didn't push me to do anything I couldn't manage and gradually I started joining in. By the time I was six or seven, I was coping pretty well but there were still times I froze completely. It wasn't until I was a teenager that I realised something had lifted and my anxiety about talking had gone.

5 What causes SM?

When children who have SM do not speak, one of two things is happening: either the prospect of speaking in certain situations fills them with such dread that they are physically *unable* to speak; or they spare themselves this intensely distressing experience by *avoiding* the need to speak. The more they experience either of these scenarios, the more their fear of speaking is reinforced.

As with other phobias, there is no single cause of SM but there are three elements that contribute to the process of 'fear conditioning': the child develops an irrational fear of talking that is triggered by specific people and the expectation to talk.

1   *A sensitive personality* – a combination of genetic (inherited) and psychological factors make individuals particularly vulnerable to developing anxiety disorders.

2   *Life events* establish a link between the need to talk and intense anxiety.

3   *Maintenance behaviour* – the reactions of other people reinforce and strengthen the child's belief that speaking is difficult, stressful and best avoided.

These three sets of contributing factors provide important clues to subsequent management of the condition. However, while it is essential to identify and address maintenance behaviour, it is not always necessary to pinpoint how or when the SM first started. Even more importantly, there is no need or value in feeling responsible or attributing blame. SM can develop despite the best intentions to provide a safe, loving and enriching environment.

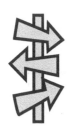

Chapter 2 A holistic view of selective mutism

Table 8.2 'Possible maintaining factors with alternative management strategies' (page 134)

Online: Form 4 'Checklist of possible maintaining factors'

Form 10 'Reactions of family/friends/staff'

6 No child of mine would behave like that. Why do parents put up with it?

SM is not caused by absent, ineffective or overindulgent parenting. Parents try their hardest to get their child to talk but nothing works. Gentle encouragement, pleading, cajoling, insistence, threats, bribes, rewards and punishments all make the child more afraid of speaking. SM is the result of a subconsciously learned fear. The only way to overcome it is to *unlearn* this fear.

> *We don't reprimand children who are afraid of the dark or force them to sleep in a dark room.*

To help understand, consider another common childhood anxiety – fear of the dark. Few children grow up with a phobia of darkness because it does not require a course in parenting to handle the situation appropriately. We recognise that offering a reward to endure a night without a light on is pointless; the incentive offered could never outweigh the child's genuine fear. We do not increase their anxiety by punishing them, telling them off, or insisting that they stay in a dark room for hours with no escape. If we did, we would soon see an increase in bed-wetting and insecurity during the day and have a fight on our hands when it came to putting the child to bed every night. Instead we leave a light on. We provide a sympathetic ear and talk openly about the child's fears. We tell them we are not far away. We find appropriate story books and tell them they won't always be scared. And, rather than keeping things as they are, we naturally implement a psychological technique called *graded exposure.* We progress from the landing light to a glow-plug and close the door a fraction, all at the child's pace, until eventually they get used to being on their own in the dark. Exactly the same techniques work for SM.

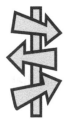

Chapter 8 Ensuring an anxiety-free environment

Chapter 9 Facing fears at home and in the community

Online: Handout 5 'Selective mutism is a phobia'

Handout 7 'Helping children to cope with anxiety'

7 Isn't this child just being stubborn?

People frequently make comments such as 'How does she manage to keep quiet for so long? She must have incredible willpower!' However, once SM is recognised as a phobia, such comments become as nonsensical as 'How on earth does she resist picking up spiders?' and 'What incredible willpower to avoid flying!' Phobic individuals do not stubbornly refuse to do the things they fear; they cannot face their fears, and cope through avoidance and more comfortable alternatives. Similarly, children who have SM may remain silent but that is not the same as 'choosing' to be silent or 'refusing' to speak. If they had any choice in the matter, they would choose not to have SM.

> Ian's father commented: 'I don't know why he won't give in. I've promised him the bike he wants when he talks to his teacher, but he simply won't do it. He's so stubborn.'

If children can find a way to avoid anxiety, naturally they will take it. If successful, they will not be anxious; just as adults with a phobia of flying are not anxious when they are not on an airplane. Consequently, children with more strong-willed personalities may be adamant that they are not going to repeat an experience which previously triggered a panic reaction, while those with more compliant personalities may dawdle or beg their parents to be excused.

When sensing the genuine distress at the root of such demands, it is tempting to allow children to opt out of activities completely. However, this is not helpful in the long term and only increases avoidance and fear of speaking. It is essential to find ways for the children to participate in non-stressful ways.

Chapter 8 Ensuring an anxiety-free environment

Chapter 9 Facing fears at home and in the community

Online: Handout 5 'Selective mutism is a phobia'

Handout 7 'Helping children to cope with anxiety'

8 The child was smirking at me. What's that about?

Just as children who have SM may be described as glaring, sullen or grumpy, they are often perceived by their teachers and other people to be smirking. These children are simply caught in a tense, frozen moment when they can neither smile nor grimace. Who knows what they are feeling? They could be trying to smile to show willing; they could be feeling panicked; they could be experiencing relief as the spotlight moves from them to another child. It is impossible to tell simply by looking …

None of us is as good at reading facial expressions as we like to think. Luckily, we usually have numerous clues: we witness the *full range of facial movement* from start to finish; and match this to *what* the individual is saying and *how* they are saying it in the context of a *two-way conversation*. However, these clues are not available when observing a silent child who has a fixed expression. Coupled with a lack of information and common misassumptions about SM, conclusions may be drawn which are detrimental to the child. Ultimately, these conclusions could make or break the quality of that child's experience of school or other social settings, as they are bound to affect the adult's attitude towards the child.

For a demonstration of how difficult it is to read facial expressions, go to http://greatergood.berkeley.edu/ ei_quiz/ and try the Body Language Quiz. Even people who achieve an above-average score are likely to make several mistakes. The quiz shows how easy it is to get facial expressions wrong and how subtle the differences are between certain expressions when there are no other contextual clues.

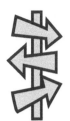

Chapter 5 Meeting and involving the child or young person

Chapter 8 'Sharing emotions' (page 126)

Chapter 10 'Talking about feelings' (page 220)

9 Is SM about having control?

Children who have SM are often said to be 'very controlling'. Control and anxiety are closely linked, as anyone with a 'control-freak' friend will know!

However, there is a difference between the control we need over our environment to keep anxiety at bay and control that is driven by power-seeking. The former is part of our basic human need to feel safe and secure. For example, we check that doors are locked, we prepare for an interview, we are reluctant to delegate if we think that mistakes will be made.

> *Children who have SM need control in order to keep their anxiety at bay.*

When she was little, Charlotte had complete control over our whole family. She wouldn't speak to anyone other than us [her parents] and her brother, so I couldn't leave her with any of my friends.

She stuck to me like a limpet and it was such a relief to find a teacher who was prepared to build a relationship with her in our own home.

In exactly the same way, children who have SM take steps to manage their anxiety about speaking. Remembering their panic in situations where they were expected to speak and the subsequent disappointment, embarrassment or humiliation when they could not, it is natural to seek damage limitation. They do this in three ways:

1 Through avoidance, as discussed in question 7.

2 By finding out every detail of what is about to happen, so that there are no surprises.

3 By stipulating changes that make the situation more manageable.

This is not manipulation or a need to dominate; it is how most people cope with anxiety. We need to give children who have SM *more* control by involving them in agreeing appropriate modifications as we work towards their full participation.

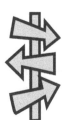

Chapter 8 Ensuring an anxiety-free environment

Chapter 9 Facing fears at home and in the community

Chapter 10 Facing fears in educational settings

Online: Handout 7 'Helping children to cope with anxiety'

10 Have children who have SM been traumatised or abused?

SM is *not* an emotional reaction to situations resulting in grief, anger or distress which affect us all, or an emotional disturbance linked to recurring memories of shocking events. Unfortunately, it is often confused with 'traumatic' or 'reactive' mutism which is a symptom of post-traumatic stress disorder (PTSD). Every popular bookshop has titles about children who have suddenly become mute after tragic events and gradually regain their speech over months or years as they come to terms with the horrors of their past. Children with reactive mutism communicate normally before the precipitating event and become withdrawn across all environments afterwards. In contrast, children who have SM only find it difficult to communicate in specific situations. The vast majority have experienced nothing out of the ordinary and, as a group, they are no more (and no less) likely to have been abused than any other child.

Yet there may well be a critical event that triggers SM, such as getting lost, being left with strangers or in an overwhelming environment, waking to find an unexpected baby-sitter or being teased about poor pronunciation. The situation is traumatic for the child but it is the child's *reaction* to the event that is extreme, rather than the event itself.

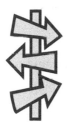

Chapter 2 A holistic view of selective mutism

Chapter 3 'Traumatic mutism' (page 55)

Online: Appendix E 'Evidence base'

11 My child can talk at school so I was told it can't be SM. Is that right?

Children who have SM are not necessarily silent at school but there will be a consistent pattern to their speaking habits. For example, they may speak to one or more adults but not children; or to children but not adults; or in the playground but not in the classroom.

A less obvious pattern occurs when children are able to give minimal responses but do not ask questions, initiate conversations or speak up when something is wrong, unless they have been specifically instructed to do so. For example, they give very short answers, or join in shared or routine activities such as singing or answering the register, or pass on a short message at someone else's request. This 'low profile' SM tends to be regarded as shyness, but the children do not respond to gentle encouragement and open up as shy children do. Instead, they display increasing social anxiety and a definite cut-off point where they cannot contribute further. These children have the same dread of speaking as other children who have SM, but their compliance and fear

> Avtar had left his consent form at home and firmly believed he would miss out on his class outing as a result. He loitered at the end of the day until his class teacher gently asked what was wrong. Finally, he spoke for the first time.
>
> After this, Avtar spoke to his teacher whenever she asked him a question, but remained unable to initiate conversation.

of breaking rules make them equally afraid of incurring disapproval. They therefore manage minimal responses to comply with adult expectation.

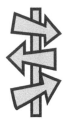

Chapter 1 'Some children are just shy. How can I tell the difference?' (page 7)

Chapter 2 'High and low profile SM' (page 31)

Chapter 4 'The child's speaking habits' (page 65)

Online: Handout 3 'Quiet child or selective mutism?'

12 My child has stopped talking at playgroup. Is it SM?

Young children who have SM generally do not *start* talking to the people they meet in new environments. If a child suddenly stops talking to one or more people they previously spoke to freely, another explanation should be sought. They have probably been criticised, physically hurt by another child, or frightened by something they have seen or heard, and lack the emotional development, expressive language or assertiveness to cope with the situation. Once they have been helped to identify or communicate the trigger, and it has been addressed with reassurance that it won't happen again, talking usually resumes fairly quickly.

However, if the situation is not dealt with, and the child goes through an extended period of silence and anxiety, during which they feel under pressure to speak, there is a danger that the child will come to link their anxiety to *talking* in the setting, rather than a specific incident. At this point, they are more likely to meet the criteria for SM and may transfer their fear of talking to other people or settings.

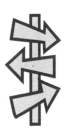

Chapter 3 'Indicators against a diagnosis of SM' (page 55)

13 My child does not talk at all. Does that rule out SM?

If your child has *never* spoken, or has regressed after an event such as a seizure, this is not SM. An expert assessment is needed to ascertain the reason for their lack of speech. Some children have physical, neurological, perceptual or cognitive difficulties which delay or prevent normal speech development.

If a child has been speaking normally in all situations but suddenly stops speaking altogether, this would be *total* rather than *selective* mutism. Any kind of shock, such as a serious accident or being evacuated from a burning house, can temporarily overwhelm a child into silence. It can take time for them to understand the event and their emotions, and feel reassured that they are now safe. If there is no obvious trigger, the situation should always be investigated because the child might have experienced or witnessed a more disturbing threat or assault – thankfully, this is very rare.

All individuals with SM speak to fewer and fewer people in the initial stages. Just as a phobia of one cat can generalise to a phobia of all cats, toy cats and pictures of cats, the child's fear of talking becomes associated with more and more people. This rarely affects the people they talk to freely. However, the process sometimes continues until they do not talk even to the close friends or family members they had no difficulty with initially. This is known as 'progressive mutism' and generally means that the SM has not been handled well or has been complicated by other events which have traumatised the child. All of the contributing factors will need to be addressed.

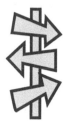

Chapter 1 'Why has my child stopped talking to the family too?' (see below)

Chapter 3 'Traumatic mutism' (page 55)

Chapter 9 'Progressive mutism' (page 170)

Chapter 13 When it is more than selective mutism

14 Why has my child stopped talking to the family too?

As discussed above, some children who have SM stop talking to family members as part of a gradual shutdown or 'progressive mutism'. The possible reasons for this are outlined below. Sometimes a sudden silence is unrelated to SM but it is assumed that the child's SM has 'spread' to the immediate family. Always look at the overall pattern of talking in all settings, together with events in the child's life around the time they stopped talking to family members.

a) Children with SM and rigid thinking patterns or autism spectrum disorder (ASD) may have an issue with conflicting 'rules'. These rules are not determined by the child; they represent the pattern of speaking that emerges after fear conditioning takes place (see page 9). For example, when home and nursery are kept completely separate, there is no issue and the child may internalise the rules 'I can talk to Mum and Dad' but 'I can't talk to my teacher'. However, as boundaries blur, there is a clash; for example, Mum comes into school and the child can't talk to her in front of their teacher. This can be an enormous shock to a child with poor reasoning abilities. The panic that is triggered by the teacher being within earshot becomes associated with talking to Mum. Rather than modify the first rule to 'I can talk to Mum when no one else is listening', some children produce a simpler rule: 'I can't talk to my teacher or my Mum'.

b) When SM is not openly accepted and addressed, fear of being overheard by anyone who might 'spill the beans' is a major concern. For example, children may stop more and more social activities, to avoid friends from their talking and non-talking circles meeting. Similarly, if children are under pressure to talk at school, they may be terrified that their teacher will increase the expectation to talk once it comes out that they have spoken to a friend or speak at home. Children in this situation often *deny* that they have spoken. It may be less distressing to stop talking at home too.

> I went to dance classes outside school and could just about speak there. Then someone from school showed up. I couldn't stand the stress of hiding my speech from the girl from school, and my muteness from the rest of the dance class. So I gave up the dance class.

c) Teenagers with SM may feel intensely pressured by their teachers' or parents' lack of understanding, disappointment, criticism or entreaties to talk. Powerless to meet unrealistic expectations, and unable to face further confrontation, complete withdrawal feels like the only option.

d) As a child's SM becomes more entrenched, they may also stop talking to a parent with whom they have infrequent contact or one who is impatient, overly critical or forceful about their talking.

e) It can be very difficult for children who have SM when a virtual stranger joins the family circle; for example, when a new partner, step-parent or live-in nanny is introduced. Initially, at least, they may be unable to speak whenever this person is present, and the reasons for this may be poorly understood. If such children are pressurised into speaking before they are ready, they may stop talking at home altogether.

f) Young children often have separation anxiety and will be particularly distressed if separated from their mother for any length of time; for example, when a relative moves in while Mum is in hospital. Children may be unable to talk to this relative, either because they are so upset about their mother or because they have SM and do not know the relative well. This can set up a pattern of not talking at home which the child finds hard to break when Mum returns.

g) Children who have SM, like all children, may be bullied at school. If they are scared to tell anyone for fear of making things worse, or lack the awareness or vocabulary to explain what is happening, they may become increasingly withdrawn at home as well.

h) A child or young person with SM may experience *additional* trauma or upset that leaves them unable to speak. For example, bereavement and illness can leave individuals too shocked, fatigued or feverish to speak to close family in the short term. Usually this would be recognised as a normal reaction and the individual would be talking again within the month that must elapse before a diagnosis of SM can even be considered. However, when there is a history of SM, the failure to speak can create considerable alarm, and parents or the affected young person probably fear or assume that the situation is permanent. Just when reassurance and calm are needed, communication becomes associated with anxiety and tension, and the individual is unable to start talking again.

Note: very occasionally, SM *starts* in the family setting when communication becomes associated with anxiety rather than pleasure. For example, when there is repeated pressure to perform whenever visitors are there or when there is overzealous correction of pronunciation.

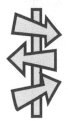

Chapter 9 'Progressive mutism' (page 170)

Chapter 13 'Autism spectrum disorder (ASD)' (page 279)

Online: Handout 13 'Easing in friends and relatives' is useful for new partners and visitors

Appendix F 'Resources': Sutton & Forrester (2015) in the book section includes an appendix 'Helping a new partner join a family where there is a child with SM'.

15 My child is getting increasingly resistant to *everything*, not just talking. What can I do?

For many children, SM is only *one* of their anxieties, all of which can be managed in broadly similar ways.

When children become increasingly resistant to trying new things, it is a sign of mounting anxiety. Usually it means that their only coping strategy is to *eliminate* rather than manage their anxiety. Often it is associated with staying with a parent rather than facing anxiety; for example, falling asleep with parents at night-time or staying at home rather than going to school. On the surface, the child is becoming more and more demanding; beneath these demands, there is a child who has learned that the world is full of terrors which must be avoided, and that it is the parents' role to protect them by removing their anxiety.

> *Avoidance strengthens fear.*

When children suggest doing something differently to help them participate or succeed, adults must listen and learn. However, when they start dictating terms, it is time to pull rank! We need to take a strong lead when children want to opt out of activities and social situations altogether. Avoidance may remove anxiety in the short term but the ensuing relief is a powerful reinforcer which makes it even harder to try again another time. Instead, we must do everything possible to keep the child's anxiety to a minimum, by understanding and addressing the cause. Once we are reassured that a situation poses no actual threat, either physical or emotional, we must explain that it is normal to worry and support the child to face their fears.

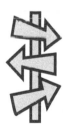

Chapter 8 Ensuring an anxiety-free environment

Chapter 9 Facing fears at home and in the community

Online: Handout 7 'Helping children to cope with anxiety'

16 Is it advisable to separate twins when one or both of them has SM?

Children who have SM *cannot* speak, so separating a child from their twin (or friend or sibling) takes away their only security and puts them in an even more stressful position. Appropriate support strategies must be put in place. These include allowing children who have SM to talk through their friends and siblings as a step towards talking independently. The only good reason to opt for different classes is because one or both twins want to spend more time apart in order to develop their own identity.

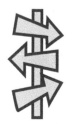

Chapter 9 Table 9.1, 'Stages 0–4' (page 151)

Chapter 10 'Talking through other children' (page 182)

17 My child found school much too stressful. Am I right to consider home-schooling?

Home-schooling is a personal decision made for a variety of reasons. If it is because a child's SM has not been handled well in the public sector, while home-schooling will provide respite, it will not *cure* SM. Like all phobias, SM can only be overcome by facing fears in the situations that create anxiety; avoiding those situations only makes the fear more intense.

All of the home-schooled children we have known have wanted to return to school in time; but, of course, they cannot be expected to return to a hostile environment. All have managed a successful transition to schools or colleges which worked with parents to understand and accommodate SM. Thankfully, the majority of UK schools know that it is their legal obligation to put in this work while children who have SM are still on roll.

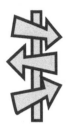

Chapter 8 Ensuring an anxiety-free environment

Chapter 10 Facing fears in educational settings

Chapter 11 Making successful transitions

Chapter 14 Examples of interventions (Lisa; page 303)

18 Why does my child talk to strangers but not people he knows well?

Uta does not speak to any of her grandparents, so we couldn't believe it when she spoke to her uncle who she's never met before and didn't shut up until he left. He's not used to young children, so he didn't make a big thing of trying to get her to talk. But he did show her how to make a dowsing rod and she got so caught up in it, she seemed to forget herself and just started talking. He had no idea what a big deal this was and just carried on as normal, which I think really helped.

We hoped this would be the turning point but, when my parents came round the following week, Uta was back to nodding and shaking her head.

Children who have SM may surprise everyone by speaking to someone they barely know. This can be very hurtful to staff and relatives who have been waiting for a breakthrough, but it has nothing to do with favouritism. In new situations where there are no past associations to influence behaviour, little need or expectation for extended dialogue, and no chance of being 'found out' by people they cannot speak to, the child's natural incentive to speak may not be suppressed by anxiety. Clinicians carrying out assessments may skilfully facilitate speech by taking children through a small-steps progression. Older students frequently explain that talking is easier with strangers because they will not be surprised to hear them speak – unlike their peers at school. Unfortunately, such successes are usually isolated incidents which do not affect the established pattern of situational mutism.

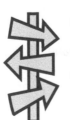

Chapters 4–6 Assessment

Chapter 10 'Talking to the child about reactions from others' (page 206)

19 My child is making progress but doesn't talk if I'm around. Why is that?

This is very common when children have got used to their parents answering for them. If the parent takes the role of speaker in social situations (albeit in response to their child's need for support), the child will automatically take the passive role of non-speaker in their company. The situation is soon turned around when parents discover ways to stop answering that are equally supportive for their child.

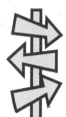

Chapter 2 'Overview of contributing factors' (page 36)

Chapter 8 Table 8.2 'Possible maintaining factors with alternative management strategies', item 24 (page 138)

Online: Handout 12 'Do I answer for my child?'

20 Should we be more protective of children who have SM?

There is no conclusive evidence to suggest that children with SM are at greater risk of harm or bullying than any other child but some important safeguards are necessary. There are two issues to consider:

1   How will the child cope in an emergency situation?

2   Is the child an easy target for bullies and predators?

Regarding emergencies, children who have SM have a good track record. Their intense fear of speaking means that they endure disappointment, frustration, upset, humiliation and even pain in silence. However, as soon as there is a *real* threat, they speak. Just as a surge of adrenalin enables a mother to snatch her baby from under the wheels of a car, children who have SM have been reported to raise the alarm when their friends were hurt; they have provided directions when they were the only one who knew the way home; they have read aloud when told they could not go home until they reached the bottom of the page. Of course, we do *not* endorse deliberately intimidating children in this way. Terrifying a child into speaking does not cure SM. On the contrary, such practice simply heightens their negative associations with talking.

> *In extreme situations, safety will prevail.*

However, while the fight–flight–freeze response is there to keep us safe, it cannot protect anyone from victimisation. Children who have SM may indeed be easy targets if it is perceived that they have no voice and 'won't tell'. It is important to remember that, although children who have SM often do not speak, they *can* speak to people they are close to. As with any other child, they need:

★   clear rules for staying safe

★   good communication with parents so they know they can talk about anything they don't feel comfortable about

★   to know they will be believed if they *do* tell.

At school, it is essential to establish a similar line of communication. Children who have SM cannot be expected to initiate dialogue – spoken or written – to report illness, bullying or teasing. This inability to initiate is part of the SM condition. They may 'report' accidents by standing near adults in the hope that someone spots them bleeding, but further explanation will usually wait until they see their parents. Therefore, it is important for a designated adult to establish a relationship with each child or young person and agree with them, and their families, a means of reporting any difficulties. Initially, at least, they will need to be *asked* on a regular basis if there is anything troubling them or that they need help with.

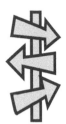

Chapter 8 Ensuring an anxiety-free environment

Online: Forms 12 and 13 'Environmental checklists'

21 How common is it?

It used to be very rare to meet a child in playgroup or nursery who did not talk. Today, many preschool workers will have encountered one or more children who barely say a word but are reported to speak freely at home. Most schools can expect to have at least one child who has SM on roll, but they will not always have been identified.

Given that SM is an anxiety disorder, it is not surprising that numbers are increasing. Anxiety conditions in general are more commonplace and experts suggest that this is linked to the increased stress in our daily lives. As a population, we have more choices, greater expectations, an unhealthy work–life balance and a protocol-bound society which takes health and safety to new extremes. Children today are exposed to stressed parents, increased family breakdown and changeable routines. There is increased pressure on schools to get children talking in order to meet educational targets. There seems to be little time for anyone to slow down and simply *be*.

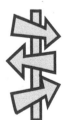

Chapter 2 'Prevalence' (page 36) and 'Implementing a prevention strategy' (page 45)

Online: Handout 3 'Quiet child or selective mutism?'

Appendix D 'Early years workshops'

Appendix E 'Evidence base' (prevalence)

22 At what age does it start?

SM can be triggered at any age from preschool to teens but it usually starts between two and four years old. However, the actual onset can easily be missed because silence is often accepted in young children as shyness. It is only when the child is repeatedly expected to speak to people outside their comfort zone that their discomfort becomes apparent and alarm bells start to ring; for example, when they start school or nursery or are introduced to a new partner or step-parent. Even then, the child's silence may be misinterpreted as shyness or resentment.

Later onset is usually triggered by an incident involving actual or perceived teasing, bullying or humiliation from teaching staff or peers. It could coincide with extreme self-consciousness on transition to secondary school and puberty. These children will already have an anxious or a sensitive nature and are likely to experience social anxiety before, and certainly after, the event.

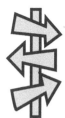

Chapter 1 'Some children are just shy. How can I tell the difference?' (page 7)

Chapter 2 'What causes SM?' (page 9)

23 Do I need an official diagnosis?

The answer is not necessarily, especially when children are young and there are no other difficulties apart from SM. The features of SM are set out in this manual. There is also plenty you can do before deciding to involve professionals or while you are waiting for an appointment.

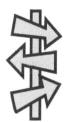

Chapter 3 'The case for lay diagnosis' (page 57)

Chapter 8 'Reaching a shared understanding' (page 116)

Online: Handout 2 'What is selective mutism?'

Handout 3 'Quiet child or selective mutism?'

24 If I need an official diagnosis, who would do it?

The primary clinicians fulfilling this remit in the UK are speech and language therapists because SM is a communication difficulty. But paediatricians, psychologists and mental health professionals are also qualified to make a diagnosis. In all cases, it is worth asking some questions about their understanding and experience of SM.

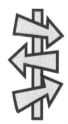

Chapter 3 'How to find a suitable professional to make a diagnosis' (page 58)

25 My child was referred to speech and language therapy. Isn't SM a psychological problem?

Speech and language therapists (SLTs) work with a wide range of communication difficulties stemming from a variety of causes – physical, developmental, cognitive, neurological *and* psychological. Those with psychological causes include psychogenic voice loss in adults, puberphonia (high-pitched voice persisting beyond adolescence) and SM. Anxiety management will be a large component in the treatment of all these conditions.

Stammering has many similarities with SM, particularly where the avoidance of speaking situations is concerned, and the experience and knowledge that SLTs use in treating stammering have a direct application in the treatment of SM.

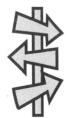

Chapter 2 'Implications for multidisciplinary ownership of SM' (page 42)

Chapter 13 'Stammering or stuttering' (page 284)

26 At what point should action be taken?

Many children take a while to settle in at their school or nursery and may not speak to new adults for some weeks. Action should be taken immediately to ensure that there is no pressure on quiet or reluctant speakers to speak, while simultaneously providing gentle support that enables them to participate at their own pace.

After a month, it helps if staff and family compare notes and begin to monitor the situation.

★ Does the child's talking vary in different situations and with different people?

★ Which activities bring out the best in them?

★ What possible explanations are there for the child's lack of speech?

This applies equally to children who are learning a second language. After two months, parents and staff should meet for an open, non-critical discussion to share their observations and concerns and agree a way forward. Remember that these preliminary investigations will not necessarily lead to a diagnosis of SM.

Once SM is suspected, there are two points to remember: don't delay, but don't rush in. These messages are complementary rather than contradictory because, although all the evidence points to *early* intervention, it is important to ensure good information gathering, liaison and planning. Intervention must be carefully tailored to the needs and capabilities of everyone involved, following a strict progression. Once a plan has been formulated, it should be implemented immediately.

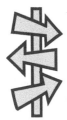

Chapter 2 'The importance of early intervention' (page 44)

Chapter 3 'Making a diagnosis' (page 53)

Chapter 7 Moving from assessment to management

Online: Handout 9 'Helping young children to speak at school'

27 Why is early intervention so important?

SM could largely be eradicated if it was identified early and managed appropriately. If ignored or mishandled, the child's anxiety is intensified and generalised and it takes longer to resolve their SM. This can lead to additional complications such as low self-esteem, escalating social anxiety, reluctance to submit written work and school avoidance.

Not only are early intervention techniques effective and non-invasive, they are also relatively cheap and easy to implement. The alternatives for older children and adults with entrenched SM include more expensive interventions such as home-tutoring, disability allowance, medication and significant involvement with mental health services.

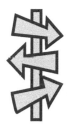

Chapter 2 'The importance of early intervention' (page 44)

Online: Appendix E Evidence base

28 Is it too late to help teenagers and adults who have SM?

It is never too late to help individuals overcome their SM and improve their quality of life.

Some young people do not need any formal intervention; they reason that their fear of speaking is irrational but, having been labelled a non-speaker, their silence was hard to break in their current setting. A move to secondary school, college or university provides the opportunity for a fresh start and, with determination to speak from day one, they have succeeded and grown in confidence with each new achievement. In the authors' experience, these are usually young people with clear goals who have managed to maintain some independence and close friendships throughout their schooling. They can communicate reasonably well in some situations outside school, particularly where strangers are involved. It is this experience that convinces them that change is possible in a new environment.

Other teenagers will need more help. Family and staff will need to address the question of why their difficulties have persisted for this long. They should consider the need for further assessment, a better understanding of the young person's difficulties, and more intense or

> Having had selective mutism all through secondary school, I knew it had to change when I went to university. I focused on building my confidence outside school with people who didn't know about my problem and set myself increasingly difficult tasks that were scary but doable. The more people I interacted with who saw me as maybe just a bit quiet, the more my confidence grew. I still couldn't speak at school however!
>
> The most freeing thing for me was seeing the SM as an unfortunate thing I suffered from (like eczema) rather than being me. Once I started viewing it like that, I could also see it as something that I could learn to live with, cope with and help myself to overcome. I am still an anxious person but it no longer controls me, I control it.)
>
> (Written after successful transition to university)

different strategies. With committed support, they too can work towards coping in a new environment by understanding their own anxiety, developing their social skills and independence, and developing the confidence to talk to key adults, peers and strangers. Meanwhile, it is the duty of their current teachers to improve their quality of life by ensuring that their needs are fully understood and their 'voice' is heard.

Adults too can change their lives through self-help, peer-support, mainstream or alternative therapies.

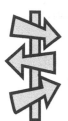

Chapter 10 'Additional considerations for adolescents and young adults' (page 214)

Chapter 11 Making successful transitions

Chapter 14 Examples of interventions (Lisa and Sander)

Chapter 15 Learning from people who have experienced selective mutism

Online: Booklet for teenagers and adults 'When the words won't come out'

29 Nothing has worked so far. Why should it be different this time?

By following the advice in this manual, you will be approaching SM as a phobia with the means to fully involve the child or young person in managing their response to anxiety triggers. In contrast, if SM is treated as a behaviour problem or control issue, no amount of intervention will be effective. Equally, if some of the strategies are lifted from this manual without due regard for the general principles of anxiety management, or the overall treatment progression, little progress will be made. There are no short cuts. Good results depend on appropriate, consistent support and *open communication with the child about their difficulties*, whatever their age.

> **I knew it was time to do things differently when my three year old said, 'Mummy, am I making you sad?'**

Many parents find the latter aspect the most difficult and either choose to keep quiet, for fear of making their child self-conscious, or comment 'He won't discuss it' or 'She just runs away if I try to talk to her'. But, often, parents have not talked to their child about the *nature* of SM or calmly put it in perspective alongside other common fears. Instead they have asked questions which the child cannot possibly answer: '*Why* don't you ...', '*When* will you ...?', 'Are you going to ...?' This makes the child feel that they are doing something wrong; it is not surprising that they don't want to listen.

Children who have SM need explanation, reassurance and confidence in the adults they look to for guidance. It will only increase their anxiety if we keep quiet and hope the problem will go away, or try to intervene without explaining what we are doing, or simply encourage the child to talk without providing any strategies. A good conversation opener would be something like: 'I can see you are trying really hard to talk to Grandad. What does it feel like when you try to get your words out?'

Communication with teenagers can be tricky at the best of times, especially when they say nothing is wrong and are apparently happy sitting in their bedroom with only their computer for company. We must recognise that extreme resistance to face their difficulties is borne out of fear of yet more failure, unreasonable expectations, anxiety and humiliation. Disengagement is a protective coping strategy after years of being let down. Again, we need to present facts rather than ask questions. We cannot expect young people to 'be ready to change' if they have no idea what help is available, what it involves and how it will work. Once they believe in the *possibility* of change, we can start to help them move forwards.

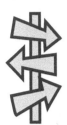

Chapter 5 Meeting and involving the child or young person

Chapter 9 'Additional considerations for adolescents' (page 169)

Online: Handout 1 'Talking to the child about speech anxiety'

Booklet for teenagers and adults 'When the words won't come out'

30 What form will intervention take?

First, we consider some types of intervention that are *not* helpful. One popular misconception is that SM children are traumatised and unable to express themselves for fear of revealing a family secret or deeper anxieties. This can lead to weeks of counselling or some form of play or art therapy. Children may enjoy these sessions, particularly if no pressure is put on them to speak. They may respond well, in terms of becoming more relaxed and communicative, in the specific setting of the therapy room but they rarely carry this over into other settings. In most cases, this approach delays, rather than facilitates, progress.

> *SM children are afraid of the sound of their voice, not of what they might say.*

The intervention approach recommended in this manual addresses anxiety at a behavioural and cognitive level. We talk openly to children about their anxiety, and about the feelings they experience when trying to talk. We look at each child within the family and school context, to ensure that the mutism is managed positively and consistently. With early identification, a few modifications to staff and parental interaction styles may be all that is required, so that communicative effort is reinforced rather than silence, avoidance or inappropriate substitutes for speech.

If it becomes apparent that a more structured approach is needed, a carefully staged programme is set up which aims to alleviate the child's anxiety by gradually facing their fears, first in very specific situations, and later on a more

Having established conversational speech with me in her home, Holly could talk to me anywhere, provided no one else was listening. We attempted to buy a drink in a café, but Holly could not tell me what she wanted until we were back in the privacy of my car.

With support, she learned to talk to strangers. After that, she could talk to anyone who did not know her, and spoke freely to me in front of any number of bystanders. At school, however, where she was well known as 'the girl who doesn't talk', she continued to experience intense anxiety and her SM remained until a school programme was implemented.

generalised basis. The programme involves working progressively towards conversational speech starting with simple participation and non-vocal communication.

Older children who are extremely anxious, angry, frustrated, despondent or depressed may also need to examine and reframe their cognitive belief system, in order to adopt a more rational and helpful approach to social communication and problem solving.

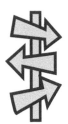

Chapter 8 Ensuring an anxiety-free environment

Chapters 9 and 10 Facing fears

Chapter 13 When it is more than selective mutism

31 What about medication?

The vast majority of children who have SM make a good response to a well-executed intervention programme without medication. As stated in Appendix E, the UK's NICE guidelines are consistent with our experience and do not recommend medication as the treatment of first choice for anxiety disorders. However, in older children with entrenched difficulties, where other methods of treatment have proved unsuccessful because of crippling anxiety or resistance to intervention, medication may be included to facilitate their engagement with an intervention programme.

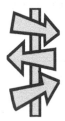

Chapter 13 'The question of medication' (page 273)

Online: Appendix E 'Evidence base'

32 Who should be involved in intervention? Do we need an expert in SM?

Much depends on when intervention starts and whether SM is the only condition to be addressed. However, in all cases, good teamwork is essential for a coordinated approach. Central to the intervention process are the child who has SM, their family and staff from the child's nursery, school or college. If there are no other complications, and parents and staff are agreed on a collaborative approach with access to the right information, it is possible to implement a successful intervention plan with no one else involved. In other situations, specialist support and advice may be provided by SLTs, psychologists or cognitive behavioural therapy (CBT) practitioners, depending on local service provision, the age of the child, and the extent and nature of additional difficulties.

Outside professionals will need to act mainly as consultants, listening to and offering advice to the families and staff who are in the best position to support the child on a daily basis. To be effective, this advice needs to be ongoing with regular reviews to monitor and update any targets and management strategies.

Equally important is a designated school or college-based keyworker, such as a classroom assistant, school counsellor, learning mentor or student support worker, who will implement agreed strategies and liaise with the family.

Building rapport with a mentor who can offer continuity and emotional support becomes especially important for older children with more entrenched SM, high levels of social anxiety and increasing social withdrawal. This could be someone from school, college or the voluntary sector, again supported by an outside specialist. As children reach their mid-teens with unresolved SM it becomes increasingly likely that mental health services will need to be involved so that the young person can access CBT and possibly a trial period of medication.

Finally, parents and siblings may also benefit from the involvement of a psychologist or mental health team to address the impact of SM and anxiety on the whole family.

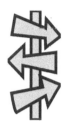

Chapter 3 'How to find a suitable professional to make a diagnosis' (page 58)

Chapter 13 When it is more than selective mutism

33 How long will intervention take?

This depends on so many factors that it is impossible to give a simple answer.

Here are a few pointers.

★ If the guidelines in this manual are followed, it can be relatively easy to establish speech with one or two key people within a month or two.

★ Reaching fully effective communication with all people in all situations takes much longer. It will depend on: the individual's particular circumstances; how long they have lived with SM; the presence of additional factors; and the availability, competence and coordinated effort of their support team (family, school staff, practitioners).

★ If caught in the very early stages, before a strong pattern of anxiety-related avoidance has been established, the ability to go on to talk fully and freely in groups and public places occurs much more easily, and often spontaneously, after minimal low key interventions.

★ At primary school, with early intervention and intensive input, parents and professionals may see good results within a year, but could still be monitoring the situation for another year or two.

★ With teenagers, the real progress is not usually seen until the students are in a new setting and free from the old associations with their last school. Even then, staff will need to monitor the situation closely and be led by the student.

★ Progress in the wider community is less predictable if support only centres on the child's educational establishment. Unless strategies from this manual are used by families in home and community settings to complement and reinforce the work done at school, difficulty talking to the extended family or strangers may persist for years after the child is talking in their school environment.

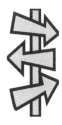

Chapter 10 'Letting go' (page 231)

Chapter 12 Troubleshooting: why isn't it working?

CHAPTER 2

A HOLISTIC VIEW OF SELECTIVE MUTISM

Introduction

Although this is primarily a practical manual, this chapter describes our thinking about selective mutism in the light of research findings, our clinical experience and the views of international experts in the field.

Selective mutism (SM) is classified as an anxiety disorder, characterised by being able to speak in some situations but not others. But this description tells us very little about the nature of SM. It is a state of almost constant vigilance; a range of intense emotions and physiological reactions affecting mind and body; a condition which influences, and is influenced by, family dynamics and the behaviour of relatives, staff, peers and even complete strangers.

This chapter therefore considers:

★ **The nature and presentation of SM**

- Reaching a shared understanding

- High and low profile SM

- Viewing SM as a phobia

- The physiology of phobia

- The influence of SM on thinking and reasoning

- The impact of SM on behaviour

- Differentiating between SM and social anxiety disorder

- The prevalence of SM

★ **What causes SM?**

- Overview of contributing factors

- Onset of SM

★ **Implications for multidisciplinary ownership of SM**

- Need for holistic assessment

- Need for multidisciplinary care pathways

- Need for training to ensure adequate recognition and understanding of SM

★ **The importance of early intervention**

- The cost of ignoring SM

- Implementing a prevention strategy

★ **Rationale and framework for our treatment approach**

There is an evidence base of research findings and references in Appendix E, in the online resource library, to support this chapter and our rationale for treatment.

The nature and presentation of SM

Reaching a shared understanding

Since the first edition of this manual in 2001, more research studies and books have been published than ever before, increasing our knowledge about the nature of SM. This was reflected in revisions of the international medical classification systems, DSM-5 (2013) and ICD-11 Beta-draft (due in 2017). SM is now categorised as an Anxiety or Fear-Related Disorder alongside other anxiety conditions affecting both children and adults. The nature of the links with anxiety remains unspecified and SM is simply defined in terms of consistent speaking habits with several exclusions, as summarised in Box 2.1. Nonetheless, understanding of the condition is much improved since it was first included in DSM III (1980) under the name of 'elective mutism'.

Box 2.1: **Essential characteristics of SM behaviour as described by DSM-5 and ICD-11 Beta-draft**

1   Individuals present a consistent pattern of speaking in some situations where speech is expected but not in others.

2   The failure to speak is persistent, lasting more than one month, but not including the first month in a new environment such as school.

3   The failure to speak has a significant impact on educational or occupational achievement or social communication.

4   Lack of knowledge or comfort with the required spoken language, or a disorder of communication or a condition like social anxiety disorder, may also be present, but is not the cause and does not explain the mutism.

Yet a remarkable level of agreement has been reached between international experts about understanding and management of the condition. Dedicated websites and treatment manuals describe SM as a *fear* of speaking, or the expectation to speak, that responds to a behavioural approach to reduce anxiety. Not surprisingly, this conclusion has led to considerable speculation: how to account for a fear of speaking in a heterogenic population that crosses all socio-economic groups, cultures and life experiences? We subscribe to the Occam's razor school of thought: the simplest explanation is most likely to be correct! While acknowledging that individuals develop this fear in different ways, we propose that only the process of *conditioning* can account for the absolute consistency of speech habits that is the central feature of SM. In other words, SM is the result of a *learned* fear or *phobia*. Established at a subconscious level, this conditioning leads to an increasingly conscious internalised rule system that enables people who have SM to recognise their pattern of anxiety triggers, and to predict situations where they will or won't be able to speak.

High and low profile SM

SM is easy to recognise when children speak to some people, or in some places, but not in others. However, things are rarely this clear cut because the individual's ability to speak is entirely context-dependent. Thus a child may be able to speak to a parent, friend or particular staff member, but only when they are sure no one else is listening. Or they may speak freely in front of strangers, but stop as soon as they see a classmate, fearing that they will be expected to talk at school. Despite these apparent variations, a consistent situational pattern can be identified where the child never speaks to certain people; this is described as 'high profile' SM in Anxiety UK's booklet *Children and Young People with Anxiety* (see Appendix F).

DSM-5 also allows for 'low profile' SM by stating 'Children with this disorder do not initiate or *reciprocally* respond when spoken to by others'. In other words, they may respond minimally but not in a reciprocal, conversational manner. This is a pattern we see in compliant children who are anxious about upsetting authority figures or looking foolish in front of their peers. We also see it in children and young people who are beginning to make progress. They manage to answer straightforward questions and comply with simple verbal routines but it will be clear that this is not without effort; they are tense and speak quietly or in a strained manner. Children with low profile SM are particularly vulnerable at school because their high anxiety levels may not be recognised. All the time they speak a little, it may not be apparent that they are unable to initiate contact of their own accord, seek help, correct misunderstandings, make friends, or report illness or bullying. Without appropriate support, many children with low profile SM say less and less until a high profile pattern is apparent or they become adults with low profile SM.

Viewing SM as a phobia

In an Association of Child and Adolescent Mental Health (ACAMH) occasional paper (Johnson & Wintgens, 2015), we describe how SM meets the criteria for specific phobia, as defined by DSM-5 (summarised in Box 2.2), but accrues additional complications over time. SM arises through the same psychological processes as specific phobia, that is, transference, modelling and direct negative association; it shares the phenomenology of specific phobia, that is, an interaction between genetic disposition and environmental factors that is more common in females than males; and it responds to the same treatment approach – graded exposure to a specific stimulus, in this case, the expectation to talk to people outside the individual's comfort zone.

Box 2.2: Essential characteristics of specific phobia as described by DSM-5 and ICD-11 Beta-draft
1 Individuals consistently experience marked and out of proportion fear of the presence or anticipation of one or more specific objects or situations.
2 Exposure to the phobic objects or situations provokes an immediate anxiety response.
3 The phobic situations are either avoided or endured with intense anxiety or distress.
4 The fear, anxious anticipation or avoidance has a significant impact on the individual's personal, educational, occupational or social life.
5 The fear, anxious anticipation or avoidance persists for at least several months.

Four factors complicate matters.

1   Speaking is central to our lives (unlike spiders for example), so SM has a far greater impact than other phobias and puts individuals on almost constant alert.

2   There is no obvious external trigger (again, unlike spiders). The individual rarely feels threatened by the people they want to speak to but, despite this, is afraid to speak. It seems both to the individual and people around them that the individual is 'at fault'.

3   Few people *realise* that SM is a phobia. So, even when trying to help, they unintentionally do the very things that make phobias *worse*.

4   In the absence of any explanation or solution, children who have SM grow up knowing that other people find their behaviour unusual at least, and intolerable at worst. Over time, it becomes increasingly difficult to separate their own identity from their behaviour and a change in self-perception occurs that is rare in other phobias: they feel rejected, unlikeable, a failure, unworthy.

The variety of presentations and 'types' of SM described in the literature are consistent with the concept of a phobia. It has been noted that children who have SM are not always anxious and it is well known that phobic individuals are only anxious when the phobic stimulus is present or anticipated.

The authors believe that the nature of SM does not change. However, it manifests in different ways according to an individual's coping skills; these, in turn, reflect a combination of personal characteristics (eg extrovert, introvert, shy, strong-willed, compliant, passive or resourceful) and the way the phobia is handled by other people. If silence is accepted in very young children, they will not feel uncomfortable. If alternative means of communication are accepted, and there is genuinely no pressure to speak, children will happily point, write or gesture instead. Conversely, if children are afraid that gestures such as nodding will increase the expectation to talk, they will be tense and immobile. If reassured that they won't be chosen to answer questions in class, children will relax and enjoy their lessons; otherwise, they will be in a constant state of apprehension. Strong-willed children will resist (and appear to 'refuse') anxiety-provoking activities; compliant children will 'suffer in silence'.

The physiology of phobia

A phobic reaction to an imaginary threat is exactly the same as the body's automatic reaction to *real* danger. It starts in the brain but instantly affects other parts of the body as the sympathetic nervous system activates the fear reflex: the *fight or flight response*. Heart rate and blood pressure increase, muscles tense, blood is diverted to arms and legs, pupils dilate and the mucous membranes dry up. We are now ready to make stronger movements, run faster, see better and breathe easier in preparation for battle or escape. Side effects include trembling, tingling, dizziness and shortness of breath as the body takes in more oxygen through shallow, rapid breathing.

When the fear reflex is triggered and we are in real danger, we don't have time to think – we don't *need* to think – if there's any way out; we take action. But if there's no escape, we *freeze* rather than fight or take flight – sudden shocks or bad news have the same effect. Our heart pounds; body stiffens; face is fixed and expressionless; throat tightens; we catch our breath and, for a moment, cannot move or speak. This freeze response is consistent with reports of SM. Parents can feel their child's heart racing as a stranger tries to engage them. Children who can describe the moment when they try to speak invariably report a sense of blocking in their throat as the muscles tighten. Observers may note a trembling chin or excessive swallowing as the child tries to speak. Adults frequently use words such as 'shock', 'paralysed' and 'freeze' when recalling their SM (see Chapter 15).

> **I had so much I wanted to say but I could never get the words out. It was like my throat seized up ...**

The major conclusion from studies of fear is that the part of the brain responsible for triggering the fear reflex, and other emotions such as anxiety, is the amygdala. The amygdala also stores memories of events which immediately precede the fear response, a feature that enables us to become increasingly alert to danger. Although eventually combined with conscious knowledge, fear memories are largely created and stored at a *sub*conscious level; unfortunately, this leaves the brain open to the misinterpretation of events and inappropriate reactions. Panic sensations can become associated with objects or events that are part of the experience, but not the actual source of fear; this process is known as *fear conditioning*. As a result, neutral objects or events can become fear-inducing triggers, capable of activating the same panic sensations as the original trigger. In the case of SM, the neutral event is the expectation to speak; individuals start to fear the *act* of speaking, rather than the person they are talking to or the possible consequences of speaking.

The influence of SM on thinking and reasoning

When faced with a threatening situation, the automatic functions of the amygdala operate 20 times faster than the thinking part of the brain, the frontal cortex. If someone with a cotton wool aversion is blindfolded and unexpectedly touches some cotton wool, their hand recoils before they even realise what it is. In short, we react first and think later. This has its advantages. As Joseph LeDoux (1997), one of the most respected researchers in the area of fear, memory and emotion, explains, when we see a snake, we don't need to know that it is a reptile, or that its skin can be used to make belts, before we take action. Maybe it was only a stick, but it is better to run away and be safe, rather than sorry!

The downside is that we have very little conscious control over our reactions. We can *tell* ourselves that a fear is irrational but, once fear conditioning has taken place at a subconscious level, logic has very little influence. When sensations of pure fear or panic are triggered, we obey a deeper instinct and feel compelled to escape.

> **When I stood in the classroom for the first time and that anxiety hit me, I had no say in the matter, it just struck. The same happened at every subsequent expectation to speak.**

However, reasoning has an important role in the changing picture of SM over time. Unfortunately, it is a role which serves the child or young person's instinct to stay safe but leads to a more entrenched and, ultimately, damaging belief system as follows.

1   Children who have SM are very aware of the situations they can and can't manage. They may fervently deny laughing or speaking, or instruct their parents not to tell other people they have spoken. This reveals a very conscious aspect of SM behaviour which undoubtedly plays its part in the shutdown we see when 'the wrong person' walks in on a conversation. This is not a simple matter of choosing when and with whom to speak. SM children do not want people to find out they can speak *when they are afraid of where it might lead*. Will this person tell others they can speak? Will more be expected of them now, putting them in the very situations they dread? It is significant that strangers pose much less of a threat in this regard, so shutdown does not always occur. Yet it is common for parents to be aware that children are speaking in fewer and fewer settings – a sign that their anxiety is not being appropriately accommodated and their fear of speaking is escalating (see 'Maintaining factors on page 38).

2   The longer young people live with the negative consequences of SM (not being chosen by peers; no longer receiving greetings or playful banter; never doing enough to gain praise or a glowing school report, etc), the more it threatens to alter their self-image. They feel increasingly unpopular and worthless and start to believe what they hear: that they are shy, rude, difficult or stubborn and should try harder. In the absence of any other explanation, they conclude that they are ignored because people find them stupid, dull or weird. At this point, SM is far more than a fear of speaking; it has affected the way individuals think about themselves and other people. Many, if not most, of these young people would now also meet the diagnostic criteria for social anxiety disorder (SAD); see the section below on differentiating between SM and SAD).

3   Even if children who have SM reject or are not exposed to the negative opinions of others, the vast majority are self-aware and intelligent, with a need to understand a behaviour which no one has explained to them in terms of a physical response to anxiety. There must be a *reason* why they hate speaking so much …

> **I don't want to speak because my voice sounds horrible.**

> **I can't talk to my teacher – she contaminates the air and I'll get her germs.**

Families usually hear these reasons, not at the onset, but once the SM is well established; and, when one reason has been negated, often another surfaces. These scenarios suggest retrospective justification rather than a true explanation for the child's silence.

The impact of SM on behaviour

While thinking and reasoning may not have much influence over the body's automatic responses, they do have a powerful effect on *behaviour*. One of the key features of phobias is that they are predictable and therefore can be managed mainly through avoidance. People with phobias cannot contemplate uncontrollable feelings of fear, so they do all they can to avoid the trigger. As children who have SM learn to predict the situations that trigger anxiety and panic, they do what they can to avoid them, as summarised in Box 2.3.

Box 2.3: Avoidance behaviour in SM

1   Physically removing self from situation; eg running away, going to another room.

2   Psychosomatic illness (subconscious avoidance); eg stomach ache, nausea, headaches.

3   Trying to become invisible; eg averting eye contact, growing a long fringe, not moving.

4   Adopting non-speaking mode; eg using only writing or gesture to communicate.

5   Using an alternative to normal voice; eg whispering, different accent.

6   Talking in a language that is not spoken by certain people present, thereby excluding them from the conversation.

7   Asking to opt out socially; eg wanting to decline a party invitation or miss school.

8   Oppositional behaviour when other attempts to opt out have failed; eg refusing to get dressed, using threatening language or actions, damaging self or property.

The ultimate avoidance strategy or 'safety behaviour' is to opt out of social situations altogether, in order to avoid the stress of silence that is beyond their control. Knowing what lies ahead, children with stronger personalities will dig in their heels and either opt out or negotiate an alternative with their parents. What seems like 'having their own way' is actually a successful coping strategy. When no escape is possible, subconscious avoidance behaviour surfaces in the form of psychosomatic illness – headaches, stomach aches and sickness. It is well documented in the literature that true oppositional disorders are rare in children who have SM and that oppositional behaviour generally reflects their need to avoid speaking in certain situations.

Sadly, when SM is poorly understood by staff, friends or relatives, the trigger for children's anxiety is almost impossible to avoid and individuals spend inordinate amounts of time feeling chronically anxious that they *might* be expected to speak. Older children learn that, even when they *can* speak a little to certain people, often it is better to remain quiet because speaking only invites extended dialogue and unwanted reactions. In the absence of a well-managed intervention programme, avoidance behaviour tends to increase, reflecting children's enhanced situational awareness and escalating anxiety, sense of helplessness and lack of control. The authors know teenagers who have taken drastic steps when they didn't feel understood or listened to.

SM also has a significant impact on other people's behaviour which is discussed under 'Maintaining factors' (page 38).

Differentiating between SM and social anxiety disorder

It has been suggested that SM is a childhood variant of SAD and a means of avoiding the stress of social participation. However, as stated in DSM-5, children who have SM 'may be willing or eager to perform/ engage in social encounters when speech is not required'. This supports our view that children are not

It's like this absolutely horrible feeling when you'd almost rather die than have to utter a word in front of certain people.

using silence to avoid participation; rather, their silence and lack of participation is the result of being unable to speak. Moreover, the core feature of SAD is a fear of negative evaluation. Individuals with SAD are therefore afraid of doing or saying anything that won't be well received and are looking ahead to the *consequences* of their actions.

In contrast, individuals with specific phobias dread the panic that their phobia triggers, rather than worry about the effect their phobia has on other people. As one adult commented, 'I have SM but I don't agree that it's extreme anxiety causing it. If anything, it's the other way round – mutism causes the extreme anxiety. It's terrifying not being able to say what you need to say.'

I desperately wanted to prove to my teacher that I could read but the words stuck in my throat.

This and numerous other testimonials indicate that SM is an irrational fear of the act of speaking itself, rather than fear of the *consequences* of speaking or not speaking. However, although SM and SAD are distinct anxiety disorders, they can coexist. Individuals with SM can develop SAD (as discussed above in 'The influence of SM on thinking and reasoning'), and vice versa. This is discussed further in Chapter 13.

The prevalence of SM

Many children receive appropriate, sympathetic support early in their school lives so, as expected, SM is more common in younger children.

Estimates of the prevalence of SM have increased over the years and most recent studies suggest that about 1 in 140 children under 8 years old are affected. When older children are included, the prevalence is lower: about 1 in 550 children. These figures are unlikely to include 'low profile' SM, however – children who give brief responses but do not ask questions or converse freely (page 31). Certainly, all primary schools and most secondary schools can expect to have at least one child who has SM on roll, and it is a condition that all teachers can expect to encounter. We therefore urge all teacher-training institutions to include SM awareness when covering additional educational needs.

What causes SM?

Overview of contributing factors

Looking at the cause of SM involves asking how individuals develop a conditioned fear of speaking. In common with other anxiety disorders, there is no single cause; SM arises from a unique interaction of genetic (inherited) and environmental factors. Although these are different for each individual, there is a combination of contributing factors as shown in detail in Figure 2.1 opposite and summarised in Figure 2.2.

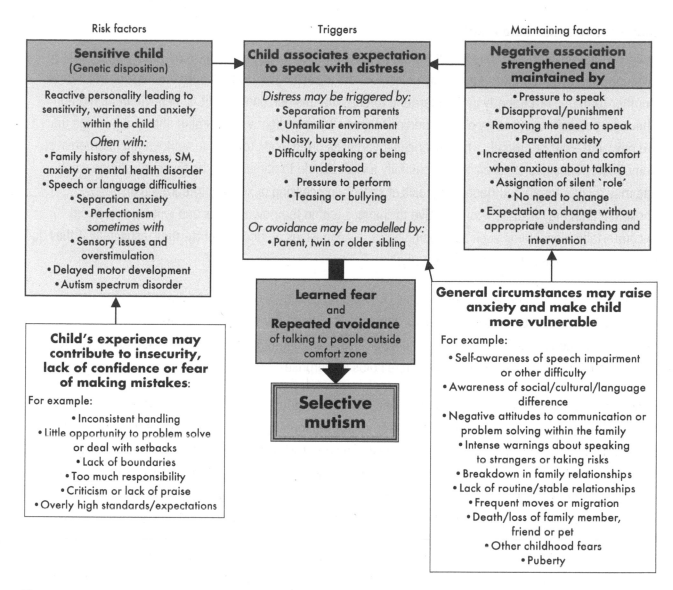

Risk factors

Sensitive child
(Genetic disposition)

Reactive personality leading to sensitivity, wariness and anxiety within the child

Often with:
• Family history of shyness, SM, anxiety or mental health disorder
• Speech or language difficulties
• Separation anxiety
• Perfectionism
sometimes with
• Sensory issues and overstimulation
• Delayed motor development
• Autism spectrum disorder

Child's experience may contribute to insecurity, lack of confidence or fear of making mistakes:

For example:
• Inconsistent handling
• Little opportunity to problem solve or deal with setbacks
• Lack of boundaries
• Too much responsibility
• Criticism or lack of praise
• Overly high standards/expectations

Triggers

Child associates expectation to speak with distress

Distress may be triggered by:
• Separation from parents
• Unfamiliar environment
• Noisy, busy environment
• Difficulty speaking or being understood
• Pressure to perform
• Teasing or bullying

Or avoidance may be modelled by:
• Parent, twin or older sibling

Learned fear
and
Repeated avoidance
of talking to people outside comfort zone

Selective mutism

Maintaining factors

Negative association strengthened and maintained by
• Pressure to speak
• Disapproval/punishment
• Removing the need to speak
• Parental anxiety
• Increased attention and comfort when anxious about talking
• Assignation of silent 'role'
• No need to change
• Expectation to change without appropriate understanding and intervention

General circumstances may raise anxiety and make child more vulnerable

For example:
• Self-awareness of speech impairment or other difficulty
• Awareness of social/cultural/language difference
• Negative attitudes to communication or problem solving within the family
• Intense warnings about speaking to strangers or taking risks
• Breakdown in family relationships
• Lack of routine/stable relationships
• Frequent moves or migration
• Death/loss of family member, friend or pet
• Other childhood fears
• Puberty

Figure 2.1: **Factors contributing to the development of SM**

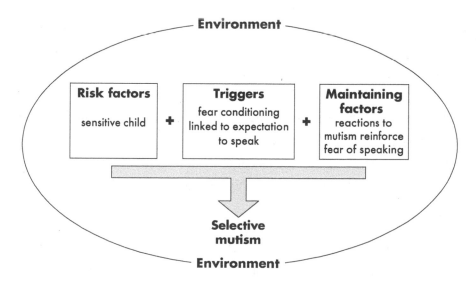

Figure 2.2: **Summary of factors contributing to the development of SM**

Stage 1: The vulnerable child

Children who develop SM have a reactive personality and can be described as sensitive, whether this involves sensitivity to other people's opinions, to life's uncertainties, to their surroundings, or to all three. Another term used frequently in the literature to describe this personality trait is 'behavioural inhibition'. Children are easily aroused by change and on the alert for any slightly threatening stimulus – things that are new, different or difficult. This enhanced awareness often leads to great insight, caring or creativity. Some highly sensitive children have a painfully low threshold to stimuli such as touch, noise and smell and may qualify for an additional diagnosis of sensory-processing or sensory-integration disorder. These children may also be very sensitive to changes within their own bodies and will want to avoid uncomfortable sensations such as a racing heart, tired muscles or stomach butterflies, especially if they do not understand what is happening and why.

Sensitivity presents in different ways. Some children are generally cautious and shy; others are very outgoing once they are sure of themselves; others have rigid or perfectionist natures. All thrive on reassurance and tend to be thoughtful, self-conscious, unwilling to take risks or make mistakes, easily overloaded and most relaxed when the future holds no surprises.

Research now strongly suggests there is a genetic link to anxiety and the body's heightened reaction to stress. This helps in understanding why children of this personality type are more prone to developing anxiety disorders and more likely to have at least one parent who shares their sensitive personality and tendency to worry. It is also known that, while this basic personality trait is genetically determined, how it is expressed in later life, in terms of general temperament and coping strategies, is shaped by early childhood experience. For example, parenting style can positively or negatively influence children's anxiety levels.

Additional difficulties with communication, learning, development or social interaction (such as developmental coordination disorder or autism spectrum conditions) put children at even greater risk of feeling anxious and self-conscious as a result of confusion, failure, comparison, teasing or correction.

Stage 2: Life events

Sensitive children are susceptible to developing anxiety disorders but whether they develop SM, or other fears, depends on the interplay and timing of ensuing life events. In the case of SM, an event or ongoing situation creates an association between the expectation to talk and intense anxiety, as discussed in 'Onset of SM' (page 40). This may occur against a backdrop of other stressors which contribute to a generally heightened state of anxiety, such as loss, bereavement, moving home, concern about a family member, or struggle to cope with different rules or cultural values. Most of the stressors and specific life events that lead to fear conditioning would not be regarded as out of the ordinary, but sensitive children feel things more deeply and are less resilient to coping with change and anxiety.

Stage 3: Maintaining factors

Childhood fears are common and usually transient. So it is important to ask why some fears, like SM, assume the intensity, persistence and life-influencing nature of phobias. The answer lies in psychological principles of reinforcement; in behaviours and events that strengthen and *maintain* the fear, to the point where no amount of reassurance or logic can dispel it.

It follows that a key component to overcoming SM is to identify the maintaining factors that are operating for each individual. We know from our casework that if this maintenance behaviour is not eliminated or significantly reduced, SM will continue or, at the very least, take much longer to resolve. Conversely, if SM is recognised in the early stages, we have found that a team approach to successfully addressing maintenance behaviour may be all that is needed for children to overcome their fear.

Therefore, we have extended our assessment procedure to include a checklist of possible maintaining factors to help staff members and families explore and identify relevant issues (Form 4 online). The different types of maintaining factors are outlined in Box 2.4, cross-referenced to items on the checklist. Overall, they create the vicious cycles of pressure and avoidance which are common to all phobias (Figure 2.3).

Box 2.4: Summary of SM maintaining factors

SM is maintained when:

a) Talking is a negative experience

Expectation to talk is linked to unreasonable pressure, anxiety, disapproval or failure.

(Items 1–18 on 'Checklist of possible maintaining factors')

b) Fear of talking is strengthened through avoidance

Avoidance brings instant relief from anxiety which reinforces the individual's conviction that there was indeed something to fear.

(Items 19–20)

c) Avoidance is a positive experience

Avoidance is more rewarding than participation.

(Items 21–22)

d) *Not* talking becomes a habit

Little or no experience of successfully mastering anxiety convinces the individual that the situation is permanent and nothing can be done; ultimately, they become resigned to a non-talking role.

(Items 23–28)

As Figure 2.3 indicates, a feature of maintaining factors is the strong, self-reinforcing, interpersonal dynamic. The individual's difficulty in speaking impacts not only on themselves but also on their family, peers and teachers, whose instinctive reactions impact on the individual, and so on. Naturally, the individual is encouraged to speak – the very thing which triggers their fear response – putting them under enormous pressure to do something that feels impossible. *Avoidance* of these situations, in itself a maintaining factor, is a natural coping strategy; not only for the individual with SM but also for friends, families and teachers who witness their distress and step in to reduce their anxiety. When 'rescued' – an adult speaks for the child, or moves on to a different child, for example – the child initially experiences great relief. This strengthens their conviction that talking is too difficult; each time this happens, their fear of talking increases.

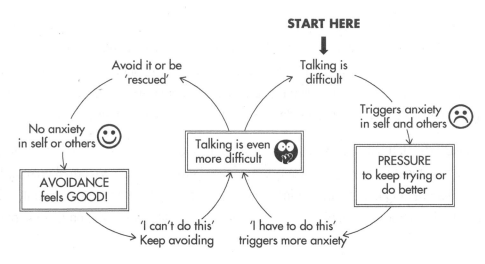

Figure 2.3: **How pressure and avoidance contribute to selective mutism**

The influence of parenting style on anxiety has been researched extensively, and is relevant when considering maintaining factors. It highlights two parenting styles which tend to increase anxiety in children, making them more fearful of trying anything new.

We have seen the first style only occasionally in parents of children who have SM: a derisive, critical style which undermines the child's sense of self-worth and willingness to take risks. The parents we meet more often report this style in their own parent, that is, the *grand*parent of the child who has SM. We often see the second style: this is labelled 'overprotective' parenting in the literature but that is not a term that we use. These are, without exception, loving parents who are responding to and being guided by their child's anxious temperament. Often they have an anxious or shy temperament themselves and may have painful memories from their own childhood of incidents which they want to spare their child from experiencing. They are tuned-in to their child's raised stress levels and understandably eager to make their child's experience of life as pleasant as possible by helping them to avoid anxiety-provoking situations.

The challenge, therefore, is to find a middle ground between putting pressure on a child to speak (however subtly) and removing all expectation to speak along with the opportunity to learn that speaking need not arouse anxiety. Enabling staff and parents to do this in a way which allows children to move forward without anxiety underpins our approach to intervention.

Onset of SM

Families are not always aware of, or able to recall, an initial trigger for SM. Parents may only gradually become aware that their child speaks to a limited number of people or has stopped speaking to people they have not seen for a while. This is not at all surprising; it is often the *impact* of event(s) on the child that is extreme, rather than the event itself. If children seem startled or shocked for a short time during normal daily events, this is soon forgotten when they return to their normal interactive selves. Moreover, onset often occurs at a very young age when silence with unfamiliar visitors or strangers would not be regarded as unusual. It may only be when the child does not speak at nursery or school that parents have a reason to become concerned.

An extensive examination of our own caseloads and other documented accounts suggests that, in keeping with other phobias, the fear conditioning responsible for SM occurs through transference, modelling or direct association.

Transference

Transference explains the more unusual phobias such as fear of buttons, kittens or hard-boiled eggs. It occurs when something causes alarm or distress and the negative association is transferred from the true source of anxiety to an accompanying object or event; in this case, the expectation to speak.

In the case of SM, transference is more likely to occur when the parent is absent and unable to provide reassurance. For example, the child has been left in an unfamiliar environment, or the child has become separated from their parent in the street. As the child inwardly panics and becomes too overwhelmed, anxious or emotional to talk, someone tries to interact with the unresponsive child, unaware that the child is effectively in a state of shock. The attempted conversation becomes a tangible part of the child's experience.

None of us can reason effectively when we are in a state of high anxiety, let alone young children. They cannot rationalise that the expectation to speak was not primarily responsible for their distress. The next time they are expected to speak in a similar situation, the same panic sensations flood back, making speech impossible. This negative association often outlasts the child's memory of the original incident.

Modelling

Fears can be learned by observing the reactions of people we normally look to for guidance. For example, if an older sibling openly demonstrates fear and avoidance of talking, a younger child may become equally convinced that talking poses a threat. Similarly, if shy, anxious or immigrant parents demonstrate a reluctance to engage with people outside their close family circle, or to speak the unfamiliar language used at their child's school, this anxiety can be conveyed to their children.

Direct association

Sometimes children directly associate talking with anxiety. Examples include being teased or criticised about the way they speak and being urged to recite or recall information when they feel uncomfortable with the task. We have seen the latter lead to children as young as 18 months becoming withdrawn and silent as soon as visitors arrive. A focus on fun, with no pressure to perform, quickly turns things around.

Literature reviews indicate that the mean age of onset of SM is 2.7 to 4.1 years, when the child begins to move independently outside the home environment. However, it can start earlier or later than this. We have found that earlier onset is often associated with illness, developmental issues and/or separation anxiety (see Figure 2.1, page 37). It seems likely that infants who depend on the comforting presence of parents become highly anxious and agitated when passed to strangers and cannot enjoy or engage with their cooing and 'babytalk'. Later onset, well after school admission, is often triggered by an incident involving actual or perceived teasing, bullying or humiliation. This could coincide with puberty when children are particularly vulnerable and self-conscious.

Implications for multidisciplinary ownership of SM

Need for holistic assessment

In 2008, an international consensus-based care pathway of good practice for SM was developed by Keen *et al*. The aim was to agree and validate the key principles underlying the assessment and management of SM through a consensus process involving 13 international experts, in order to create a local care pathway. One of the key principles agreed by the majority was the need for early assessment of possible associated conditions and social and family issues.

We would support this recommendation but our experience indicates that it does not go far enough. The nature of 'early assessment' needs defining, along with the role of screening. It is evident that not all children present a complex picture of SM and should not have to undergo unnecessary direct assessment. This is discussed further in Chapter 3.

Much of the rationale for the early assessment of coexisting problems is backed up in the literature. Research analyses of populations of children who have SM invariably find significantly higher rates of additional problems than would be expected in the general population. The most common ones are other anxiety disorders (especially separation anxiety, SAD and other phobias), communication disorders (especially expressive language and speech disorders) and developmental motor problems (affecting movement, coordination and balance). In other words, there is a greater than average chance that children who have SM will also be struggling to master other anxieties or the skills needed for language, social or motor development. This is covered further in 'What causes SM?' (page 36), where we note that additional problems can impact on confidence and therefore increase a child's general vulnerability and ability to function confidently within group settings. Therefore, it is extremely important that a child's response to treatment for SM is not compromised by a failure to identify or address other difficulties where these exist.

With this in mind, Figure 2.1 (page 37) highlights the essential components of holistic assessment and shows the importance of identifying:

★ contributing factors to general vulnerability and the onset of SM

★ factors which cannot be changed but may need to be explored and discussed in the context of overall anxiety (eg the individual's personality, loss of loved ones, migration)

★ maintaining factors which can be changed and must be addressed as a first step towards overcoming SM.

Multidisciplinary care pathways

Given the wide range of possible contributing factors and the changing presentation of SM over time, a number of people from several professional groups will be needed to carry out whatever assessment might be necessary for children with SM and address the various aspects of intervention. Speech and language therapists, psychologists, psychiatrists, paediatricians, occupational therapists and physical therapists may all have a part to play. They should also be ready to liaise with, and refer on to, other agencies as appropriate, following agreed guidelines, to ensure a coordinated approach.

No single discipline 'owns' SM but a speech and language therapist's skills in communication assessment and small-steps treatment planning, and a psychologist's skills in contingency management, graded exposure and cognitive reframing are particularly relevant. We urge these disciplines to liaise with local health and education services in order to agree a multidisciplinary care pathway and avoid a situation where parents or teachers are passed from agency to agency as a result of ignorance about SM or confusion over professional boundaries. For more information, please see the chapter 'Effective Care Pathways' by Johnson *et al*, in *Tackling Selective Mutism* (2015). Figure 2.4 summarises the recommendations in that chapter and the components of an effective care pathway.

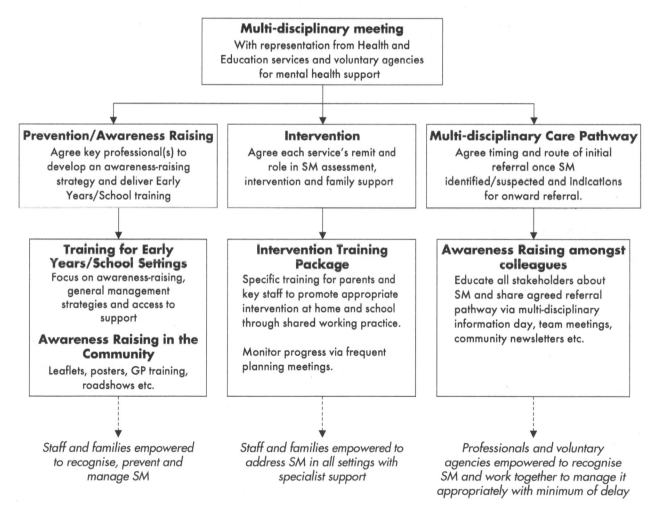

Figure 2.4: **Development and implementation of an effective multi-agency care pathway for selective mutism**

(Source: Smith & Sluckin, 2015, p191. Reproduced with the kind permission of Jessica Kingsley Publishers.)

Training to ensure adequate recognition and understanding of SM

Ideally, everyone who assesses a child who has SM for possible associated difficulties and issues, and certainly everyone who is involved in specific intervention and daily management, needs to recognise and understand SM adequately. The situation is definitely improving. Public and professional awareness has increased, more speech and language therapists, teachers and psychologists are receiving specialist training, and mental health practitioners are beginning to diagnose the condition in adults as well as children. But local expertise and service provision currently varies from excellent to non-existent, both within and outside the UK.

An effective care pathway will include training sessions on a universal basis, so that professionals, families and schools can access information about SM as part of a local network of provider services and service users. The content of a typical training session is outlined in Appendix D. One important aim is to equip families and schools to make a lay diagnosis of SM, as discussed in Chapter 3, in order to agree and implement appropriate management strategies without further delay.

Ironically, the need to channel resources into SM provision is often masked by a lack of referrals in the first instance. However, as would be expected from the prevalence rates cited earlier, it is our experience that, once it is known that a service or multi-agency team is available to support children who have SM, there is no shortage of referrals or uptake for information sessions.

The importance of early intervention

The case for early intervention is overwhelming; it is the most efficient, cost-effective and compassionate way forward.

The cost of ignoring SM

With long-term outcome studies indicating improvement in most cases, there is a danger that children will be left to 'outgrow' the disorder. However, no one 'outgrows' anxiety disorders as such; it takes sympathetic handling and appropriate support or determination and self-belief to work through them. Moreover, complete remission of the core features of SM is noted in only 39 to 58 per cent of subjects in long-term outcome studies using post-DSM-IV criteria. With no guarantee of a successful outcome, recovery cannot be left to chance and, in a caring society, there can be no justification for allowing children to live with SM any longer than necessary. Every extra year represents another year of intense anxiety for the child and considerable anguish or frustration for the family members and teachers who don't know how best to support them.

Furthermore, although the core features of SM may resolve, living with SM into adolescence and beyond is associated with a range of psychosocial issues that are not seen when the disorder is treated early. For example, low self-esteem, poor social communication skills, social anxiety, depression, underachievement and general dissatisfaction have been noted in 'recovered' adults. Looking at our caseloads, all students who were referred in their mid to late teens present with one or more of the following:

★ school refusal

★ self-harming

★ SAD

★ social withdrawal from immediate family

★ low mood treated by antidepressants

★ progressive mutism.

Of these, only school refusal is evident in pre-teens. Therefore, we are in no doubt that early intervention for SM is essential to protect children's health and well-being.

There is, of course, an economic argument for early intervention. When handled inappropriately, the pattern of non-speaking becomes more entrenched and, as discussed earlier in this chapter, the individual develops unhelpful thinking patterns. So a behavioural approach alone is no longer sufficient to turn things around. What may have been fairly easy to manage in a single class at primary or elementary school becomes a networking issue for 10 or more subject teachers as the child gets older. For some individuals, the prospect of intervention becomes too scary to contemplate. A young person may only be able to engage with the therapy process after a course of anti-anxiety medication. Consequently, the longer selective mutism lasts, the longer and more complex it is to resolve. Early intervention offers a relatively quick, non-invasive and inexpensive solution.

Implementing a prevention strategy

Given that a diagnosis of SM cannot be made for two months after admission to playgroup, nursery or school, early years staff are in the unique position of having, in effect, a two-month period for *prevention* rather than intervention. The human drive to socialise and communicate is extremely powerful so if children speak only a little, or not at all, it should not be ignored. We recommend that all staff in early years settings are made aware of SM and are ready to provide appropriate support as soon as they spot a quiet child.

The aims of a prevention strategy are to:

★ help the child work towards talking without placing undue pressure on them to speak before they are ready

★ value all forms of communication and encourage participation rather than avoidance

★ involve and support parents, providing appropriate information in a non-judgemental and non-alarmist manner

★ follow clear guidelines for onward and timely referral to local health and educational services, having considered a range of possible explanations for the child's reluctance to talk.

Early years training is a feature of the care pathway recommendations discussed earlier. It aims to avoid a situation where children are left for 12 weeks or more before taking action. This is a period where the very efforts teachers make in helping new children to 'settle in' can actually have the effect of maintaining and reinforcing SM (Cline & Baldwin, 2004). Handout 9 in the online resource library, 'Helping young children to speak at school', could be a helpful starting point. It gives guidance for supporting all quiet children and reluctant speakers on school admission, not just those with SM.

Rationale and framework for our treatment approach

The literature generally agrees that the effective management of SM points to:

★ early identification

★ involvement of the child, family and teaching staff

★ elimination of any maintaining factors

★ introduction of a behavioural programme of desensitisation and graded exposure.

In addition, older children may be offered cognitive behavioural therapy (CBT) or pharmacological treatment in conjunction with an intervention programme.

However, it is evident from long-term outcome studies and the re-referrals to our own services that a holistic view of SM is needed to ensure a comprehensive approach to intervention and recovery. SM cannot be treated in a single environment or in relation to one or two people with the hope that progress will transfer to other people and other settings. Similarly, it is not enough that a child simply speaks; the quality of the child's interactions, social functioning and general well-being must be considered.

In the first edition of this manual, we used two progressions to support the development of small-steps treatment programmes: the stages of confident speaking and the progression from a low to high communication load. Over the next 15 years it became clear that this sequential approach was too linear a framework. We have replaced it with a circular model to embrace all aspects of our programme and to encourage a more balanced approach to intervention (Figure 2.5).

Using this model as a framework for intervention, confident talking is defined as:

The ability to talk freely with a range of people in a range of places, both one to one and in a larger group, to meet all conversational needs without undue fear of negative judgement.

The original progressions are retained within the new model as interaction on a one-to-one basis, and conversational content. There are additional progressions for a range of conversational partners, group interaction, talking in public places and social purpose. All of these aspects are summarised in Table 7.1 (page 108). They are also described in more detail in Part 3 Management.

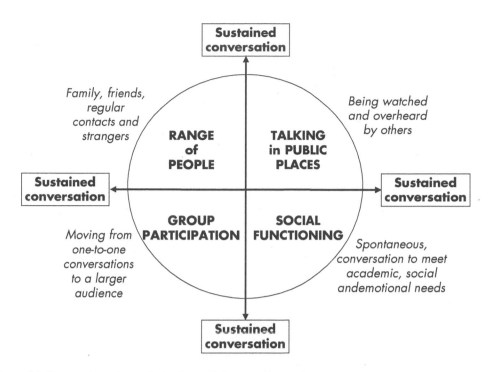

Figure 2.5: **A multidimensional model of confident talking** (also in Handout D1, Appendix D)

We believe that a collaborative approach involving home and school, supported by other agencies as appropriate, is the most effective way to work through all four quadrants of the circle. By setting out all of the components of a successful intervention programme, we hope that everyone can find a useful starting point, whether working alone or in partnership with other people. The message from research evidence is clear: *do not delay intervention*. Therefore, we encourage everyone involved with the child to:

★ make a start in following the approach in this manual

★ keep track of progress

★ use their findings to support their resolve to build a team around the child.

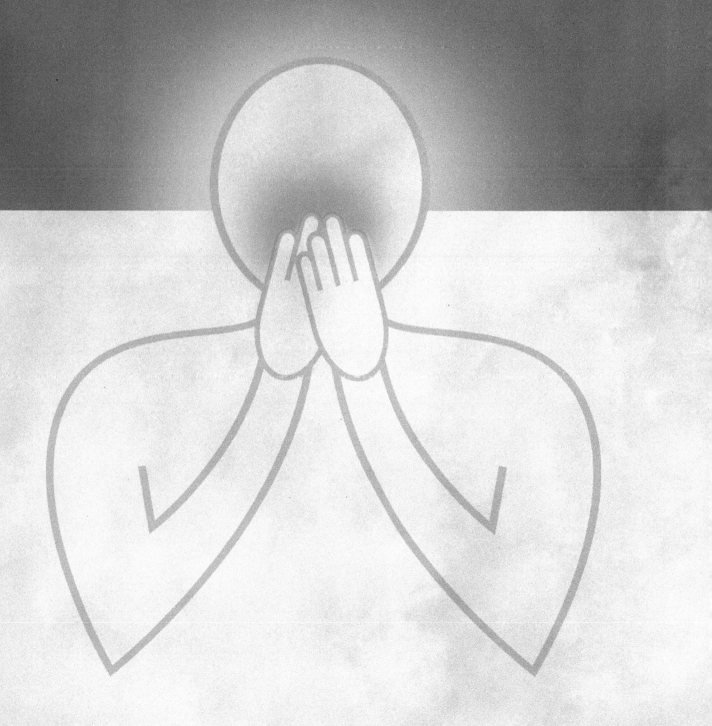

PART 2

GUIDELINES FOR IDENTIFICATION AND ASSESSMENT

CONTENTS

Chapter 7 Moving from assessment to management

CHAPTER 3

MAKING A DIAGNOSIS: WHAT WE NEED TO KNOW AND WHY

Introduction

This chapter looks at the following topics.

★   How to reach a diagnosis of selective mutism.

★   Who can make a diagnosis.

★   How to find a suitable professional to make a diagnosis.

★   The case for lay diagnosis.

★   What makes for a good assessment.

★   The assessment framework.

★   The two possible levels of assessment.

★   Whether to carry out a core (simple) or extended (detailed) assessment.

Together with Chapters 4 and 5, this is probably a chapter that most clinicians will turn to at an early stage. However, it is equally important for parents to understand the essence of assessment and diagnosis if they are to work in partnership with professionals or, in some cases, to take the lead in their child's management.

How to reach a diagnosis of selective mutism

When assessing children with mutism, first we need to decide whether their symptoms fit the diagnosis of selective mutism (SM).

Indicators towards a diagnosis of selective mutism

★   The child has a consistent pattern of not speaking to, or in front of, certain people.

★   The child talks comfortably to at least one other person, but stops talking, whispers or becomes visibly tense when aware of anyone else approaching.

★   Even when it is clearly in the child's interests to speak or cry out, they do not.

★   The child has described, in the absence of stammering, a sensation of 'freezing' or their voice getting stuck or not coming out.

★ Although SM can exist *alongside* other diagnoses, the child's mutism *cannot be better explained* by one of the following: speech or language difficulties; social communication difficulties; hearing loss; developmental delay; learning difficulties; cultural influences (including additional languages); or psychiatric conditions. In other words, even if the quality of the child's speech or language is affected by another diagnosis, there is still a consistent pattern of speaking to some people but not others.

As part of the diagnosis, we have to decide whether it is low or high profile SM and whether there are any other difficulties in addition to the SM. As speech and language therapists (SLTs), we have found it useful to categorise children who have SM as follows.

1 'Pure' selective mutism (low or high profile)

2 Selective mutism, plus speech or language impairment or learning a new language

3 Selective mutism, plus other diagnoses such as autism spectrum disorder (ASD) or social anxiety disorder; additional major concerns (medical, environmental or emotional); or progressive mutism.

High or low profile selective mutism
High profile SM is easier to spot: the child does not speak at all to certain people.

With low profile SM, the child manages to speak a little when absolutely necessary (fear of the consequences of *not* speaking outweighs the fear of speaking) but does not spontaneously initiate conversation or make requests. Low profile SM is less obvious but not less serious. It is likely to be overlooked, so there is a risk of it becoming entrenched, with the development of high profile SM, social anxiety disorder or school avoidance. With both profiles there is always a consistent pattern of speaking habits, with body tension, wariness and tendency to freeze.

Progressive mutism
The child started with a clear pattern of low or high profile SM but has gradually stopped speaking, even to people they once spoke to freely. This can occur for a variety of reasons, including:

a) in addition to the anxiety experienced in certain situations where speech is expected, there are considerable gains for *not* speaking or there is little need to speak

b) the child has a relatively inflexible or rigid thinking style and has found it hard to make sense of the 'rules' around situations where they can and can't speak

c) after many years of being misunderstood, older children may withdraw from communication completely, unable to cope with the associated stress any longer.

In keeping with SM, individuals with progressive mutism can speak when alone (although rarely have a reason to) and may find some respite in talking to animals or babies who have no expectations of them.

See question 13 in Chapter 1 (page 14) and 'Maintaining factors' (page 38) for more information.

Indicators against a diagnosis of selective mutism

There are many reasons why children don't talk and SM is just one of them. In any assessment we must therefore look carefully at the child's history and speaking patterns for other explanations which would indicate a different diagnosis and support strategy. The findings below are not consistent with SM.

★ The child shows the same limited speaking habits across all settings.

★ The child shows inconsistent speaking habits (eg talking to the teacher on some days, but not on others), in *identical* circumstances. This could relate to other anxieties or emotional issues such as worries about home, school performance or being teased.

★ The child does not talk in any setting, with the exception of 'progressive mutism' (see above).

★ Abrupt cessation or reduction of speech in a particular setting indicating a need to investigate and address possible triggers (eg bullying, criticism or seeing another child reprimanded for talking).

★ The child has indicated an acute self-consciousness about a speech difficulty or different accent and is afraid that they will be teased, corrected or unable to get their message across. There are indications that their anxiety has a reasonable foundation which is likely to respond to reassurance at an emotional or a practical level.

There are three important points to consider which are described further below.

a) SM must not be confused with 'traumatic mutism'.

b) It is unrelated to 'psychogenic voice disorder' or 'conversion disorder' which generally occur in adults.

c) Some children are better described as 'reluctant speakers'.

(a) Traumatic mutism

This is sometimes called 'reactive mutism'. It comes under the umbrella term post-traumatic stress disorder (PTSD) and is usually managed by psychologists or Child and Adolescent Mental Health Services (CAMHS). It is characterised as follows.

★ A sudden reduction of speech with an identifiable trigger, although the child may not disclose this immediately.

★ Speech withdrawal is evident to some degree across all environments, and the child may be totally mute.

★ There may be some variation in communication depending on mood.

★ The child may have associated images or flashbacks and nightmares.

(b) Psychogenic voice disorder

This total or partial loss of voice (in spite of a normal larynx) is caused, or maintained by, emotional or psychological factors and conflict. The person can mouth words or whisper freely but cannot produce a normal voice. It is managed by a speech and language therapist specialising in voice disorders, working in close collaboration with an ENT (ear, nose and throat) surgeon and possibly a psychologist.

(c) Reluctant speakers

Most people recognise times when they are reluctant or unwilling to speak. Children may also have good reason to hold back for the following reasons.

★ General discomfort or wariness in unfamiliar or group situations. The child is shy or overwhelmed and needs time to 'warm up'; they prefer other people to initiate contact.

★ Complexity or ambiguity of language used. The child needs simpler, more explicit input and help to develop their language skills.

★ Lack of confidence in expressive language skills (eg second language, speech disorder).

★ Personality and style of conversational partner. The child will respond better to a non-confrontational, non-directive, affirming style of interaction.

★ Fear of consequences (eg cultural influences, other people's reactions). The child may need overt permission or reassurance before being able to speak freely. If they fear being corrected for speech errors or being told to slow down when they speak, they will benefit from more helpful strategies such as modelling, and showing interest in *what* the child says rather than *how* they say it.

★ Lack of interest in conversational topic or social interaction (bear in mind a possible ASD diagnosis).

Whatever the reason is for being reluctant to speak, communication should *never* be an unpleasant or anxiety-provoking experience; otherwise, there is a risk that talking will increasingly be avoided and SM will develop. Many of the suggestions in Chapter 8 (Ensuring an anxiety-free environment) and Handout 9 'Helping young children to speak at school' are, therefore, equally appropriate for reluctant speakers; that is, providing permission and opportunity to speak with no uncomfortable pressure or unreasonable expectations. In addition, we have outlined particular areas above where support may be indicated, rather than addressing the specific fear of speaking which characterises SM.

Who can make a diagnosis

Unfortunately, the world is not full of SM specialists. Also, SM is not the speciality of one specific profession. So it may not be easy for a parent or teacher to find a suitable professional to assess and diagnose the child if there is not an obvious person known to the school or the family doctor.

In the UK, the primary clinicians responsible for diagnosis are usually speech and language therapists who have a clear professional remit to address SM because it is a communication difficulty. However, paediatricians, educational psychologists and mental health professionals with experience and knowledge of SM may also make a diagnosis.

The case for lay diagnosis

This may seem controversial but there is a case for families to decide themselves, perhaps along with school staff, that their child has SM. There are certainly many examples of parents and teachers who have

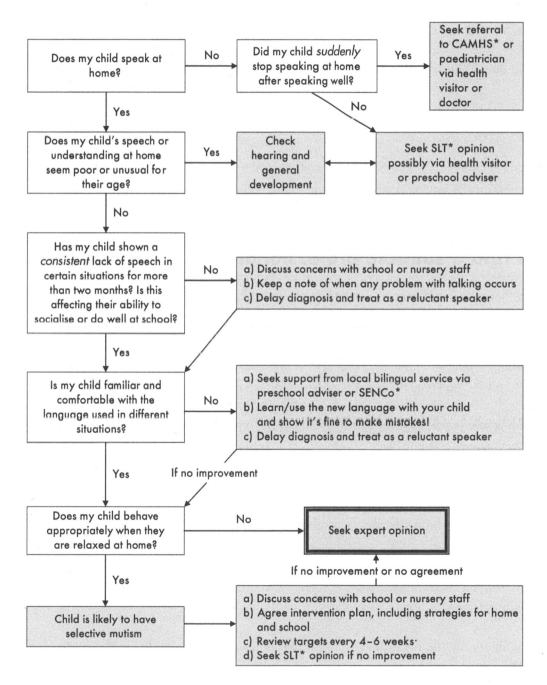

Figure 3.1: **Flow chart for lay diagnosis of selective mutism**
(*CAMHS = Child and Adolescent Mental Health Service; SLT = speech and language therapist; SENCo = Special Educational Needs Coordinator)

successfully used their own resources, often with no previous experience, to diagnose and manage a child's SM. There remains a considerable lack of knowledge about SM within the medical and educational profession. Lay diagnosis may avoid misdiagnosis (eg suggesting it is a part of ASD); or misinformation (eg advising 'Don't worry, she'll grow out of it'; or ruling it out because the child spoke to the mother in front of the doctor or briefly answered the therapist's questions). Furthermore, the time it takes to find an appropriate specialist to diagnose SM can delay the start of intervention unnecessarily.

Lay diagnosis is recommended as a starting point if parents and school staff agree that:

a)   the child's pattern of communication is consistent with SM (see diagnostic indicators on page 53)

b)   there are no additional issues with speech or language development or other major concerns

c)   they have access to information about appropriate intervention and are willing to work together to implement it.

The flow chart in Figure 3.1 may be helpful if starting down the lay diagnosis route. It could also be used in conjunction with the screening questions on the parent interview form (see Chapter 4, online resource).

How to find a suitable professional to make a diagnosis

If there are other significant concerns in addition to the child's inability to speak freely, an appropriate specialist should be consulted for an assessment and diagnosis. The same applies if parents and teachers cannot reach agreement, or the child does not begin to improve within six weeks of implementing an intervention plan. Specialist opinion is particularly important when there are several issues and the timing or manner of intervention may need to be modified to take into account additional diagnoses.

In any case, it is worth asking a few questions about the professional's experience and interest in SM. A practitioner is needed who:

a)   is familiar with SM and views it as an anxiety disorder

b)   will not confuse SM with shyness, autism, depression or behavioural problems such as a need to control other people

c)   will start with an exploratory interview about the child's upbringing, early development, lifestyle and social relationships

d)   will investigate alternative explanations for the child's mutism, if needed, and refer the child on to other disciplines, if indicated

e)   can identify a range of contributing and maintaining factors to support the diagnosis and indicate the starting point for appropriate intervention

f)   understands that SM requires a small-steps approach to enable the child to master their fear of speaking in a range of situations and different environments.

Parents might therefore ask:

a)   What is your experience of SM? Is that experience of assessing children or managing their SM or both?

b)   Can you tell me a little about how you understand SM? (How it arises; how it relates to other difficulties; and how it should be managed.)

And if the professional has little experience or understanding of SM:

c)   Given that SM is a recognised anxiety disorder (DSM-5, 2013) treated by speech and language therapists or psychologists in other parts of the UK, would you be interested in reading the information I have and finding out more about it?

Professionals may not have firsthand experience of SM but be keen to learn more. In this case, we recommend the following online resources: Handouts 2–5 or the booklet for teenagers and adults 'When the words won't come out'.

What makes for a good assessment

Good assessment is essential as a basis for effective management. Although it is important to see whether the diagnosis fits, you are not just ascertaining whether the child does or does not have SM. You may guess that either from the referral; or the features that you witness on first meeting the child; or those that are described to you by a teacher or parent; or your own observations as a parent or teacher.

Assessment is needed to:

★   work out the pattern, severity and effect of the SM

★   find out if there are any other significant or relevant concerns

★   establish how well the SM is understood and being managed by the people who are closely involved

★   know enough about the child's development, interests and friendships in order to start implementing successful intervention.

All SM assessment should cover four key assessment areas:

1   the pattern of the child's SM (speaking habits)

2   how the SM is managed by home and school (to identify relevant maintaining factors)

3   the child's speech, language and cognitive profile

4   the child's emotional and social profile (including any other factors which might be undermining the child's confidence).

The child's speaking habits and the presence of any maintaining factors in managing the child (points 1 and 2) must be explored in depth with all children. However, the information from points 3 and 4 can be gained either at a simple screening level or, if there are concerns, from a more detailed, extended assessment.

The assessment framework

Figure 3.2 shows the assessment framework; the four key assessment areas are in the centre. There are various ways of collecting comprehensive information from home, school and the child. These feed into the four areas and help to build up the picture. Chapters 4 and 5 provide various tools, such as checklists, interview forms and questionnaires. However, evidence of ability as shown in written work, computer literacy, artistic skills, problem solving, organisation and reported conversations are as relevant as more formal methods.

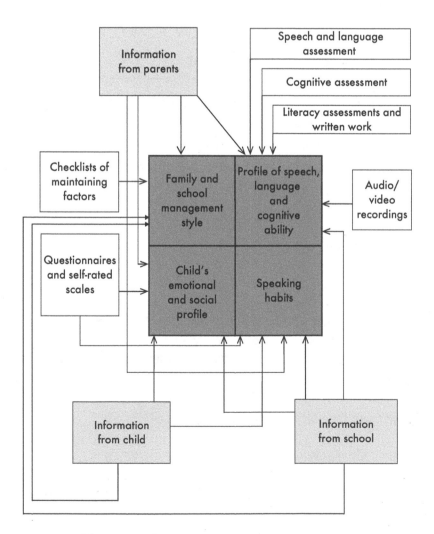

Figure 3.2: **The assessment framework**

The two levels of assessment

1   The *core assessment* comprises information from the parents and the school, to establish the child's speaking habits, as well as the general levels of the child's language, learning and reasoning abilities to eliminate significant developmental difficulties. Chapter 4 includes proformas for interviews with parents and the school, and a section on the child's speaking habits. The family and school management style must be assessed to determine the extent of any factors that reinforce or maintain the SM.

2   The *extended assessment* includes more in-depth information about various areas of the child's development, emotions and behaviour. It may also include specific assessments of speech and language, cognition and literacy skills, as discussed in Chapter 6.

The core and extended assessments involve the child, through interaction or observation; and, of course, a young person may be able to participate more directly. These aspects of assessment are covered in Chapter 5.

Deciding on a core or an extended assessment

We don't believe in overassessment or pathologising the problem more than is needed. Children who have SM are anxious and stressed about having to speak, or even perform, in unfamiliar situations, in front of people they don't know. So it is best to avoid putting them under increased pressure if it is not necessary, especially as the results are likely to be unreliable because of anxiety.

However, we do believe that professionals should be rigorous and skilled in their information gathering. They should also be wise enough to discern when they need to go further with their investigations or seek help from other professionals.

It may be helpful to consider the following factors.

★   **The stage at which the need for an assessment has been identified.**

For most children, a core assessment will suffice initially, particularly if the mutism has recently been identified and at a young age. Children referred for a second opinion, or where previous treatment has not been effective, may require an extended assessment.

★   **The existence and extent of other concerns.**

Parents or teachers, who know the child best, may have picked up other difficulties that need addressing as well as the mutism. An extended assessment is indicated where additional concerns about cognitive, emotional, social or physical development emerge.

CHAPTER 4

THE CORE ASSESSMENT: INITIAL INFORMATION GATHERING

Introduction

This chapter looks at:

★ information from parents

★ information from schools

★ the child's speaking habits

★ maintaining factors at home and school.

The online resource library includes several forms to supplement the areas discussed in this chapter.

Information from parents

There is much to recommend meeting or speaking to the parents first, without the referred child or teenager being present. This allows freedom for discussion away from an already self-conscious child. It also enables the parents to express their concerns fully without exacerbating the problem. At the meeting, the clinician will want to hear about the child's strengths, interests and difficulties, especially about speaking freely, and to ask the parents some questions.

The parent interview form

There is a short parent interview form (Form 1a) in the online library resource. It covers:

★ *presenting problems* – mutism, its background and other problems or concerns

★ *family* – history, household, significant members, losses

★ *speaking pattern*

★ *screening questions* – consideration of additional difficulties.

We recommend using it at the initial meeting to gather basic information and to determine whether a core or an extended assessment is indicated. The form is designed to make sure that the child has no other difficulties besides selective mutism (SM) which warrant further investigation and possible inclusion in an overall intervention plan. It is most likely to be used with the parents but could be used with anyone who spends time with the child regularly. If nothing significant arises, continue with the other assessment areas (school report form, speaking habits, and maintaining factors), then move on to Chapter 5 'Meeting and involving the child'. If there are other concerns, use Form 1b 'Extended parent interview form' to get more detailed information.

Information from school

It is often through starting school, playgroup or nursery that a child's mutism comes to light. School represents a major threat to most young children who have SM. Here the child and parents have to separate; it is a large, strange place and it is full of unfamiliar people. Although not necessarily unfamiliar for older children or teenagers, school or college is where they spend most of the day. Therefore, it is very important to gather comprehensive information about the child's past and present functioning in school.

Overt observation of the child or young person in school, whether in the classroom or the playground, is *not* recommended. Children who have SM are acutely self-conscious and wary of being 'spied on'. They need to develop trusting relationships and this type of observation is counterproductive. However, classroom observation can be valuable for the purpose of observing classroom practice and the child's interaction with others. We have seen children very frozen in class but school staff members were unaware of the child's high anxiety level. Classroom observation works particularly well if the observer is unknown to the child and sits with a group of other children and appears to be participating rather than writing notes.

The school report forms

There are two versions of a school report form online: Form 2a (up to 11 years) and Form 2b (11+ years). We suggest that it is a routine part of professional assessment for all children. The form could be sent to the school as a questionnaire to be filled in by the teacher who knows the child best. Better still, and time permitting, it could be used as the basis for a school interview visit. A telephone interview with the teacher might be an alternative, if it is timetabled in advance.

The areas covered on the primary school form are:

★ Background information

★ Present school (starting date and concerns)

★ Speech, language and communication

★ Social interaction, temperament and behaviour

★ Ability, attainment and interests

★ Additional assessment and help

★ Siblings

★ Parents

★ Staff training and experience.

The secondary school form has an additional section, 'Coping with the school day'.

Once again, the areas to be covered are set out in a logical sequence, with a main heading which can be used as a general introduction to lead into the questions. After this, there are some questions in **bold type**, which can be used to elicit specific information. Small *italic type* is used for ideas that need to be kept in mind when gathering information, and the aims of probing each area.

The child's speaking habits

One primary focus of assessment is to establish a clear picture of the child's or young person's speaking habits – that is, to know how comfortably they speak to whom, in which locations, and under what conditions. This information will come from the following online resources:

★ the parent interview form

★ the school report form

★ the young person's interview form (Chapter 5)

★ the communication rating scales (Chapter 5).

The information will give an insight into the child's anxiety triggers (their internal 'rule' system, as explained on pages 15 and 30) and indicate the starting point for intervention. For example, the child may:

★ talk in a large supermarket but not in the local corner shop

★ talk to the family in the school building if they think no one else is within earshot

★ not talk directly to visitors to the house but talk to the family in their presence

★ talk to a friend at home, but not at school, and only in the friend's house when other people are out of the room

★ be more conversational with female relatives

★ talk to Mum in the car but stop in the street

★ talk to a friend when walking to school or college but stop at the gates

★ answer their teacher's questions but never initiate conversation or ask for help

★ talk to children or adults individually but not in a group.

It can be helpful to assemble the information into some form of visual representation. This has the following advantages.

★ To check that all of the relevant information has been gathered.

★ To check with the informants that the information is accurate.

★ To provide a format for explaining the therapeutic process in terms that can be easily understood.

★ To provide a format for explaining the child's difficulties to other people (eg staff members at school or playgroup).

★ To establish a baseline for planning intervention and monitoring progress.

★ To allow families and young people to see how far they have come when progress seems slow.

★ To gauge when the child may be ready to be discharged.

Record of speaking habits

There are various ways to summarise speaking habits visually. We suggest a grid as shown in Form 3 (online). There is a completed example of Form 3 on page 67. People the child needs to talk to are recorded down the side, according to their familiarity – family and friends, regular contacts, and strangers. Across the top there are the situations where speaking is expected, with the emphasis on who else is present. A further distinction is made about whether the child can initiate conversations as well as respond to questions or prompts.

Comments can be written in the relevant boxes and a large or small tick can indicate speaking at normal volume or in a quiet voice, as illustrated in the example on page 67.

We have found that the grid provides a helpful baseline, which can be added to in different colours as progress is reviewed. As an alternative which is accessible to younger children, we suggest making a talking map (see Chapter 5).

Maintaining factors at home and school

Sometimes it is hard to know how to support an anxious child who has SM and not easy for parents and teachers always to react in the most helpful way. As explained in 'Maintaining factors' in Chapter 2 (page 38), some patterns of responding can inadvertently impede or delay a child's progress. This is not a criticism; it's a fact of life. So, it is essential to investigate how the child's SM is being managed at home and in school, in order to identify any potential factors that might need addressing.

There are several ways of doing this. Some people may choose to use the short book *Can I Tell You about Selective Mutism?* (Johnson & Wintgens, 2012) as a basis for reflection or discussion. It contains sections on how teachers and parents can help a child who has SM. It is written from the perspective of Hannah, a young girl who has SM, which can be an effective and powerful way of recognising and addressing the

Form 3 RECORD OF SPEAKING HABITS Name: **Binky** Age: **6; 3** Date: **3/12/2015** (Completed example)

PEOPLE	One-to-one, no one else around (eg at home, in empty classroom with no fear of interruption, deserted park)		One-to-one, others in background (eg in shop, classroom or waiting room)		Group conversation (eg family meal, car journey, class discussion, play activities)	
	Responds	Initiates	Responds	Initiates	Responds	Initiates
Family and friends						
Parents Mike & Sue Siblings Jess & Tom	✓	✓	w		✓ just family	✓ just family
Mike's parents	✓	✓	w		✓ with family	✓ with family
Sue's parents (B. rarely sees them)	just starting to nod, smile					
Best friend Sara	home ✓ school ✓	home ✓ school ✓	possibly in playground		✓ only at home	✓ only at home
Gemma (Binky often asks for G to come and play but doesn't talk to her)	lots of laughter	makes needs known by pointing, pulling				
Regular contacts (eg teachers, peers, friends' parents, youth group leader)						
Doesn't speak to anyone else but has good relationship with: Sara's Mum, Mrs Banks, teaching assistant, Jojo, child minder						
Strangers (eg staff in shops and restaurants, visitors to house)						
never speaks to strangers						

Note: large tick = speaks at normal volume; small tick = quiet voice; w = whisper issue of management and maintaining factors. Parents or teachers might check on the helpful things they are already saying and doing; also make a note of some things they might do differently.

Checklist of possible maintaining factors

This online checklist will help parents and school staff to identify the factors which have a role in maintaining the child's SM. Again, this could be used as a basis for discussion with a clinician. Alternatively, parents and school or nursery staff could consider the list themselves and decide whether there are any items that they could address, and how.

Using this checklist, staff and parents often recognise a particular style or approach towards handling SM that is *strengthening* the child's fear of speaking. This delicate subject can be understandably distressing and must be handled sensitively so that no one feels they are being blamed or criticised. Most maintaining factors are a direct and natural *response* to the child's silence and represent a genuine attempt to improve the situation. It is important to reassure parents and staff that, once identified, maintaining factors can be eliminated or significantly reduced, with an almost instant impact on the child's or young person's well-being. Table 8.2 in Chapter 8 (page 134) gives suggestions for more helpful ways to support a child who has SM.

Online resources for Chapter 4

The forms accompanying this chapter are available at www.routledge.com/cw/speechmark for you to access, print and copy.

CHAPTER 5

MEETING AND INVOLVING THE CHILD OR YOUNG PERSON

Introduction

This chapter looks at:

★ **Meeting the child for the first time**

   Preparing for the meeting

   Reassuring the child

   Offering the opportunity to talk but with no pressure

   Introducing appropriate activities

   Facilitating participation

   Talking openly about speech anxiety

   Finding a special incentive

★ **Adaptations and additions for young people**

   Consent to treatment

   Engaging with a more withdrawn young person

   Email correspondence

   Use of questionnaires and rating scales

   Talking openly about speech anxiety

   Learning about phobias

   Information from the young person

   Assessing the young person's speaking habits

   Assessing the young person's perception of maintaining factors

   Establishing the young person's priorities

   Checking how the young person sees themselves

The online resource library includes several forms, a handout and a booklet to supplement the areas discussed in this chapter.

Meeting the child for the first time

How often have you heard that first impressions make a big difference? This is particularly true when a clinician is meeting an anxious child, so the first meeting needs to be carefully planned with clear aims. Whether the purpose is to play with the child informally, carry out formal assessments, or talk to the child about their speech anxiety, the most important aim of the first meeting is to get the child or young person on board. In other words, to reassure and encourage them and try to engage them, while keeping their anxiety to a minimum. Success will depend on *what* is said to them and *how* it is said. If a diagnosis of selective mutism (SM) has been made, you want to start helping them to understand SM and to explain a little about your role. With older children, it is important to be completely open, getting across to them that you want to understand a bit about their hopes and fears and to work out with them a way to help them move forward.

Meeting strangers is stressful for children who have SM. So a parent or member of staff with whom the child has good rapport should be present at the first meeting, except with teenagers who are often more self-conscious with an audience. It may then be useful to have initial introductions and explanations with the familiar person present, before seeing the older child alone if they are comfortable with this. Offer the choice of meeting at home, in school or at the clinic if you have this flexibility. Also, be prepared to make an exception if the child cannot face a trip to your usual workplace. The advice on 'Home visits' in Chapter 10 (page 239) may be helpful.

Preparing for the meeting

It is important to be honest about the purpose of the meeting but the parents may be unsure how to explain this to the child. Something about meeting someone who knows how difficult it is 'to talk comfortably at school or with new people' may do. It is essential to give reassurance that they are going for help to enjoy the situations they worry about, not to see someone who will try to make them speak. This can be linked to something at home or school which you know they are anxious about (eg '[X] wants to help you because you're worried about going to college').

Have a private word with the parents beforehand about how they should act during the session.

★ They should not put pressure on the child to speak because this could raise the child's anxiety unnecessarily before the meeting.

★ You are used to children not speaking and will find other ways to communicate during the session.

★ It would be helpful if parents could talk to their child during the session to put him or her at ease, but not to worry if the child doesn't answer.

★ Parents should not answer questions which you specifically direct to the child but they may repeat unanswered questions to the child after a few seconds. This should be in the form of a question, so that the child can answer the parent, rather than encouragement to tell you the answer.

Parents may also need to be warned that you will be talking to their child about their speech anxiety. If parents have not done this before because they fear making the situation worse, it will be important to explain why this is such a vital step (see page 73, 'Talking openly about speech anxiety').

Reassuring the child

Five points can be made during the meeting, taking into account the age of the child and your existing knowledge about them. These are particularly useful to balance any anxious comments that parents may express in front of their child.

1   *There is no pressure to speak.* Say you know that they sometimes find it hard to speak comfortably with new people. If speaking feels comfortable that is great, but there is no need. Put a pen and paper on the table for an older child and say they may prefer to write things down, it's up to them.

2   *They are not alone.* Explain that you have seen, or you know of, other children who find it hard to speak at school; they are not the only one experiencing these difficulties.

3   *Their difficulty in talking will not last for ever.*

4   *It's not surprising they found it hard to speak* when they went to school – schools are big and very different from home.

5   *If appropriate, add that it must have been especially hard* not speaking English very well, or being in a strange country, or having difficulty talking clearly, or whatever applies.

Offering the opportunity to talk but with no pressure

It can be daunting to be faced with a silent child for the first time, especially when you are anxious not to make the situation worse. Even the most confident adult can be surprisingly tongue-tied or overcompensate by prattling on without pausing. Remember that the child is much more nervous than you and will respond best to a calm, friendly approach, a sense of humour and the reassurance you have given them that you don't mind if they don't talk. Don't be afraid of pauses but maintain a relaxed facial expression and focus on a shared activity rather than watching the child to see if they respond. Position yourself alongside, rather than opposite, the child so that they don't feel scrutinised.

At first, avoid asking the child direct questions. It is best for the clinician to adopt the role of commentator, rather than questioner, starting sentences with 'I wonder ...' or 'That looks ...' or 'I like the way you ...'. Don't expect speech and then it will be a bonus! If you do ask a question, don't wait more than a few seconds for an answer. If there is no response, move on smoothly or invite the child to answer by pointing or writing.

Introducing appropriate activities

If you are meeting the child at home, ask the parent to involve him or her in a favourite activity before you arrive, so that you can gradually show interest and join in. Similarly, in a clinic setting, young children will benefit from a general play session with you and their parent, so they get used to you and the room. You might have a few things out on a table or the floor, or let the child look in the toy cupboard and point out something of interest. Link the choice of toy or activity to what you learned from the parent that the child likes to play with.

However, it can be very difficult for children with SM to make choices, which may lead to further expectation to interact, even if you are only asking which toy they prefer, or where they would like to sit. A particularly 'frozen' child may only want to sit or stand and watch or listen. If their parent starts playing, they may gradually join in. If necessary, you can distance yourself a little with general tidying up or paperwork, allowing the parent to relax the child before you join in the activity. Older children will not want the distraction of games. They need to hear straight away why they are there and what you would like them to do.

Here are some ways in which you might initially approach the child, depending on their age and the activity you want to introduce:

I like to help children when they're having a difficult time at school

These look fun! I wonder which one you'd like to do first?

It's my job to help children like you who find it very hard to talk, even when they really want to

Your Mum told me you like ...

Don't worry. When you're here, you only ever have to do things that you feel OK about

I know you're not always happy at school, so I want to help your teacher make school fun for you

I know you're having a hard time talking to people. If you could look at these things with me, it would help me find the right way to make things easier for you

First, I need to find out a bit more about you, like what you enjoy doing and what you find easy or difficult at school

Facilitating participation

The first meeting with the child gives you the opportunity to observe the extent of their communication with you and how they interact with their parent in public. Remember that the most important thing is to allow the child to be as relaxed as possible; and that you will be offering opportunities for participation without any pressure to speak. Table 5.1 overleaf gives a framework to underpin observations about the child's level of participation, with suggestions of appropriate activities to introduce at each stage. When children are at their most anxious at stages 0 and 1, they need reassurance that you are happy for them to watch or listen and to only join in if they feel comfortable. As their anxiety decreases, they can be offered activities with an increasing expectation to communicate.

Move slowly from Stage 2 activities which require simple participation to those where a response is indicated. Note the extent of the child's involvement in the activity, their reliance on their parent to communicate for them and how at ease or tense they are. Tension may be noted as stiff or agitated movements, averted eye gaze, a hand over the mouth or a strained or distorted voice (eg nasal or high-pitched). See if the child can use gesture, with or without encouragement (nodding, pointing, using fingers for numbers). Note any vocalising in laughing or coughing, any whispered or voiced noises (eg vehicle noises if you are building a train track or a roadway), or any other sounds or words. A voice-activated toy may be helpful. As the child relaxes further and speaks to their parent in your presence, they are more likely to respond to simple 'X or Y?' choices (eg 'I'm not sure what Billy's got there. Is it a leopard or a tiger?') or a Stage 6 single word activity such as 'Pairs'. See Appendix A (online) for appropriate activities at different stages. Chapter 6 describes how these stages relate to more formal assessment procedures.

Talking openly about speech anxiety

Many children get the message from well-meaning adults that talking is easy. This is borne out by the fact that no one else in their nursery, school or street appears to be having this difficulty. To have no understanding of why they are different is confusing and scary in itself. Dreading the feeling of panic that takes over when they try to speak, they say (and often convince themselves) that they don't *want* to speak. Dispelling this myth can be a tremendous relief and helps children to believe and trust in you and any suggestions you might make to help. Even very young children can recognise the difference; they do *want* to talk, but they don't want to feel *scared* about talking.

The Pep Talk

Once a diagnosis of SM is made, it is important to talk directly to the child about their speech anxiety. This should be done in a relaxed, open way, so that the difficulty is acknowledged and there is no misunderstanding or stigma to interfere with the intervention process. Everyone who takes a key role in helping the child overcome their fears will need to have a quiet word with them, to convey the same messages and show the child that they can be 'trusted' not to move things on too quickly. We call this the 'Pep Talk' and it is a key step on our management checklist (see Chapter 7). Handout 1 'Talking to the child about speech anxiety' (online) may help staff and parents to grasp the main points they need to convey to the younger child. Draw simple faces as you talk to illustrate the emotions of feeling relaxed and happy, versus anxious, panicky or worried (see the examples in the activity below and in Chapter 8, Figure 8.3).

Table 5.1: **Confident talking – the stages of one-to-one interaction** (also in Handout D3, Appendix D)

Stage	Child's presentation	Example of behaviour
0	Absent	Child or young person stays in the bedroom, hides behind a chair or observes activity from a distance.
1	Frozen	Child sits passively or accepts help without moving (eg does not take a ball that is offered; stands motionless while coat is buttoned up).
2	Participates without communication	Child participates silently in activities such as board games or jigsaw puzzles; takes items that are offered (eg a biscuit or crayons); and complies with requests which do not require an answer (eg deals out cards or draws a picture).
3	Uses non-verbal and written communication	Child responds to questions and may even initiate contact through: pointing; nodding or shaking head; tapping; gesture; drawing or writing. Child is relaxed and responds to the adult with a variety of facial expressions.
Talking bridge	Tolerates voice being heard by a bystander	Child talks to or laughs with parent without hiding their mouth in a visitor's or the therapist's presence; talks to other children in the same room as their teacher; talks to family member using a telephone in a public area. Voice may be quiet but is audible rather than whispered.
4	Talks through another person	Child answers when the parent repeats the therapist's question; asks the parent if a person present can play a game with them; talks in a structured activity with an adult but looks at their friend or parent when they speak. Voice may be quiet but is audible rather than whispered.
5	Uses voice	Child vocalises an audible rather than a whispered sound to express emotion, accompany shared play, participate in an activity or directly communicate (eg laughter, humming, sound of police siren, animal noises, letter sounds, 'mmm' for 'yes'). Child reads familiar material aloud on request (reading is a vocal exercise for proficient readers, rather than communication).
6	Communicates with single words	Child says a single word in response to questions or choices or in structured activities such as games. Voice may be very quiet but is audible rather than whispered.
7	Communicates with sentences	Child uses sentences in response to questions or in structured activities such as games or play readings. Child may: • occasionally offer a spontaneous comment • only ask questions during structured activities. Voice may be very quiet but is audible rather than whispered.
8	Conversation	Child has an adult-led, two-way conversation, provided no one else is perceived to be listening. Child: • volunteers spontaneous comments but questions may be limited • may not initiate contact or seek help outside planned sessions.
Note		Whispering is not included in this progression because it is an avoidance of using voice. For the purposes of keeping records, whispering can be regarded as stage 3+. When the child is completely comfortable, 8+ may be observed, for example: unplanned conversation on most topics; child-initiated questions and requests; social language and conversation-fillers (words and phrases that add no meaning but feature in relaxed, uninhibited conversation).

Initially, no response is necessary from the child, but they often listen intently. Then, in time, as the adult repeats key messages for reassurance and encouragement, they will begin to use the same vocabulary to identify and express their feelings to the people closest to them.

Very occasionally, children are so averse to meeting strangers that they hide behind a chair or door. In this case, we deliver the Pep Talk messages by addressing their parent or carer, knowing that the child is listening. Having received the necessary reassurances, albeit indirectly, these children begin to engage and accept help.

Some parents may be reluctant to give SM a name, fearing that this will label their child and create more anxiety. In our experience, the opposite is true. These children have already been labelled – but incorrectly. They have heard other people label them as shy, difficult, naughty, rude or stubborn and labelled themselves as different, unlikeable or a failure. Not understanding that SM is a fear which they can overcome and not part of their personality, they will grow up believing what adults say about them and feel helpless to do anything about it. The Pep Talk is their turning point. By labelling their anxiety as 'selective mutism' or 'feeling scared of talking' or 'a phobia of talking', they now have something tangible *and separate from themselves* to focus on; a challenge like learning to swim.

> **The most freeing thing for me was seeing SM as an unfortunate thing I suffered from (like eczema) rather than being me. Once I started viewing it like that, I could also see it as something that I could learn to live with, cope with and help myself to overcome.**

> **I put off mentioning SM to my child for years, fearing it would make her even more self-conscious. But it was clearly a relief to her and, finally, we are making progress.**

There is further advice about this issue in Chapter 1, FAQ 29 (page 24) and in Chapter 8 'Ensuring an anxiety-free environment'.

Acknowledging speaking habits

A talking map is a useful tool to openly acknowledge talking patterns with a child of about 5–9 years old, as well as to create a baseline record of the child's speaking habits. Activity 1 shows how to make a talking map. It is usually facilitated by a parent's presence, but can also be attempted with the child alone. It is essentially a drawing activity, representing significant places in the child's life and the people with whom the child can talk freely in these places. Depending on the child's routine, it may be appropriate to include some of the following places.

★ School (can divide further into playground, classroom, hall, after-school club, etc at a later date)

★ Library

★ Shops/restaurants/cafés/fast-food outlets

★ Organised group activities (eg Brownies, Cubs, gym club, Sunday school)

★ Homes of friends and relatives

★ Place of worship

★ Doctor's/dentist's surgery/hospital

★ Play areas (eg park/adventure playground/swimming pool)

★ Holiday activity centre

Ask the parents and teaching staff about relevant places in advance because it is essential to begin this activity already knowing the child's speaking habits. You will be *sharing* this information with the child, rather than asking them who they can and can't talk to.

We suggest that you make and keep a copy of the original talking map. Then encourage young children to add people to their map as their talking circle widens.

Activity 1: How to make a talking map

Step 1

Take a large piece of paper and draw the child's house in the centre. Describe their home as a place where it's easy to talk because they are relaxed and full of a nice, warm, happy feeling. Place a picture of a happy face next to the house (see Figure 5.1). Draw the child inside (Picture A) or try to engage the child by seeing if they would like to draw themselves inside the house. Some children are too frozen to join in initially, but they may write their name above your stick figure or add more people later. Add other family members and friends to whom the child speaks comfortably at home.

Step 2

Add simple representations of other places in the child's community or further afield which are or have been significant in terms of offering opportunities for communication (Picture B). At each place either draw, or ask the child to draw, the people you know they talk to in that setting (Picture C). Place a picture of a worried face beside locations where they never talk, explaining that when people there ask them questions, this worried feeling stops them talking. You want to help that worried feeling to go away.

Step 3 (optional)

Discuss links between home and other places on the map. Again, represent the communication pattern by drawing, or inviting the child to draw, people they talk to when travelling by car, public transport or on foot (Picture D). *This final step can be added at a later stage as required.*

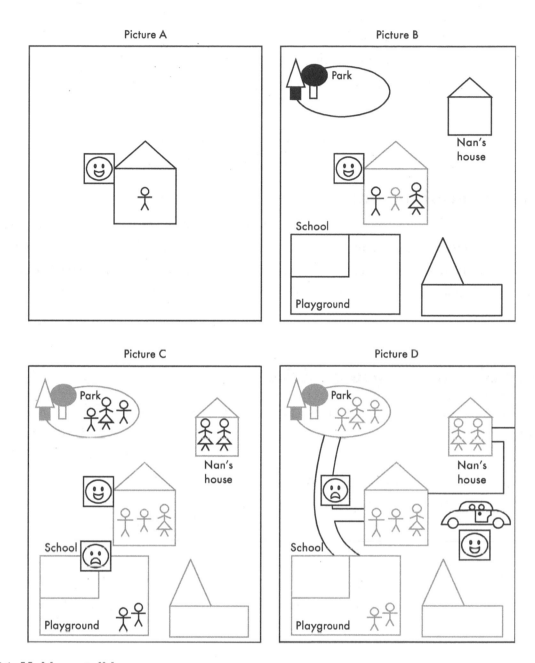

Figure 5.1: **Making a talking map**

Information from the child

As the talking map activity shows, it is important for the child to know that we are more interested in how they *feel* than how much they speak. If the child is relaxed after the Pep Talk, and able to communicate non-verbally (for example, when the assessment is carried out by someone they have already built rapport with at school), they can be asked how they feel with certain people or in certain situations.

Activity 2: Linking feelings to different situations

Show the child photographs or simple pictures of different people (eg staff at their school) or pictures of different situations or times of day (eg playtime, having lunch, circle time, various lessons, assembly, PE and reading to their parent at home). Using two emotion symbols as in the preceding activity, ask the child to place them beside each person or situation, to let you know when their worried feeling appears. By 6 or 7 years old, the child may be able to use the full range of emotion symbols as shown in Chapter 8 (Figure 8.3, page 126), to represent different degrees of anxiety.

This activity may be replaced by Form 8a 'Primary communication rating scale' or Form 8b 'Secondary communication rating scale' (online) for older children.

Finding a special incentive

Facing your fears takes courage and determination. It is always helpful to discover a particular incentive so that intervention programmes can be steered in that direction. Sometimes children openly share their disappointments with parents, for example: 'I didn't get to stroke the puppy because I couldn't tell him to sit.' But often they either cannot express how their life would be improved if they could talk or they find the question too abstract.

Activity 3: The miracle question

This technique comes from *solution-focused therapy* (de Shazer *et al*, 2007). It can be adapted as a drawing activity for young children, enabling them to visualise a life without SM. Say something like: 'Imagine you went to bed one night and, while you were asleep, a fairy [or magician] waved a magic wand and wished you the best, happiest day ever. So when you woke up and went to school, you had the best time ever. It was the best school in the world. Can you draw me a picture of you having a good time at school?'

Figure 5.2 shows an example drawn by a seven year old, showing how important it was for her to have friends and be included at school. Her programme subsequently prioritised

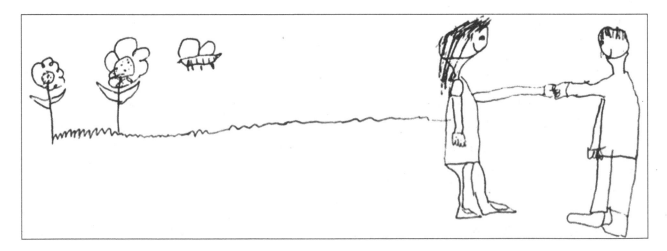

Figure 5.2: **'The best school in the world'**

talking to other children, rather than her teacher, and was introduced as a way of making friends.

Activity 4: Picture this!

This is another way for children to visualise and share their hopes for a future without SM. Form 5 (online) can be used with children of about 8–9 years old after personalising it by selecting age-appropriate situations. For example, one girl, aged 8 years 10 months, wrote that it would make her happy if she could tell grown-ups that she needed help with class work. This provided an excellent focus for her intervention programme.

Adaptations and additions for young people

The assessment of older children and young people needs to cover the same four key areas:

1   speaking habits

2   maintaining factors

3   speech, language and cognitive profile

4   emotional and social profile.

In addition, it is important to establish:

5   The young person's immediate concerns and views of a good outcome, in order to tailor intervention to their aspirations.

6   Their familiarity with the concept of phobias as a basis for understanding the nature of their difficulties and rationale for treatment.

7   Their ability to make an informed decision about engaging with a trial period of intervention.

Consent to treatment

Factors 5–7 above have a crucial role in securing the engagement and consent to a trial period of intervention of young people who are withdrawn and resistant to outside support. Consent is not a one-off event that precedes an initial meeting. It is a process of information sharing, discussion, decision making and review (Mental Capacity Act 2005). At 16 years and above, young people in the UK are entitled to refuse treatment but this must be an *informed* decision. If they refuse treatment because they are too anxious to take any risks, or too depressed to care, they lack the capacity to make this decision. Equally, if they refuse treatment without knowing exactly what they are turning down, and the understanding that change is possible, they are not in a position to either consent or opt out.

Therefore, we recommend that, for young people who are despondent and unwilling to engage with outside services, two or three meetings are planned with the sole aim of enabling them to make an informed decision.

Engaging with a more withdrawn young person

For many young people, it may already be clear from discussions with parents and staff that SM is an appropriate diagnosis. The initial meetings may be more about establishing a therapeutic relationship and assessing the impact of SM on their well-being. The young person might have said that they don't want or need help but *this must not be taken at face value.* Many young people, by the time they are in their mid-teens, have become worn down by their SM and the lack of understanding and appropriate help from the people around them. They may appear to be uncommunicative and unmotivated; to have given up hope of change and to be withdrawing from contact with others. So it may be a challenge to break into their rather enclosed world and show them that things could change for the better.

We need to show the young person that we care enough; we believe they have hopes and dreams; we want to listen to them and find out what are their priorities. You can do this as follows.

★ Meet them at home, or possibly school.

★ Be clear about your expectations, eg 'I've got some information I'd like to share with you if you could give me 20 minutes to go through it'; or 'I'd like to tell you a bit about what I do and give you a chance to think about what *you* would like'.

★ Explain that you will be doing most, if not all, of the talking and that it's entirely up to them if they say anything or just listen.

★ Explain your role in simple terms, eg 'I work with people who find it hard to say what they want to say'; or 'I work with teenagers who've had a tough time at school or college'.

★ State your aims, eg 'My work is to help young people enjoy themselves socially and educationally, so that they can get the most out of life'; or 'My job is to identify the barriers or obstacles which might be standing in the way'.

★ Reassure them, eg 'I will not make you do anything you don't want to do'; or 'I won't pass on any information you give me without your permission, unless I'm worried about your safety'.

★ Move on as appropriate to 'How do you see yourself?', or 'Establishing the young person's priorities', or 'Talking openly about speech anxiety' (see below).

★ Use screens (eg a laptop or tablet) or written activities to reduce eye contact and avoid appearing too confrontational.

★ Avoid direct questions and use non-verbal means of communication to learn how the young person sees things and what is important to them.

★ Suggest a trial period of intervention after which the young person will evaluate the assisting *adult*, rather than the other way round!

Email correspondence

It may help to build some rapport by email or text before the initial meeting and to make email or text contact between sessions. The majority of older children will be able to express more of their true selves when they are not face-to-face with you. Initially at least, this may be the only way they can handle more 'risky' topics such as making requests, expressing preferences or dissatisfaction, or revealing personal details. Some clinicians may, therefore, choose to carry out some assessment by email or offer the young person a choice about how aspects of assessment are completed.

Using questionnaires and rating scales

Questionnaires are relatively non-threatening because it is clear that there is no pressure to speak. But, as with verbal communication, written open-ended questions are harder to respond to than closed, factual questions. Open-ended questions require more information from the young person and they need to be physically relaxed in order to think clearly and write freely. Therefore, self-rated *scales* are a particularly useful way of collecting information about feelings and attitudes. This is because there is no right or wrong answer and the young person is simply required to write down a number or circle their response.

Talking openly about speech anxiety

Young people will no doubt have heard others talk about their mutism in front of them. However, they probably have not had the subject discussed openly and constructively *with* them. Most of them will either not have heard of the term 'selective mutism' or not have understood much about it. Yet this is crucial in helping them face and overcome their fear of talking. In addition to the points that need to be conveyed in the Pep Talk (page 73), it is important for children aged about 10 and above to understand the nature of fears and phobias in general.

The timing of this conversation is crucial. Many young people are crying out for an explanation for their struggle with talking over the years and need one as soon as possible. Indeed, the relief of discovering that they have been experiencing a phobia rather than a personality trait, and meeting someone who wants to inform rather than judge them, often facilitates their involvement in the assessment process. Others may need longer to build rapport before they are ready to reflect on their difficulties in this way.

Older teenagers and adults who have a good grasp of the nature and irrationality of phobias can be given the online booklet 'When the words won't come out' . This explains SM in the context of phobias and how to overcome them. It also provides a good basis for reflection with any young person who is experiencing low self-esteem and severe social anxiety in addition to their SM. It can help them identify the impact of SM on their life and would form an important part of assessing their readiness for intervention.

Viewing selective mutism as a phobia

Many young people are already conversant with the concept of phobias. For example, a 10-year-old, who had seen a television programme about people who were afraid of flying, beamed when told by her mother that SM was another type of phobia and commented: 'I *thought* I couldn't be shy! It didn't make sense.'

See also the description of Sander in Chapter 14 (page 306) for an account of a 16-year-old who made rapid progress once he knew what he was dealing with.

Young people with little or a hazy understanding of phobias may benefit from doing the activity below. It usually helps to include their parent, sibling, friend or familiar mentor. This person will not only gain a better understanding of SM and the young person, but also they could have a valuable role in keeping the conversation going and putting the young person at ease.

The main points to get across are:

★ fears are different for different people

★ how scary things are is all in the mind

★ an intense fear of something that is not a real threat is called a phobia

★ they have a phobia of talking

★ phobias can be overcome!

Activity 5: Learning about phobias

Step 1

Give everyone some cards or sticky notes displaying the same single objects or events. Ask the participants to sort them into two columns for things they personally find 'frightening' and 'not frightening' (Figure 5.3, box 1). Explain that the 'frightening' column is not for things they simply don't like much; the items there could actually make them feel real fear or panic. Use the list of items in box 1, or compile your own, making sure that it includes things that are both likely and extremely unlikely to arouse fear.

Step 2

Reflect together on the resulting columns, making it clear that there are no right or wrong answers (Figure 5.3, box 2). The same item can be threatening or non-threatening, depending on different circumstances and whether or not the person is, for example, a good swimmer or a trained animal handler. Using common fear triggers such as 'spiders' or 'clowns', it may be possible to eke out individual differences between friends or family members, to acknowledge how the same things can affect different people in very different ways.

Step 3

Now focus on items in the 'not frightening' column that the young person could never find scary. Point out that, even though *they* are not frightened by these things, there are people in the world who find them *terrifying*. This gets across the concept of phobia; the fear is real but the trigger

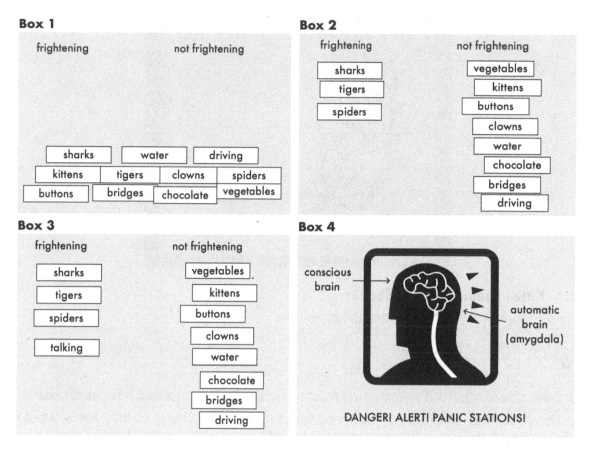

Figure 5.3: **Learning about phobias**

poses no actual threat. It helps to find examples to support this such as Greg Sherrer's wonderful illustration in Figure 5.4 overleaf. A quick internet search will provide the young person with the official names for phobias of cats, buttons, chocolate, and so on, together with personal accounts of these and other unusual phobias. Explain that there is always a good reason for acquiring a phobia. For example, the smell of egg sandwiches at a loved one's funeral can trigger a phobia of hard-boiled eggs; or getting a button caught in a fence when trying to escape can trigger a phobia of buttons. Establish the idea that, when panicking about one thing, the fear can become linked to another object or event in the immediate vicinity. Challenge the young person to think about how someone might develop a phobia of their favourite food!

Step 4

Add a new card for 'talking' to the 'frightening' column and explain that SM is also a phobia (Figure 5.3, box 3). Using your knowledge of the young person's history, explain how their phobia started or talk more generally about the fact that many young children associate talking to strangers with the panic of being in a new or uncomfortable situation without their parents. Emphasise that phobias are common and can happen to any bright, sensitive individual – they are nothing to be ashamed of. Most importantly, they can be overcome! As 'homework', the young person could ask their family members and find out who else they know has a phobia.

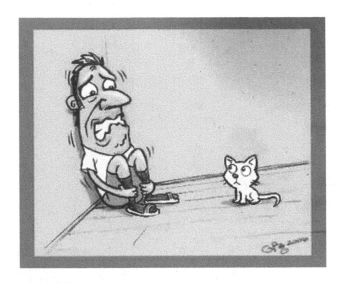

Figure 5.4: **'Kitten phobia' by Greg Sherrer**
(Source: Grog's Bleg, August 2006, http://grogsbleg.blogspot.co.uk)

Step 5

Now for the science bit! Of course, you must use your discretion about how much detail you go into. We find it helpful for young people to visualise anxiety, so they know what is going on as they learn to manage and control it. Box 4 in Figure 5.3 introduces the idea of the automatic functions of the amygdala which we have little control over, and how we can *teach* the amygdala that talking is perfectly safe so that it no longer triggers a panic reaction. For example:

> The **amygdala** controls your fear reflex. It tries to keep us safe and, whenever it senses danger, it automatically sets off an alert which gets your body ready to protect itself. So even though you feel really afraid, you're ready to fight back, run away or just freeze and hope the danger goes away. Your heart beats really fast and your muscles tense up, even in your throat. No wonder you can't speak!

> When you were younger, your amygdala remembered how you hated it when … so it got the idea that talking to … was something to be afraid of. When you had to talk again, it set off the alarm and your heart started racing and you felt that horrid panic again – even though this time there was nothing to worry about. The more people tried to get you to talk, the worse it felt so, of course, you tried to get out of talking, even though you didn't want to upset anyone.

> So, we just need to teach your amygdala that there's no danger. If you show it that talking is safe, it will stop raising the alarm, your body and throat will stay relaxed and words will come out easily again. But don't worry – you can teach it gradually in tiny steps so you stay in control and stop the big panic reaction.

The final point paves the way for intervention.

Information from the young person

Here we describe some forms and questionnaires that have been useful in working with young people who are able and willing to engage in the assessment process. In most cases these would supplement the information from parents, carers or staff but, depending on the circumstances of the referral, they could be the main source of information. They can be completed before, after or during the initial meeting with the young person.

All of the resources can be adapted for individuals and used on-screen rather than as paper documents, if preferred. Introduce questionnaires by explaining that the information will help you get to know the young person and find the best way of helping. Where appropriate, explain the rating scale and the method of responding. It may help rapport to read out the statements to the young person, rather than leave them to complete the form in isolation.

Young person's interview

Form 6 (online) is the teen or young adult equivalent of the parent interview. It enables a young person to give a wide range of information about themselves, especially:

★ speaking habits

★ speech, language and cognitive profile

★ emotional and social profile

★ the way their SM is handled by other people.

The form can be completed in an interview either orally, if the young person feels comfortable speaking to the clinician, or on-screen with keyboard input from the young person. However, when given the choice, young people often prefer to fill in the form on their own, knowing they can seek clarification if necessary, before bringing it to the initial meeting or returning it by email. Their answers then provide a good structure for further discussion or examples.

All about me

Form 7 (online) is a less formal questionnaire which gives information about a young person's interests and attitudes. It is a good starting point for getting to know their tastes and likely motivators, and can be followed up by more detailed questions in particular areas, if required.

Primary communication rating scale

Form 8a (online) is a questionnaire which looks at anxiety levels in different talking situations. It is particularly suitable for children aged about 8–11 years. It provides a useful baseline measure which can be repeated at intervals.

Secondary communication rating scale

Form 8b (online) is like the primary one but suitable for older students.

Worrying thoughts

Form 9 (online) is useful when the young person has become increasingly isolated or anxious; or is not making progress; or is just as worried about saying the *wrong* thing as being unable to get their words out. It helps to identify negative thoughts which may need to be addressed alongside or separately from SM. There are some notes for interpretation on the back of the form.

Assessing the young person's speaking habits

When meeting the young person, the professional can assess their speaking habits in three ways.

1   Using the information from the young person's interview or communication rating scale (see above).

2   Asking the young person to fill in the record of speaking habits (Form 3 online).

3   Discussing with the young person how freely they can speak with certain people in certain situations.

The young person's level of participation during the session (see page 73) is also significant but it must be noted in the context of a range of situations, rather than in isolation.

Assessing the young person's perception of maintaining factors

When considering their talking, young people will be very aware of what other people do that is both helpful and unhelpful. This information can be taken from the young person's completed interview form (Form 6, items 6 and 7). Alternatively, the relevant items from the form can be presented to the young person separately, along with the usual assurances of confidentiality.

However, some young people find it difficult to respond to open-ended or personal questions in the initial stages of building rapport. They may find it easier to complete Form 10 'Reactions of family/friends/staff' (online). This is the student version of Form 4, the parents' 'Checklist of possible maintaining factors', described in Chapter 4. It is a good working document because it will show the young person that you believe the onus is not simply on them to change; everyone has a part to play. With the young person's permission, parents and teachers will be asked to provide support in ways that alleviate, rather than exacerbate, their anxiety.

Establishing the young person's priorities

When SM has become entrenched, young people need a very real incentive to face their fear of talking and risk exposing themselves to the high anxiety they have been doing their best to avoid for years. Therefore, it is important to tailor intervention to personal goals by establishing their priorities. When a young person seeks or is ready to accept help, they can be asked directly what they hope to gain from intervention (see item 10, on Form 6 online). However, it is not always easy for anxious students to think clearly about anything other than their immediate survival. Many get into a habit of answering questions with 'I don't know' because this avoids further conversation. Some find the future too scary to contemplate; and some, sadly, have given up hope of a better future.

The following activities show various ways to help young people clarify their thoughts. It may help to use this information in assessment reports and say, with [N]'s permission, that '[N] has identified the following priorities …'. This can be an eye-opener if the young person has previously been regarded as uncommunicative and unmotivated.

Activity 6: Formulating specific goals

This solution-focused therapy technique (de Shazer *et al*, 2007) is helpful when a young person generates goals which do not provide a clear end-point to work towards. By helping the young person shift from feelings and relative concepts to how they would like to see themselves behaving in the future, their wishes are converted to specific, achievable targets which provide a focus for intervention.

For goals such as:

- I want to be more confident
- I want to be happy
- I want to be less shy
- I want to speak more clearly

ask the young person questions such as:

- What would being more confident look like? Describe yourself being confident.
- What sort of things would make you feel happy?
- How will you know you are less shy?
- Why do you want to speak more clearly? What happens now that makes you want to change?

to arrive at goals such as:

- To buy my own drinks/food/tickets when I go out with friends.
- To be included in school activities *or* To find a course I will enjoy and get a place at college.
- To have a natural posture, so that I don't stand out.
- To be comfortable about repeating myself when people don't understand me the first time.

Activity 7: Pooling ideas

This group activity involves parents or other young people and can open up or improve channels of communication within the family.

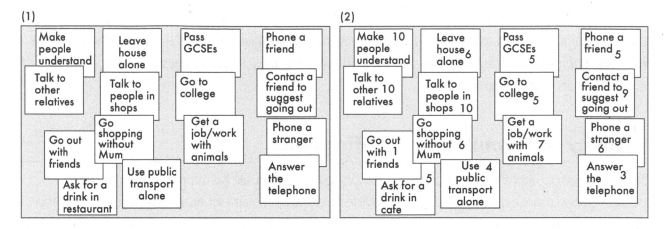

Figure 5.5: **Establishing a young person's priorities**

a)   Give each participant, yourself included, some blank sticky notes or index cards and a pen. Ask everyone to think about a few things that they (in the case of a group session) or the young person (in a family session) might like to change, in order to make their lives better; things they wish they could achieve or do more of; or things they would like to happen. Get them to write each wish (goal) on a separate card or note and put them face-down on the table when they have finished.

b)   When everyone has run out of ideas, take it in turns to turn over and read out the cards, grouping them together as appropriate, and discussing how they might be linked (see Figure 5.5, box 1). This will show the similarities and differences in people's thinking. Discard any repeated ideas and combine similar ideas as appropriate (eg 'talk to relatives' and 'talk to my grandparents'). Make a mental note to do Activity 6 with any non-specific wishes such as 'Be popular' in a later session.

c)   Ask each young person to think about how much they want or need things to change and to rate the goals in terms of importance to them, on a scale of 0 to 10. Zero indicates that achieving the goal would make no difference to their lives and is therefore not a priority; 10 is high priority and something they would like to achieve immediately if they could. Emphasise that there is no right or wrong answer and different things are important to different people.

d)   Later, these goals can be ranked in order of priority, to assist in personal target-setting (page 89).

Activity 8: Picture this! (2)

Form 5 'Picture this!' (online) is useful for young people who have engaged with assessment but don't readily express a desire to change or find the idea of doing things differently too challenging or stressful to consider. The form can be adapted to suit a variety of environments and modes of communication. Based on the miracle question technique (page 78), the young person is helped to think about their ideal world – a relatively concrete way of visualising a life without SM.

Activity 9: Establishing priorities using sorting and ranking

This activity is particularly useful if the young person is disengaged, or resistant to intervention, and is not yet ready to think in terms of facing their fear of talking. It is also a good way to identify priorities when time is at a premium or when the young person struggles to generate their own ideas. Before the session, prepare a selection of possible goals, and tailor their suitability to what you have learned from parents, interview forms or checklists.

Start the activity by saying, 'I want to make sure we work towards things that are important to *you*' or 'Can we think about what's important to *you?*'.

a) Present the possible goals as text boxes on a screen, or written on index cards or sticky notes and ask the young person to sort them into three columns according to importance (see boxes 1 and 2 in Figure 5.6). Avoid non-specific goals such as 'being happy' or 'feeling confident' (see Activity 6). Always include a couple of blank boxes or cards, inviting the young person to add things you didn't think of. However, don't press the young person if they leave them blank (they usually do!).

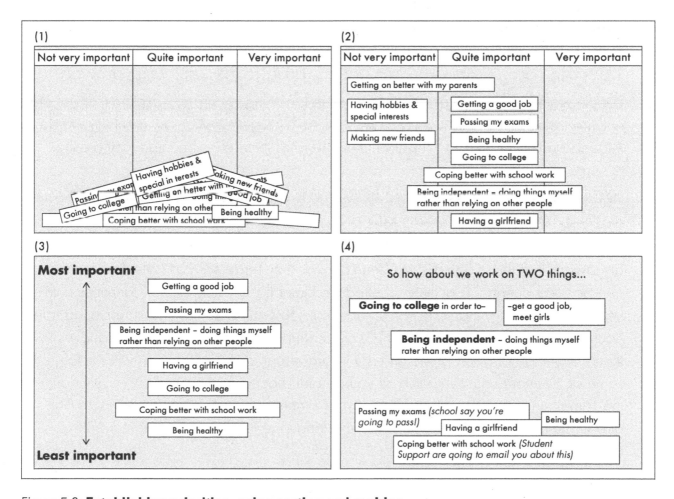

Figure 5.6: **Establishing priorities, using sorting and ranking**

b) Ask the young person to look at the items in one column and rank them by moving the most important one to the top. Repeat with the remaining items in that column until they have been reordered (see box 3). Repeat with the other columns, using your discretion. For example, there is no need to reorder two or three items in the 'Not very important' column when there are plenty of other items to be working on in the other columns.

c) This information allows you or other people to consider your own contribution before agreeing with the young person appropriate things to work on (box 4).

Checking how young people see themselves

The final activity in this chapter has been used with young people who resent perceived interference, want to be left alone, or say there is nothing wrong with them. It is designed to help find a point of agreement as a foundation for building rapport and investigating further. But it also demonstrates how relatively sensitive subjects can be discussed with apparently non-communicative young people. Thus, it can be adapted to any subject you would like to explore and is a good basis for modifying traditional talking therapies.

Activity 10: Using a rating activity to explore the young person's self-perception

a) Using the young person's words where possible (eg as reported to their parents), thank them for meeting you, especially when they must be fed up of being assessed, or wish people would leave them alone, or know there is nothing wrong, etc. Explain that you are only interested in their point of view and working out together what they would like to do. A good starting point is to think about how they see themselves because they are the experts.

b) Using an on-screen presentation, index cards or sticky notes, present some terms, as shown in Figure 5.7 (box 1), selected with the young person's particular circumstances in mind. For example, include autism spectrum disorder only if they are aware that this diagnosis has been considered. Terms such as 'selective mutism' can be used during this activity or introduced later if the young person identifies with freezing and being unable to speak. Say that you would like the young person to rate each term or description from 0 to 10, according to how much they think it applies to them, 0 being not appropriate and 10 very appropriate. Add that you will explain some of the more unusual words as you go along because they don't always mean the same things to different people. Have a simple one- or two-sentence explanation of each term to hand, being careful to use language that is as non-medical and destigmatising as possible.

c) Start by saying something like, 'For example, if I was doing this, I'm definitely not a "typical teenager" so I'd give that zero. But I am quite sensitive. I tend to notice how other people are feeling and get hurt quite easily if I think people are having a go at me, so I'd maybe give that a seven or eight.' Write down the numbers as you talk and then cross out or delete them as you invite the young person to have a go.

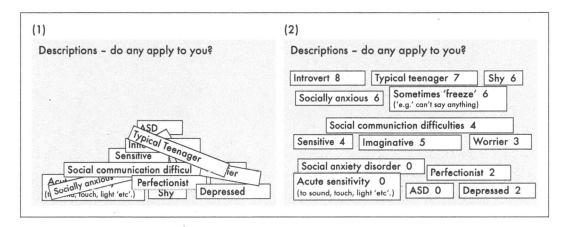

Figure 5.7: **Exploring the young person's self-perception, using a rating activity**

d) At the end of this activity you will, we hope, be able to agree some words you will *not* be using to describe the young person (move these to the bottom, as in box 2), as well as some words that the young person is fairly comfortable with (move these to the top).

If you get this far, you may like to follow up with establishing the young person's priorities using Activity 9 (page 89).

Online resources for Chapter 5

The handout, forms and booklet accompanying this chapter are available at www.routledge.com/cw /speechmark for you to access, print and copy.

CHAPTER 6

THE EXTENDED ASSESSMENT: FURTHER INFORMATION GATHERING

Introduction

You probably turned to this chapter because you are involved in a variety of ways with a child or young person who might have more than selective mutism (SM). You want to check this out; or you may be wondering who to turn to for further investigations and how to get the best out of an onward referral. If you are an assessor, you may be wondering how to approach the assessment of a child who has SM.

This chapter therefore looks at:

★ The extended parent interview

★ Speech and language, cognitive and literacy assessments

    – Is it really necessary and what are the dangers of formal assessment?

    – Is the assessor familiar with SM?

    – Presenting the assessment materials

    – Training parents to carry out some formal assessments

    – Assessing a bilingual child who has SM

    – Making adaptations to the formal assessments

★ Making effective onward referrals when needed

The extended parent interview

This comprehensive parent interview is recommended where there are additional concerns beyond pure SM. It may also be used if the child or young person is not progressing with SM intervention. It provides a framework for the detailed questioning of developmental, emotional and behavioural issues. Later, professionals may adapt the format to incorporate their own style and, with experience, they will know which parts are more or less crucial for their work situation and for individuals who have SM. The standard format can be accessed from the online resource library accompanying this manual.

The form covers the following basic areas.

★ *Presenting problems*: mutism, its background and other problems or concerns.

★ *Family*: history, household, significant members, losses.

★ *Developmental history*: pregnancy and birth, feeding, sleeping, toileting, gross and fine motor development.

★ *Speech, language and communication*: development, home language(s), speaking pattern, past therapy.

★ *Attachment and separation.*

★ *Temperament.*

★ *Play and peer relationships.*

★ *School life.*

★ *Social history.*

Before interviewing the parents, prepare them by explaining the need to ask a range of questions. Emphasise the importance of getting a full picture of the child and their family, and their history, experiences and relationships, if you are to understand their situation and how best to intervene. Reassure them about confidentiality, with the usual exception of anything that threatens the child's well-being. If you are not working in a school setting, it may be important to check whether certain information divulged to you has been told to the school. If you feel the school should know certain facts, discuss this with the parents and ask their permission.

The areas to be covered in the interview are set out in a logical sequence, with a main heading that can be used as a general introduction to lead into the questions. Then there are some questions in **bold type**, which can be used to elicit specific information. Small *italic print* is used for ideas that need to be kept in mind during an interview, and the aims of probing each area.

Please note: the online resources for Chapter 5 include a young person's interview form to use with older teenagers and adults.

Speech and language, cognitive and literacy assessments

It is known that SM often occurs alongside difficulties of speech and language; and there may also be other concerns about a child's level of cognitive and literacy skills. Therefore, at some stage, it may be appropriate to carry out formal (standardised) language, psychometric or literacy assessments. Before you start, some vital questions need to be asked which are explored further below. First:

1   Is it really necessary and what are the dangers of formal assessment?

2   How else might the information be gained?

If you decide to go ahead, ask yourself:

3   At what stage should formal assessments be done?

4   Is the assessor familiar with SM?

5   How is it best to present the assessment materials?

6   Could parents, or other people the child talks freely with, be trained to carry out some formal assessments?

7   Can formal assessments be adapted for children who have SM?

Is it really necessary and what are the dangers of formal assessment?

In our view, formal assessment should be avoided, unless the information sought is considered vital to the understanding of the child and can only be gained in this way. The very nature of the condition means the formal assessment of a child who has SM poses a challenge to an 'assessor'. This is regardless of whether they are SLTs assessing speech, language and communication, psychologists considering psychometric assessments, or teachers wanting to carry out literacy tests. Children who have SM are particularly sensitive in situations where there is an expectation to perform. Formal assessment, unless very carefully managed, is bound to raise their anxiety level. Anxiety affects people's ability to think, move and speak freely, so there is a real risk that the assessment results will not give a true picture of the child's skills, especially tests involving spoken or written language.

How else might the information be gained?

The other ways of gaining evidence of a child's skills in communicating, learning and reading include reliable reports from parents or teachers, home recordings, and written school work. These are certainly recommended for screening and a good starting point. Speech and language therapists may follow up concerns about delayed speech and language by using audio or video recordings from home to screen for impairment of speech or syntax (grammar). Videos are also useful for screening social skills and general communicative competence. Psychologists may get more information about play and cognitive abilities from detailed questions to the parents and teachers and looking at work samples. Teachers may first hear the child reading by asking the parents to make a recording at home.

At what stage should formal assessments be done?

You may feel there are possible deficits in underlying language, literacy or cognition that have not been adequately recognised and cannot be identified in any other way. You may also feel they could be reinforcing the child's anxiety about talking. When the need for further assessment becomes apparent, it may not be necessary to do this immediately. More reliable results may be achieved once parents and school staff have created a more relaxed environment for the child in school. Given that formal assessments cannot be repeated in less than a year (sometimes two years), they could be delayed until a later stage of the programme when the child is talking more.

Is the assessor familiar with selective mutism?

If formal assessment really is required, the assessor must have a basic understanding of SM and be thoroughly aware of the stages of one-to-one interaction (see Table 5.1, page 74). Assessment tasks can then be based on the level of confident talking that the child has reached with the assessor. Table 6.1 overleaf shows the possible progression, taking into account the child's anxiety level and the type of response they can make comfortably at each stage. The assessor should begin at Stage 2 or 3 and gradually progress to the highest stage that is comfortable for the child. By introducing activities which only gradually increase the child's need to communicate, the assessment procedures themselves may contribute to eliciting gesture or speech for the first time.

Table 6.1: **Confident talking – the stages of one-to-one interaction related to assessment**

Stage	Child's presentation towards examiner	Strategies for assessing speech and language, cognitive or literacy levels
0	Absent	Assessment procedures will involve mainly parents and significant others:
1	Frozen	• Parental interview assessments • Samples of the child's typical utterances, from written, audio or video recordings • Observations from other people involved with the child (eg school report form) • Tasks completed by the child in the parents' or carers' presence while you are out of the room (eg draw a person, complete a jigsaw puzzle, sequence magnetic letters, or sort picture cards into family groups), provided you check the level of assistance involved • Assessments administered by parents after suitable training, while the examiner leaves the room, or later on at home. These are supported with an audio or a video recording whenever possible
2	Participates without communication	Assessment tasks in which the child can indicate understanding or competence non-verbally but is not trying to answer a question or convey a message, so does not feel 'tested'. The child participates in activities, either with the examiner or with friends or family while observed by the examiner: • Free play • Puppet play • Letter/picture/pattern matching, copying and grouping • Completing form boards or jigsaw puzzles • Sequencing tasks • Drawing or writing activities • Silent reading as part of a game (eg follows written instructions to move round a board)
3	Uses non-verbal and written communication	Assessment tasks where the child is required to indicate appropriate items to the examiner or carry out instructions by: • Pointing • Nodding or shaking head • Using fingers to indicate number • Passing the correct object/picture/word/letter • Moving shapes or objects to a requested position • Matching words to pictures • Ticking off an item on a checklist • Circling or underlining the correct answer • Sequencing sentences to tell a story • Drawing or writing • Tapping or clapping syllables
Talking bridge	Tolerates voice being heard by examiner	Assessments *conducted* by parents, or other people the child speaks freely with, in the same room as the examiner: • Assessments requiring letter sounds or names, numbers, reading aloud, single-word answers or simple phrases • The parent works with the child while the examiner averts eye contact and appears otherwise occupied

(Continued)

Stage	Child's presentation towards examiner	Strategies for assessing speech and language, cognitive or literacy levels
4	Talks to examiner through another person	Assessments *supported* by parents or other people the child speaks freely with: • Assessments requiring letter sounds or names, numbers, reading aloud, single-word answers or simple phrases • The examiner presents the task and suggests the child reads to or tells the *parent* the answer • The parent repeats the examiner's question if no answer after five seconds, and the child answers the parent
5	Uses voice with examiner	Assessment tasks requiring vocalisation but limited communication: • Use of letter sounds or speech sounds • Reading aloud
6	Communicates with examiner using single words	Assessment tasks requiring: • 'Yes' or 'no' answer • Picture naming • Single-word answers (including letter names). This could be in response to questions about a passage the child has read aloud
7	Communicates with examiner using sentences	Assessment tasks requiring: • Imitation of sentence, digit sequence or word list • Sentence completion (phrase required) • Picture description • Sentence formulation • Supplying a reason for answer • Answering questions about a passage the child has heard or read aloud
8	Conversation	Assessment tasks requiring: • Storytelling (extended narrative) • Social use of language to request, direct, question, inform or challenge the examiner
Note		The information gained will not reflect true ability if the child is tense or anxious. Parents may be present at Stages 5–8 but to observe rather than support activities. Do not repeat activities at Stages 5–8 if they were already done with the support of a parent or another talking partner. The child will probably only respond if they feel confident that their response is correct. So, for example, they may not respond to a challenging Stage 5 or Stage 6 activity but be happy to participate in an 'easy' Stage 7 activity.

Presenting the test materials

If the child has been pointing or nodding, see whether a simple, single-word response can be achieved. During an assessment at Stage 3 (eg a receptive vocabulary test), tell the child it will save you time if you don't have to look up while you write, so could they tell you the number instead. Don't look at the child while waiting for responses. If they are averse to guessing, you could give them the option of saying 'I don't know', 'Not sure' or 'Three or four'. If the child freezes at any stage, quickly remove the pressure by saying 'I'm sorry, I'm going much too quickly, aren't I? Let's go back to how we were doing it before.' However, if the child can start using single words in this way, you might be able to move on to some of the Stage 6 assessments, perhaps a word-finding vocabulary test.

Reading reduces the risk of error and often provokes less anxiety. So, provided that children are confident readers, they may move more easily to reading tasks than those requiring picture naming or answering with short phrases or sentences.

Training parents to carry out some formal assessments

When children are very reluctant to engage with strangers, or when time is at a premium, it may be possible to obtain useful information by asking parents to carry out certain assessments. Alternatively, a member of staff who the child speaks to freely at school could be trained to carry out simple assessments which are later scored by the assessor.

Some people might be a little cautious about these suggestions. Certainly, some warnings are needed:

★ It is not suitable for every child and parent to do 'home assessments' – it would put too much of a burden on some of them.

★ Many assessments state who is qualified to administer them – check if this is so, and do not use them if specific training is required.

★ If standardised assessments are done by another person, they should be recorded so that the professional can listen to the process of assessment.

★ Standardised assessments carried out in any form other than that described in the assessment manual are best described in reports as an 'indication' of the child's skills. If any resulting data is quoted, it should appear in brackets with an explanation about the process.

★ Always ask if the child seemed relaxed or inhibited during the assessment. Some children are particularly sensitive to any form of scrutiny and start to 'freeze' when feeling 'tested', even by their parents. This is likely to become more apparent as the risk of error increases, resulting in children saying less than they could or being very reluctant to hazard a guess.

Formal assessments done at home

Some parents can do simple assessments involving picture naming, picture description, storytelling, reading aloud or simple question–answer formats effectively at home. First, practise with the parents using appropriate materials, such as a pile of picture cards. Give advice about encouragement, prompts and acceptance of the child's attempt; for example, 'good try' is useful. Lend the parent similar materials to take home and try out with their child. Then, having listened to the 'home practice assessment', and made any necessary requests to the parent, you could lend them the actual assessment.

Formal assessments done in the clinic or school

If the child is talking within earshot of a 'new' person but not directly to them, parents may be able to carry out the types of assessment described above in the clinic or school setting alongside the assessor. This gives the assessor more control over how the test material is presented. It has the further advantage of removing the pressure to speak directly to the examiner in the initial stages of getting to know the child. The assessor should explain the procedure to both parent and child and leave them at one table while recording unobtrusively from another. They should stay in view of the child rather than out of sight, but avoid looking directly at the child.

Assessing a bilingual child who has SM

The assessment of a bilingual child who has SM is similar to that of any bilingual child, coupled with the assessment of any child who has SM. It is important to assess bilingual children's competence in both their home and school language on separate occasions in an appropriate environment, which may require the help of an interpreter. Tempting though it may be to use a family friend or relative who the child speaks with comfortably, a professional interpreter should always be engaged, to ensure full and accurate communication and translation.

It may be possible to use the interpreter's assistance to train the parent to carry out and record assessments in the home language; or to ask the parent to make a recording for later translation while playing with the child. The professional should meet separately with the interpreter to discuss the results.

Making adaptations to formal assessments

Adapt how the child can respond

In certain sub-tests of standardised assessments, the child need not necessarily speak to demonstrate that they have the required language or cognitive skill. They may be able to point or write down their responses instead. For example, if they are asked to listen to a list of four words and say which is the 'odd one out', you could point to four coloured bricks or the numbers one to four as you name each item (it would invalidate the assessment to present the written words or illustrations). The child could then point to the corresponding brick or number. Obviously, an adaptation of any standardised assessment must be considered carefully in line with the directions for administration in the manual, and recorded appropriately as such, in a report.

Accept the child speaking spontaneously to a parent, rather than the assessor

This fits in at Stage 4, when the child will speak (or whisper) to the parent in front of the assessor and can be encouraged by saying, for example, 'You can tell Mummy if you like'. However, at the point when the child tells the parent the answer, rather than use the parent as a go-between, maintain a natural flow of communication whenever possible by saying, 'Oh, would you prefer Mummy to do this with you? That's fine – Mummy can show you the pictures/ask you the questions' and hand over the test materials.

Making effective onward referrals when needed

Some children will need referring to specialists who may not have seen a child who has SM before or come across this manual. For example, children may have additional physical or sensory problems and need to be referred to an occupational therapist or a physiotherapist or a paediatrician.

It may be your role as a parent or fellow professional to explain that the child has SM, before the appointment and out of the child's hearing. You could either send a leaflet about SM (there are some in the online resources for Chapter 8) or make a phone call. The key message is that SM is an anxiety condition – a phobia of talking – so the child cannot talk freely with certain people.

The following tips about how the specialist might approach the child and adapt their assessments may be helpful.

★ Welcome the child but avoid prolonged eye contact.

★ Explain to the child what you are going to do.

★ Try to allow a little time for young children to familiarise themselves with your room or any equipment you will be using. This gives parents a chance to help the child relax.

★ Where possible, avoid asking direct questions.

★ If the child needs to respond, suggest that they tell their parent the answer.

★ If this is not possible, use another method of communication: point to a card; write down the answer; or use gesture (eg use fingers for numbers).

★ Don't remark on it if the child talks; respond as you would with any other child.

It may be helpful to adapt this advice for other situations, such as visits to the dentist or optician, music exams, and so on.

Online resource for Chapter 6

The handout, forms and booklet accompanying this chapter are available at www.routledge.com/cw /speechmark for you to access, print and copy.

CHAPTER 7

MOVING FROM ASSESSMENT TO MANAGEMENT

Introduction

This chapter forms a bridge between assessment and management. Specifically, it looks at:

★ selective mutism assessment and management checklist

★ assessment summary

★ discussion of the diagnosis and cause of the child's mutism

★ overall management progression

★ planning intervention

★ formulating an action plan

★ putting the management programme into practice

★ looking ahead: a balanced approach to intervention

★ management summary

Selective mutism assessment and management checklist

Once an assessment has been completed, we suggest that clinicians note it on one form, so that what has been done and the outcome can be seen at a glance, along with the plans for management as they emerge. It may work best to record the different parts of the assessment as you go along, so that you can see what is outstanding. Parents may find it useful to go through the checklist at any stage with the person coordinating their child's programme. It is also a comprehensive format for case discussion in supervision, and may be a useful reference in review meetings.

This checklist is Form 11 in the online resource library. It has two pages: the assessment summary on one and the management summary on the other.

Assessment summary

The assessment summary covers the various aspects of assessment described in the previous chapters. Although not all of the suggested materials need to be used, each section represents an important part of any comprehensive assessment. Having completed page 1, it will become clear whether sufficient information has been gathered in the various assessments, or whether you need to return to the previous chapters and fill in any gaps. This will then be a good base on which to plan management, discussed later in this chapter.

Discussion of the diagnosis and cause of the child's mutism

After any assessment of a child's development or difficulties, there needs to be some feedback about the resulting diagnosis and an outline of what will happen next. How and when this is done may vary; but there is no doubt that time spent on this feedback will lead to the successful management of selective mutism (SM).

An important consideration is who is present at the feedback session.

★ Parents will no doubt need the fullest explanation and usually have the most questions to ask the assessor. We strongly recommend a meeting without the young child who has SM being present.

★ Feedback of the assessment to younger children will be covered in the Pep Talk; they will also need a simple explanation of the next step. There is no need to look too far ahead at this stage. For example, it could be sufficient to reassure the child that you and their parents will be talking to their teacher to work out a plan to help them.

★ Older children and young people need to be given feedback from assessments, mainly in the form of 'This suggests to me that it would be a good idea to ...' or 'Perhaps we could think about ...'. They may like to meet with their parents or separately for this and should be given the opportunity to ask questions in writing if this is more comfortable, perhaps by email after the session.

★ Some feedback of the assessment and diagnosis, and discussion about the next move, is also needed by other people who are closely involved with managing the child. If the parents are not present, a brief outline of what staff members will be told should be agreed with the parents in advance, to maintain trust and confidentiality.

The assessments will point to whether the child has SM, how it presents and whether there are any other additional difficulties that need to be taken into account, as discussed in Chapter 3. Discussion is also needed to help parents and young people understand how the SM arose. The detailed information that has been gathered will indicate the extent to which temperamental, developmental, linguistic, cultural, parental and other family factors may have played a part, as discussed in Chapter 2, 'What causes SM' (page 36). The main benefit for most families is a sense that there was nothing they could have done differently to avoid the onset of SM – such is the nature of phobias. However, while knowledge of the cause of the child's SM can be helpful in terms of making sense of the whole thing, and dispelling incorrect beliefs or assumptions, it is not essential and, indeed, may not be conclusive.

Overall management progression

Box 7.1 outlines the contents of an effective management programme. The word 'progression' is important: the first four points A–D are essential and must precede direct work with the child. Some people are tempted to jump in at point E with a programme to establish speech, but this has little chance of succeeding if points A–D have been ignored. Furthermore, with very young children, it may only be necessary to cover the first four points before the child is noticeably more relaxed and starting to speak freely.

Box 7.1: Overall management progression

A   Educate home and school about SM.

B   Plan and implement appropriate modifications at home and school.

C   Acknowledge the difficulty with the child – whatever their age.

D   Build general confidence and independence at home and school.

E   Establish speech with key individuals, using a parent whenever possible.

F   Generalise speech to other people and places, including the wider community.

G   Ongoing social skills, confidence building and assertiveness training as appropriate.

Planning intervention

Once assessment is complete, an initial planning meeting needs to be set up with the parents and the key people who will be involved. Team building is crucial to effective management of SM, so it is important not to leave anyone out. Staff from nursery, school or college are usually invited but, if the child is home-schooled, the parent may like to invite someone else involved in the child's care; for example, a friend, relative or someone from a local community organisation. Of course, it will be helpful to include someone who has a good working knowledge of SM management. If the meeting follows a formal assessment, this would be the speech and language therapist or psychologist who did the assessment. If parents and the school are working and learning together, using this manual, it may help to agree who will take the lead in acquiring and sharing this knowledge.

The purpose of the initial meeting is to:

★   agree the nature of SM and the implications for intervention

★   identify who will take the various necessary roles (see Figure 7.1)

★   decide on appropriate targets for home and school

★   agree an action plan

★   set a date for a review meeting to evaluate progress and update the targets and action plan.

At this stage, the main focus is points A–D of the overall management progression. It is particularly important to ensure that people know how to build rapport with the child without insisting that the child speaks, and to identify someone to befriend and look out for the child in their educational setting with a back-up member of staff to cover absence. This person could potentially become a more formal keyworker when points E and F are discussed at subsequent planning meetings.

Formulating an action plan

Even in the absence of a joint planning meeting, parents or staff members are advised to write an action plan which they implement, update and share as soon as is viable. The action plan provides an objective way to review and plan for further progress. It should include:

★ current goal(s) for the child (eg to be happy to attend school and family occasions)

★ realistic targets (specific behaviours, results or reported information that demonstrate progress is being made towards achieving a goal)

★ the strategies or interventions necessary in order to achieve these targets (after each planning meeting, there may be some finer detail of agreed strands of intervention to be finalised by the people who are directly involved)

Most schools use their own documentation for educational plans, but if needed, Form 14 'Target sheet and action plan' (online) provides a possible format. There is a completed example in Chapter 8 (page 140).

Putting the management programme into practice

In our experience, regular documented review meetings are the only way to achieve consistency of practice and ensure that momentum is maintained. We suggest telephone contact within two weeks of agreeing a programme; the first review after four weeks; then reviews every six to eight weeks for the first year. By the second year, a review meeting three times a year is usually sufficient but informal contact can be maintained between meetings as needed. It is best to fix the date of the following meeting at the previous one; it can always be cancelled if not required or replaced by a telephone or an email 'check-up' at the school's or therapist's discretion.

The flowchart in Figure 7.1 (opposite) summarises this process within the overall structure of planning intervention. As well as introducing the management section of this manual, it may be a helpful starting point for formulating a local care pathway.

Looking ahead: a balanced approach to intervention

Using a simple but comprehensive framework to underpin intervention provides a clear focus for everyone involved. The multidimensional model of confident talking, introduced in Chapter 2, provides this focus for collaborative working. Figure 7.2 replicates it for intervention.

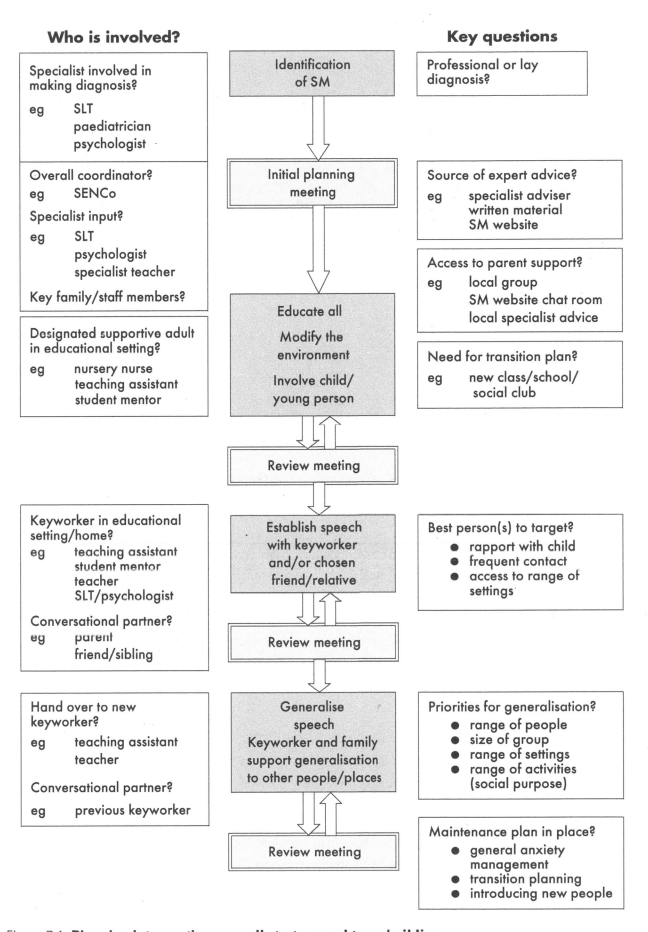

Who is involved?

Specialist involved in making diagnosis?

eg   SLT
          paediatrician
          psychologist

Overall coordinator?
eg   SENCo

Specialist input?
eg   SLT
          psychologist
          specialist teacher

Key family/staff members?

Designated supportive adult in educational setting?

eg   nursery nurse
          teaching assistant
          student mentor

Keyworker in educational setting/home?
eg   teaching assistant
          student mentor
          teacher
          SLT/psychologist

Conversational partner?
eg   parent
          friend/sibling

Hand over to new keyworker?

eg   teaching assistant
          teacher

Conversational partner?

eg   previous keyworker

(centre flow)

Identification of SM

Initial planning meeting

Educate all

Modify the environment

Involve child/ young person

Review meeting

Establish speech with keyworker and/or chosen friend/relative

Review meeting

Generalise speech
Keyworker and family support generalisation to other people/places

Review meeting

Key questions

Professional or lay diagnosis?

Source of expert advice?
eg   specialist adviser
          written material
          SM website

Access to parent support?
eg   local group
          SM website chat room
          local specialist advice

Need for transition plan?
eg   new class/school/
          social club

Best person(s) to target?
- rapport with child
- frequent contact
- access to range of settings

Priorities for generalisation?
- range of people
- size of group
- range of settings
- range of activities (social purpose)

Maintenance plan in place?
- general anxiety management
- transition planning
- introducing new people

Figure 7.1: **Planning intervention: overall strategy and team building**

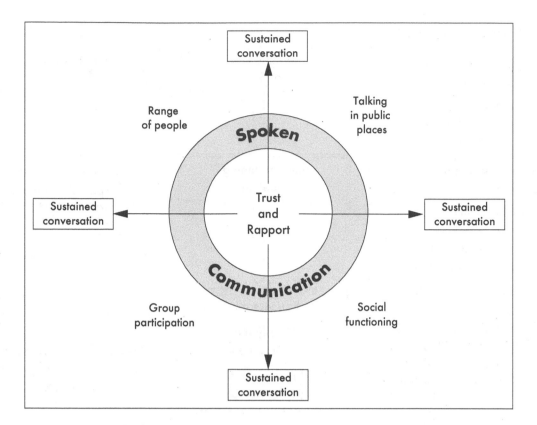

Figure 7.2: **Confident talking – a model for balanced intervention**

Using this model, steps are taken to work through five progressions in order to:

a)   reduce the child's overall anxiety, as represented by the centre of the circle (see Chapter 8)

b)   build rapport and establish sustained conversation with key people in the child's life, as represented by the spokes of the circle (see Chapters 8–10)

c)   generalise talking across four main areas, as represented by the quadrants of the circle (see Chapters 9–11).

We recommend that, before starting intervention, everyone involved becomes acquainted with this model to ensure that the following happens.

1   Consideration of their unique contribution to the overall programme. Figure 7.3 (opposite) helps families and other agencies to be clear about their role, including their limitations, and to liaise as appropriate in order to support generalisation and 'complete the circle'. This should be done in a balanced way, rather than focusing on one quadrant at a time.

2   Consideration of all aspects of confident talking in a coordinated and systematic approach to intervention, as summarised in Table 7.1 on the following page. The progression to establish sustained conversation with key individuals is in the first column. This should be complemented by four types of generalisation activity to add more people to the child's comfort zone; increase the number of people who can be addressed at any one time; reduce anxiety about being overheard in public; and facilitate general spontaneity and freedom to communicate.

Range of people

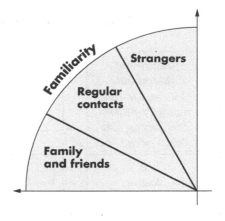

This quadrant is tackled at home and school to ensure children include both familiar people and strangers in their talking circle. The aim should be to expand the talking circle fairly quickly to avoid dependency on any one person.

Talking in public places

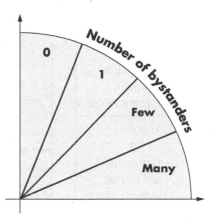

This quadrant is tackled mainly at home and in community settings by people in the child's comfort zone (people the child speaks to fully and freely when no one else is listening). By helping children increase their tolerance of being heard to speak by visitors, and in public places such as shops, parks and waiting rooms, progress is accelerated in all other areas.

Group participation

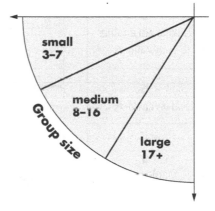

Although applicable to all settings, this quadrant is tackled mainly at school where there is more opportunity for children to routinely address large groups. Group size includes the child who has SM and often a supportive adult.

Social functioning

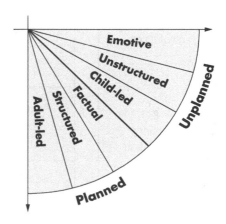

This quadrant is covered by gradually extending the type and content of activities and expectations in all settings. `Safe´ structured activities, where the child feels in control, gradually give way to spontaneous interaction, where the child takes the lead or makes a more personal or 'risky' contribution. Improvement here depends on multiple factors, especially the setting.

Figure 7.3: **Confident talking – the generalisation process**

Table 7.1: **The progressions of confident talking** (also in Handout D2, Appendix D)

One-to-one interaction — Moving towards relaxed, sustained conversation with each individual	GENERALISATION
	Note: *all aspects are tackled together in a coordinated manner, but at a different rate for each progression*

increasing demand (vertical, left axis)

One-to-one interaction	
0 Absent	**Range of people** — People the child can talk to on a one-to-one basis
1 Frozen	**Family and friends** — Immediate and extended family and close friends. This group is most likely to include the people with whom the child talks freely
2 Participation without communication	**Regular contacts** — Familiar people with whom the child is in regular contact, eg teacher, classmates, neighbours, friends' parents, babysitter
	Strangers — People the child is unlikely to see again or sees only fleetingly, eg shop assistants, librarian, school visitors, school crossing patrol, dentist

increasing demand →

Talking in public places
Presence and proximity of bystanders and possibility that talking will be disclosed to other settings

No chance of being overheard	May be overheard by one person outside comfort zone	May be overheard by a few people outside comfort zone	May be overheard by many people outside comfort zone

increasing demand →

Group participation
Group size includes the child and a facilitating adult, if appropriate

3–7 eg group work, sleepover, family meal	8–16 eg tutor group, football team	17+ eg class, party, stage performance

increasing demand →

Social functioning
Moving towards spontaneous conversation to meet the child's needs

Planned		Unplanned	
Adult-initiated	Child-initiated	Adult-initiated	Child-initiated
Structured	Unstructured	Structured	Unstructured
Factual content	Emotive content	Factual content	Emotive content

One-to-one interaction progressions (left column):

0 Absent
1 Frozen
2 Participation without communication
3 Non-verbal and written communication
4 Talking via another person
5 Using voice
6 Single words
7 Phrases and sentences
8 Sustained conversation

3   An appreciation of why individuals with SM can do some things but not others. For example, it may seem illogical that a child can speak in front of the whole school in their end-of-term production, but not approach a familiar adult to ask for help. However, as the social functioning progression in Table 7.1 highlights, the second activity exposes the child to a much higher level of uncertainty and risk. The first activity is planned, structured and rehearsed with a clear end-point in sight. The second relies on the child to initiate interaction on an ad hoc basis. This requires careful timing, with no guarantee that the request will be well received, and it may invite further conversation for which the child is unprepared.

Management summary

Page 2 of Form 11 (online) lists the key areas that will need to be addressed and are described in later chapters. Using this plan, the coordinating clinician can check that everything is covered and in the right order. This includes some important tasks that can easily be forgotten, for example, giving out information about national support organisations such as the Selective Mutism Research and Information Association (SMIRA) and local support groups, where they exist.

Online resource for Chapter 7

The form for this chapter is available at www.routledge.com/cw/speechmark for you to access, print and copy.

PART 3
MANAGEMENT

CONTENTS

Chapter 11 Making successful transitions

CHAPTER 8

ENSURING AN ANXIETY-FREE ENVIRONMENT: THE STARTING POINT FOR HOME AND SCHOOL

Introduction

This chapter looks at:

★ reducing the child's anxiety to a manageable level (in all environments)

★ reaching a shared understanding of selective mutism

★ talking to the child about speech anxiety

★ confidence building

★ building rapport

★ home and classroom modifications (including alternative forms of communication and enabling children to seek help)

★ formulating an action plan

★ moving on to specific talking targets.

The online resource library includes a range of handouts, checklists and a target sheet to supplement the areas discussed in this chapter.

Reducing the child's anxiety to a manageable level

The first step towards overcoming selective mutism (SM) is ensuring that the child's anxiety is controlled and manageable in all environments. It is tempting to push ahead with a treatment plan, as detailed in Chapter 10. However, this will not succeed if common practices at home or school are inadvertently strengthening and maintaining the child's anxiety and fear of speaking.

Therefore, it is essential to share information with everyone, in order to increase understanding, eliminate any maintenance behaviour and promote behaviour that both encourages and reinforces more verbal communication from the child. Everyone in contact with the child has a part to play in this; it only takes one person to undo everyone else's good work.

Using the information in this chapter, the aim for each setting is to provide:

★ an understanding that the child will speak when their anxiety has been reduced to a manageable level

★ opportunities for the child to speak but no uncomfortable pressure to do so

★ full inclusion in all activities, while boosting confidence and self-esteem

★ monitoring to ascertain the child's readiness for specific talking targets.

If you are closely involved in supporting children who have SM, we recommend drawing up a table with three simple columns, as suggested in Figure 8.1. This will help you to reflect and make notes as you read this chapter, perhaps over several sittings.

At the end of this chapter there is an opportunity to take the information gained from assessment to further customise this action plan.

☺	☹	Personal action plan
(Things that are helpful and need to continue)	(Things that are not helpful and need to change)	(eg changes you will make, handouts to pass on/discuss, questions to ask, further reading)

Figure 8.1: **Drawing up an action plan**

Reaching a shared understanding of selective mutism

Parents and staff members in school need information early on, so that the nature of SM can be discussed, fully understood and agreed before formulating and reviewing a treatment plan. In many countries, including the UK, initial concerns about a child's progress will lead to a series of meetings, in line with special educational needs legislation.

Parents must also get friends and relatives on board who do not have the same obligations to listen and meet their child's needs. This should be as simple as saying 'My child has a real fear of dogs. We're working on this with him but, meanwhile, he needs you to make some allowances for him please.' Unfortunately, replacing 'fear of dogs' with 'fear of talking to certain people' does not always have the desired effect. There are still many people who do not take a fear of talking seriously and feel that all the child lacks is discipline or time to 'get over' their shyness.

It is natural to be wary of upsetting relatives or professionals by challenging their views or treatment of a child, but it is unlikely that anyone would keep quiet if a child was being routinely terrified by an unleashed dog. No child could enjoy a visit from their grandparents or pay attention to instructions if constantly fearing the dog might approach. *In the same way, it is essential to educate other people about how to manage SM.* If people refuse to acknowledge these children's high anxiety levels, or the need for appropriate intervention, they must be made aware of the increased risk of additional mental health issues when SM is mishandled or ignored (see Chapter 2, 'The cost of ignoring SM', page 44, and Appendix E online).

These are sensitive issues and parents and young people often feel that they are being judged unfairly by others. There are various Facebook groups which provide chatrooms for parents, young people and professionals who want to find and share both practical and emotional support, for example, SMIRA (the Selective Mutism Information and Research Association) and SM Space Café.

Education sessions

Some local authorities provide information sessions for staff members and families, so this should be investigated through local speech and language therapy clinics or education services. There is an outline of the content of such sessions in 'Educational support' in Appendix D (online). These sessions make an excellent forum for dispelling myths and misassumptions about children who have SM and teaching the principles of management. Alternatively, the contents can be adapted around an individual child and key points shared at a meeting with parents and relevant staff members.

Having accessed suitable information, many families and schools will be able to successfully liaise and agree an action plan. Where those involved with the child cannot agree on the nature of his or her difficulties, or the principles of SM management, professional advice should be sought to mediate a discussion. Ideally, this should be done through the forum of a multi-agency review meeting. See Chapter 3, 'How to find a suitable professional to make a diagnosis' (page 58); Chapter 7, 'Planning intervention' (page 103); and Appendix D, 'Legal support' (online).

Written information

★ Two introductory information sheets are provided online: Handout 2 'What is selective mutism?' and Handout 3 'Quiet child or selective mutism?'. Handout 2 sets out the key facts and characteristics of SM. Handout 3 explains that children do not have to be completely silent to meet the diagnostic criteria for SM. This one is particularly useful for staff, friends or relatives who dispute a diagnosis of SM and see the child as simply quiet or shy.

★ There are a few simple explanations and ready replies in Handout 4 'What to say when …', to accompany the written information available in this chapter.

★ Chapter 1 'Frequently asked questions about SM' may be useful to address any specific queries that arise.

★ Other information sheets can be downloaded from several dedicated websites. In the UK, SMIRA is the main contact point for families.

★ In the UK, health and education authorities are increasingly making leaflets available as they develop services for children who have SM and their families (see the sample leaflets in 'Educational resources' in Appendix F online).

Audio-visual information

Sometimes an audio-visual presentation has more impact than written material, see below for examples:

★ The BBC documentary *My Child Won't Speak* (2010) is available on YouTube. It follows the progress of three girls with SM. Parents report that this has been particularly helpful in educating friends and relatives, and showing children and teenagers with SM that other people experience the same difficulties.

★ A 24-minute DVD – *Silent Children; Approaches to Selective Mutism* – is available from SMIRA. It gives an overview of the nature and management of SM from the perspectives of several children, parents and professionals. SLT departments may consider lending this to parents and schools to increase their understanding of the condition in the early stages of management. Short extracts may also be useful to include in education sessions (see 'Educational support' in Appendix D and 'Audio-visual resources' in Appendix F online).

Educating other people – a time and place

Parents and professionals must initially do all they can to educate staff members, friends and relatives about SM and appropriate management *without* the child present. This enables any differences of opinion to be fully aired and, it is hoped, resolved, without creating further anxiety and confusion for the child. Teenagers tell us they hate it when they hear their parents explain to other people that they have difficulty speaking and are not being rude. They would prefer this to be established beforehand, to ensure that no one makes a big deal of it if they do or don't manage to talk.

Many young people don't want *anything* to be said because they are trying to make a fresh start (see 'Making a fresh start' in Chapter 11, page 247, and Box 11.3, page 245). Some young people have found a reassuring standby in simple business cards bearing a few sentences of explanation, either to hand out themselves if they are unable to speak, or for their parents to discreetly distribute on a 'need-to-know' basis (see the examples in Figure 8.2 and 'Support for communication' in Appendix F online). It is important to discuss such scenarios with older children to establish their preferences and agree on wording they are comfortable with.

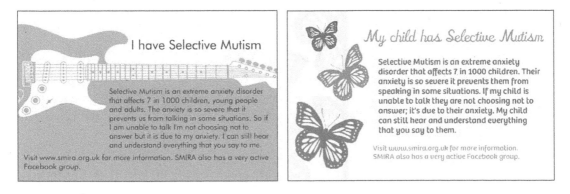

Figure 8.2: **Selective mutism awareness cards (designed by Lizzie Helps)**

Describing the child's difficulties in suitable language

When talking among adults, it is easy to get caught up in comments about whether a child who has SM 'can't talk' or 'won't talk'. As discussed in Chapter 1, neither is an adequate description. It is important for everyone involved to use terms which clarify other people's perceptions and provide the appropriate language to use. For example, you may say children 'want to talk, but cannot always speak out freely', 'find talking easier in certain situations than others', 'talk in situation A but not yet in situation B', 'are trying really hard to be brave about talking'. Or you could say that the child should be allowed to join in little by little until they feel comfortable, better or less anxious about talking.

Understanding the rationale for providing appropriate support

Adults typically build rapport with children by asking them questions; but this immediately puts children who have SM on the spot or makes them feel tested. Taking up a challenge along the lines of 'I've never had any child who refused to speak to *me*' or 'I'm sure *I* can get [N] to speak' is just as unhelpful. Removing privileges in order to 'motivate' the child to speak is pointless too. For example, if a child is terrified of dogs, they don't need motivation; they need patient support. However, although it is counterproductive to pressurise children into speaking, equally there is a danger of oversympathising, excusing the child or removing the need to speak. Any type of sustained avoidance diminishes children's confidence in their ability to change and actually *increases* their fear of speaking.

Faced with such a fine balance, it is understandable for staff members and parents to feel confused about the best action to take. The handouts in the online resource library give sound advice but cannot replace a firm grasp of the rationale behind them. Therefore, it is advisable for everyone involved to remind themselves how much they already know about phobias and how they have successfully helped children to work their way through other fears without any specialist training. Handout 5 'SM is a phobia' (online) sets out the basic principles of phobia management and is a good starting point for establishing team commitment to the treatment approach recommended in this manual. There are six key messages:

1   **Phobias can be overcome.**

2   **The first step is to talk about and understand the phobia.**

3   **Applying pressure makes phobias worse.**

4   **Gradually facing fears is the key to success.**

5   **Avoidance is not an option.**

6   **Confidence has a ripple effect.**

So, although it is indeed essential to remove all pressure to talk initially, especially in group situations where the child feels most exposed, this must be accompanied by the gradual introduction of planned situations to help the child face their fears *at their own pace*. At the same time, talk to the child and reassure them that everyone understands that talking is difficult for them at times, and no one will mind if they don't talk straightaway. The earlier you start applying these principles routinely and consistently in all environments, the sooner SM will be a thing of the past.

The online handouts accompanying this chapter and Chapters 9 and 10 'Facing fears', address the six key messages outlined above. All are equally useful for parents and professionals, both for guidance in an informing or advisory capacity, or as topics for group discussion with parents or staff members. We recommend ongoing parent discussion groups facilitated by a professional with experience of SM and knowledge of general anxiety management, to complement school intervention programmes and reinforce the rationale for providing appropriate support in home and community settings. As you might expect, it is the parents themselves who provide the success stories, encouragement and mutual emotional support in these parent meetings.

Talking to the child about speech anxiety

As any adult with a phobia will appreciate, you can only contemplate facing your fear if you feel confident that the steps taken will move at your own pace. It is essential to have a sense of being in control. It is the same for children; we see more rapid progress when the child can talk about their anxiety and take a small-steps approach. Many parents report that their child refuses to discuss it, but this usually means that the child does not want to answer *questions* about their difficulties (see 'Nothing has worked so far', in Chapter 1, page 24).

We propose an *explanation* rather than a discussion. There is guidance for families and staff in Chapter 5 (see 'The Pep Talk' on page 73 and 'Learning about phobias' on page 82) and in Handout 1 'Talking to the child about speech anxiety' (online). It is important to identify a member of staff in each setting who will befriend and talk to the child in this way, possibly with the parent present, as part of building rapport.

If parents find that their child won't sit still long enough to listen, we recommend trying any of the following strategies.

★ Children may listen better if a staff member does the talking with a parent present.

★ Casually slot the main points from Handout 1 into daily conversations, linking your child's fear of talking to other fears they or other children may display. For example, 'You know

Cheryl was finding it very difficult to talk to her daughter about SM until she saw the similarities with the Disney film *Frozen* (2013). This is how she put the key messages across.

- Princess Elsa doesn't want to freeze things around her; just like you don't want to freeze inside and stop talking. She can't help it can she? It's not her fault.

- Elsa feels free when she runs away to her ice castle in the mountains. She can be herself at last; just like you can be free at home where it's easy to talk. But staying away from everyone doesn't fix anything, does it? You end up being alone.

- Anna didn't let her sister hide away, did she? With Anna's love and understanding, Elsa learned how to control her power. And you've got people who love you and understand too. We know you get worried about talking sometimes and the words won't come out. But you'll learn to control that worry so you don't freeze any more. Talking will be easy!

how Tilly didn't come round because she's afraid our dog might jump up? It's the same with your talking; you get scared that you'll have to talk to people you don't know very well. But it's OK, you and Tilly will both get braver and you won't be scared any more. Maybe you could help Tilly get used to our dog, and Tilly could help you with your talking'.

★ Long car journeys are great for difficult topics – eye contact is easily avoided and there is no escape!

★ Stories can provide a safe setting for children to identify, acknowledge and discuss their own feelings. See Appendix F for examples of children's books about general anxiety and SM.

★ Invite your child to watch documentaries with you about other children who have SM (see page 118).

★ Take your child to a dedicated local or national parents meeting where they will meet other children who have SM.

Confidence building

Although it is tempting to focus purely on communication when supporting children who have SM, remember that it is an anxiety disorder and that the child's emotional well-being and resilience is paramount. The attitude of staff members and daily support that parents provide are instrumental in building and maintaining confidence, self-esteem, independence and a positive attitude towards problem solving and risk taking in general, so that the child is in the best frame of mind to respond to more specific intervention.

★ Handout 6 'Firm foundations: building confidence, courage and self-esteem' (online) provides general guidance for building confidence while ensuring that children's self-esteem is not affected as a result of their SM.

★ Handout 7 'Helping children to cope with anxiety' (online) is useful for all anxious children. It outlines how parents can help children develop anxiety-coping mechanisms which will see them through adolescence and into adulthood. Some children who have SM only have fears associated with speaking, but others are 'born worriers' with more general anxiety. SM intervention is not going to change their cautious nature, but the strategies these children adopt to tackle SM can be successfully applied to other fears alongside the principles on this handout.

★ When studying Handouts 6 and 7, parents may recognise that by trying to spare their children anxiety, they are actually making them more anxious and delaying their independence. This can be an extremely difficult concept to deal with, let alone change. Some staff members and parents may recognise that their unrealistic expectations are setting up the child to fail. Practitioners need to be ready to support teachers and parents in adapting their behaviour through open discussion from a non-judgemental standpoint. Many unhelpful management strategies will have been adopted in good faith, so it is important that neither staff members nor parents feel guilty or criticised.

Dealing with unhelpful comments

Teachers and parents need to be ready to deal with comments and questions from other children, staff and family members because they can undermine confidence if not handled appropriately. Classmates are inquisitive and adults probably lack information and experience of SM. The aim is to talk openly, in a matter-of-fact and positive way about the child's anxiety,

> It was excruciating having people ask me why I don't speak. I used to wish I had someone sitting beside me with a gun to my head telling me not to speak so it was obvious to them.

without making the child feel self-conscious or ashamed if they are present. Therefore, it may be necessary to have a quick response ready (see Handout 4 'What to say when' online), while making a mental note to provide more information in private when the child is not around (see 'Reaching a shared understanding of selective mutism' on page 116 and 'Involving the child's classmates' in Chapter 10, page 207).

Having the confidence to make mistakes and have a go

Teachers and parents may notice children doing less and less as they become increasingly afraid of getting something wrong. This is not the case for all children who have SM, but it is a common pattern as children get older and for those with more generalised anxiety. They may become reluctant to submit work, for example, and shrug or 'freeze' whenever they are asked to guess. Fear of making mistakes will compromise their ability to show their true colours socially, emotionally and academically. This is addressed on Handout 8 'Mistaeks Happen!' (online). Further resources are listed in Appendix F (online), in 'Tackling fear of making mistakes'.

Ironically, children who have SM may also hold back because of the praise and attention that good work attracts. They may dread the expectation to discuss or share their work or being sent to the head teacher for a reward sticker. As part of being open with them about their SM, it is important to reassure them privately that their work will secure good marks but there won't be any additional expectation to talk. For more on praise, see Handout 6 (online) and item 15 in Table 8.2 (page 134).

Building rapport

All staff and relatives should be aware of how to put children at their ease using 'commentary-style talk', as detailed below. Children and young people who have SM can easily become isolated, spending many family occasions sitting in the corner and whole days at school with no one talking to them. It is hard to communicate with someone who doesn't answer back so, after a few attempts, many people give up, aware that the situation has become uncomfortable. Changing this to ensure that all children feel included and appreciated is one of the simplest and most beneficial things we can do.

Commentary-style talk

The secret is to talk to the child without asking any direct questions that require an answer. This does not come naturally to most people, so it is worth practising on friends and family! If it helps, imagine that you are with an exchange student who cannot speak English but understands enough to keep up. You want to make sure they feel welcome, so you are open and friendly and smile a lot. You don't ask them questions because all you get is a blank look, so instead you show them around, talk about what you are doing, make light-hearted comments and get them involved in a practical activity. You are prepared for the fact that they *might* say something but, until they do, you are perfectly happy to do all the talking, rather like a one-sided commentary.

The same approach works for individuals with SM. Keep talking but don't be afraid of silences! It's good to pause and leave gaps but, when you do, look anywhere but at the child's face, or they will feel you are waiting for a response. Tag questions are useful, as in 'That looks good, *doesn't it*?', as are openers such as 'I expect …', 'I bet …', 'I wonder …' and 'You might like/have/want …'. These provide the *opportunity* to respond but don't demand an answer. It's also OK to ask *yourself* questions such as 'Oh no, where have I put my glasses?' and 'I wonder where this goes?' As children realise that you are not fazed by their silence, and don't mind if they talk or not, they will relax and begin to react by smiling, nodding and shaking their head. Be patient and genuinely enjoy their company and some children may even feel comfortable enough to talk.

> In commentary-style talk:
> ✓ Adult does all the talking
> ✗ Direct questions
> ✓ Instructions
> ✓ Chatty comments
> ✓ Rhetorical questions that need no answer
> ✓ Pauses

Encouraging participation

In addition to the above strategy, at least one member of staff, and any friends or relatives who are keen to help the child eventually talk to them, should gently build rapport with the child, as outlined in Table 8.1 on the next page, choosing activities that they know the child will enjoy (see Stage 2 and Stage 3 activity suggestions in Appendix A online). In this context, rapport is defined as the relationship which develops when the child or young person senses that the adult is understanding and will not expect them to talk before they are ready. Table 8.1 sets out target behaviours that demonstrate progressive relaxation and engagement, until the child communicates easily without talking, using an appropriate form of non-verbal or written communication (Stage 3).When the child's readiness to move up to the next stage is correctly judged, the process of building rapport often leads to higher stages of interaction. These are covered in the next chapter (Table 9.1).

Families and staff may like to use the online Progress chart 1 'One-to-one interaction with a range of people' to keep a record of how the child progresses with the various people they see regularly. This may highlight issues with particular individuals which need to be addressed. Children who have SM instinctively feel more comfortable with a certain type of person, which can be hurtful for other staff and relatives who are trying, unsuccessfully, to forge a relationship. Often it is their very efforts that the child finds overwhelming: perhaps they are talking too much or too loudly; asking questions; sitting too close; touching or organising the child. These children need their personal space with a focus on shared activity rather than themselves if they are to relax and engage.

Table 8.1: **Confident talking – building rapport on a one-to-one basis**

Stage	Child's presentation	Target behaviours (select as appropriate for different settings)
0	Absent (eg child does not want to go to school or hides behind parent or furniture)	For the parent to: • reassure the child that they will be welcome whether they talk or not. Everyone just wants them to have fun and enjoy themselves. • hold the child's hand and position themselves at the child's side, rather than pick up or shield the child. This enables the child to observe their surroundings and learn that there is no threat.
1	Frozen	For adults to reinforce the parent's message: • greet the child warmly but quietly and calmly, respecting their personal space • talk to the parent rather than the child[1] • make positive statements about the child • explain tasks and activities clearly in advance, so that the child is aware they can be done without talking. For the child to: • feel valued and know they are doing well • watch as others demonstrate a game or activity • feel unpressured and look forward to attending the setting.
2	Participates without communication	For adults to: • use commentary-style talk[2] rather than ask direct questions • use 'I wonder' statements and pauses, eg 'I wonder where this goes?', 'I wonder if you've come across these before?' • focus on materials rather than look at child for a response • respond in a natural, unsurprised manner if the child talks. For the child to: • participate happily in non-verbal activities and be guided by the adult • take turns with the adult • help the adult prepare or tidy up after an activity • take an item when offered a choice • appear at ease when listening, walking, running, etc.
3	Uses non-verbal and written communication	For the adult to: • say 'Show me …' rather than 'Tell me …' • provide items to choose from and ask 'Which one?' • offer choices followed by a gesture which the child can imitate, eg 'Yes' (*adult nods or gives a thumbs up sign*), or 'No' (*adult shakes head or gives thumbs down*); 'Where's Sam? Is he upstairs (*adult points up*) or did he go outside (*adult points out of the window*)?' • occasionally ask 'yes/no' questions which the child can respond to by either nodding or shaking their head. For the child to: • smile responsively and appropriately • use gesture (mime, nod, shake head or point) without body tension to communicate, eg indicate a choice; agree or disagree; put hand on head to indicate 'hat' • use pictures or text to answer a question, eg point to, write, tick or circle the answer.

(Continued)

Table 8.1: **Confident talking – building rapport on a one-to-one basis** (*Continued*)

Stage	Child's presentation	Target behaviours (select as appropriate for different settings)
Talking bridge[1]	Tolerates voice being heard	For the adult to make the child feel comfortable by: • not watching the child closely when with family or friends • appearing to be occupied with other things • not reacting when the child talks to family or friends. For the child to talk or laugh with a parent or friend in an adult's presence (voice is audible rather than whispered).
Note	1. This step is possible only if the parent or another talking partner is present and can be bypassed on other occasions. 2. See page 122.	

Home and classroom modifications

Adjustments at home and school

Handout 9 (online) is specifically for staff in early years settings and relevant families. The aim is to create an environment which allows all quiet and anxious children to settle in at their own pace. It should be possible to distinguish shyness and SM within a few weeks and prevent the development of SM in reluctant speakers who might otherwise feel pressured to talk before they are ready.

Handouts 10a and 10b set out general 'dos and don'ts' for other people and settings where the child does not talk freely. These strategies do not facilitate speech; they pave the way by ensuring that the child feels welcome and included, whether they talk or not. The strategies need to be maintained until the child is ready to take their talking programme to the next level (as discussed in Chapters 9 and 10), or until the child begins talking spontaneously. For example, a child's SM will need to be accommodated within the classroom setting so that they can participate in lessons *without talking* initially, and this must continue while they work towards talking to adults and children in the privacy of a separate room. In time, the child's programme will generalise to the classroom. Similarly, relatives need to be patient and understand that they are facilitating the child's recovery by initially allowing them *not* to talk.

Handouts 10a and 10b have roughly the same content for younger and older children. They are useful for:

★ any staff the child might meet in educational establishments or smaller gatherings such as swimming lessons or youth clubs

★ friends or relatives either visiting the home or hosting activities such as parties or sleepovers.

Select the handout which seems more appropriate but, as a guide, Handout 10a is suitable for children up to 10 or 11 years old. Relatives and other adults outside the school setting could be given an edited version which includes just the first few items from each section.

Older children and young people who relate well to a supportive staff member or practitioner can be actively involved in tailoring the advice given to different teachers. Handout 11, 'Enabling quieter students to communicate', can be distributed to members of staff as it stands but, ideally, it will be edited beforehand by the young person with a particular teacher or lesson in mind. The student is asked to highlight the strategies they would currently find most helpful and to delete unhelpful strategies.

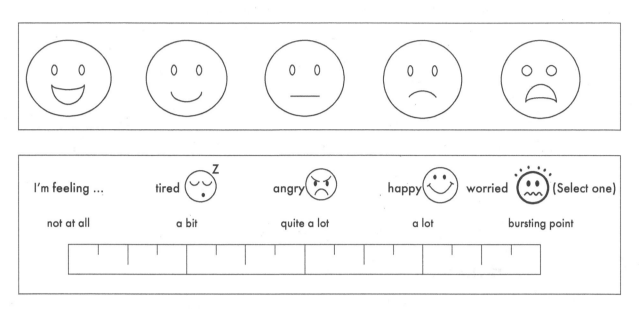

Figure 8.3: **Examples of pictorial rating scales to express emotions**

Sharing emotions

Letting people know how you feel is vital to feeling secure and supported in any environment but children who have SM find this very difficult. This is not necessarily because they cannot share their feelings. It is often a reflection of their difficulty approaching adults or the complex language involved (one word will rarely suffice, leading to unwanted questions). We recommend adopting a simple five-point rating scale early on, to give adults a way of checking how the child or young person feels (their facial expressions may not give anything away) and to provide them with a means of communication. The scale can be in the form of a simple row of faces (as in Figure 8.3), lines on a ruler or thermometer, or the numbers 0 to 5. The same rating scales can be used for a variety of emotions so that children and young people can indicate how happy, worried, upset, confused, hurt, ill, excited or calm they feel in different situations. For example, 0–5 could represent 'no anxiety' through to 'panic stations' or 'no help needed at the moment' through to 'I've totally lost the plot'. Depending on the child's age and aptitude, parents might like to use the chosen rating scale at home first to make sure the child understands it and can use it confidently and reliably.

You can also ask children how they are feeling by providing options in writing. For example, 'Which of these words best describe how you feel about this activity? Scared, excited, bored, pleased, fine, or something else?' See the sorting, ranking and rating techniques in Chapter 5 (Figures 5.6 and 5.7) for other ways to enable children and young people to share their emotions without talking.

Using alternative forms of communication

People often question the use of alternative forms of communication. By allowing a child who has SM to communicate through writing, gesture or pictures, or to record themselves reading their poem or presentation at home, are we condoning their lack of speech and removing the need to change?

Certainly, this could be the case if the child looked at the alternative as a permanent replacement for speech and received no support to move on. But denying children these alternatives robs them of a 'voice' and excludes them from full participation in social and academic activities. We regard alternatives as part of the natural progression towards speech. Explain to children that they are a good way to communicate *at the moment*, while talking is difficult, or a good back-up in case their confidence disappears at the last moment. Don't forget that these children *want* to speak! No one chooses to rely on less effective alternatives unless they genuinely believe talking is impossible. For example, a 15-year-old girl had her phone app 'Emergency Chat' ready in case she lost her nerve during her interview (see 'Support for communication' in Appendix F online), but answered all of the questions without needing to text. A 7-year-old child, who could talk easily to her teaching assistant (TA) when no one else was listening, used the communication chart in Figure 8.4 to let her TA know when she needed help in the classroom. A term later, she didn't need the chart because her TA had helped her to speak to most of her peers and she could now talk in the classroom.

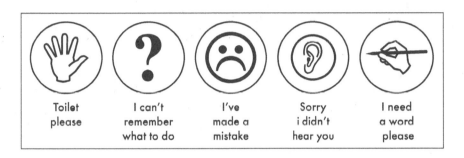

Figure 8.4: **Communication chart**

Given the temporary nature of alternative forms of communication as part of an ongoing intervention plan, we advise that only systems which are quickly adopted by the child and easily understood by other people are used; for example, pointing to words, pictures or symbols, writing, simple hand gestures, or a text display on a mobile phone or tablet. It is not worth investing time in teaching a whole new language of signs or symbols, for example, when that time could be better spent helping the child to face their fear of talking. Similarly, we do not recommend the use of high-tech communication aids which can be costly and may actually set apart the child from their peers. Of course, there are always exceptions, such as when the child has additional communication difficulties which could benefit from such a device, or is educated in a school where sign language is routinely used by everyone. Apps such as Proloquo2go® may also be useful when SM is longstanding and entrenched, either as a back-up when talking is difficult, or as a longer-term solution to enable young people or adults to participate in their local community.

Helping children to make the first move and seek help

Note that there are no guarantees that children will use any alternative forms of communication provided. For example, young children may like to keep some pictures on a key-ring, to let staff members know when they feel thirsty, ill or happy, want a turn, need the toilet, and so on. But the key-ring may stay in their pocket. This is because generally most children with SM have difficulty initiating contact. It is especially hard at school where there are many other children vying for the same adult's attention. Some children will need to work towards making the first move, one step at a time, starting with the adult approaching the child. This is shown in Figure 8.5, which gives two examples of how children might gradually gain the confidence to approach a staff member.

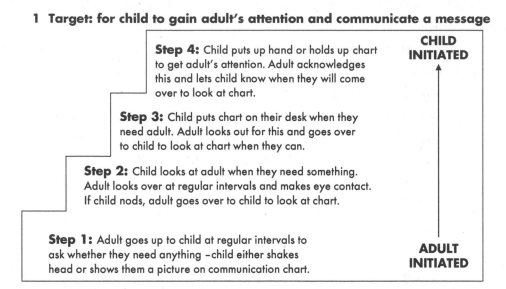

1 Target: for child to gain adult's attention and communicate a message

CHILD INITIATED

Step 4: Child puts up hand or holds up chart to get adult's attention. Adult acknowledges this and lets child know when they will come over to look at chart.

Step 3: Child puts chart on their desk when they need adult. Adult looks out for this and goes over to child to look at chart when they can.

Step 2: Child looks at adult when they need something. Adult looks over at regular intervals and makes eye contact. If child nods, adult goes over to child to look at chart.

Step 1: Adult goes up to child at regular intervals to ask whether they need anything – child either shakes head or shows them a picture on communication chart.

ADULT INITIATED

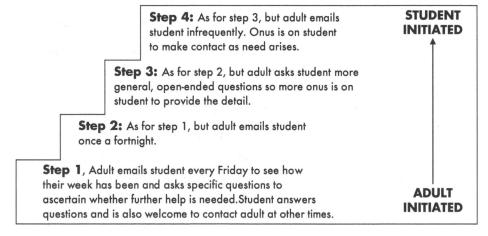

2 Target: for young person to email mentor and request support as need arises

STUDENT INITIATED

Step 4: As for step 3, but adult emails student infrequently. Onus is on student to make contact as need arises.

Step 3: As for step 2, but adult asks student more general, open-ended questions so more onus is on student to provide the detail.

Step 2: As for step 1, but adult emails student once a fortnight.

Step 1, Adult emails student every Friday to see how their week has been and asks specific questions to ascertain whether further help is needed. Student answers questions and is also welcome to contact adult at other times.

ADULT INITIATED

Figure 8.5: **Working towards initiating contact at school**

First, however, it is important for staff, or anyone looking after a child who has SM, to give the child explicit *permission* to make their needs known – a parent's say-so is rarely enough. Children need to know that they are allowed to say that they feel hungry or unwell or need help, and be told exactly how to get the adult's attention with an agreed signal if talking or a physical approach is difficult. It will also help for them to know what will happen next because most children will avoid contact if this risks a barrage of questions or the need to explain themselves in public.

Going to the toilet

We refer to various ways of dealing with daily situations, such as the attendance register, in the handouts accompanying this chapter. However, we feel that accessing the school toilets deserves special mention because a lack of access is associated with medical and psychological risks. Common issues among children who have SM include infections caused by holding in urine; dehydration through deliberately not drinking to avoid needing to go; and the humiliation of enuresis (wetting). These children usually have a fear of either using the toilet or asking to go there. The first point is discussed in Chapter 13 (pages 274–276) and the section above mentioned using a picture or symbol to request being excused.

It is also worth considering that, sometimes, there are solutions that suit the whole class. Very young children can be routinely escorted to the toilets in groups at regular intervals. School-aged children can be trusted to go to the toilet without asking first, as long as they let the teacher know where they are by putting a toilet symbol by their name on a signing-out board (this is also useful for popping to the library or school office, for example). Reminders on individual or class timetables to go at break and lunch-time, whether it's needed or not, are particularly useful for children who are either not aware that they need to go until the last minute or avoiding eating or drinking.

Providing a choice rather than seeking permission

It is important to find a way for children and young people to participate in different environments with the minimum of anxiety. With familiarity and repetition, this anxiety will reduce and they will be able to participate for longer or more fully. We firmly believe in giving children a choice in how they participate. This is because only they know what is manageable for them in different situations, but opting out is not one of the choices we offer. So, rather than ask questions like 'Are you ready to join in?' or 'What do you want to do?', which create too much uncertainty for many children, it is better to present a few options and ask the child which one they think is best.

For example, you don't want to leave out the child from sharing their news on Monday mornings. You might be tempted to give them the opportunity to speak each time, and move on to the next child when they don't take it. However, this is rather like giving a child in a wheelchair the opportunity to walk. It emphasises their difficulties, puts them on the spot and escalates their anxiety and frustration. As a result, they start to dread going to school.

Instead, have a private chat with the child and say you know they have lots of good ideas, but they haven't got used to talking in front of everyone else just yet. You want to find an easier way for them to join in. Give the child a few considered options written on sticky notes or in their home–school liaison book, and ask them to choose one. Then:

★ they could write down what they did at the weekend in their book and pick someone to read it out in class

★ their parent could write it down and the teacher could read it out

★ they could bring in a clue and nod or shake their head as the other children guess what they did

★ they could record a message at home on a tablet or Talking Tin (see Appendix F 'Talking resources' online).

Depending on the age of the child, you could also include a blank option in case they have a better idea, or invite the child to take the choices home to discuss with their parent.

Dealing with difficult behaviour and stress

Schools and families may try their utmost to create anxiety-free environments, but it is impossible to completely alleviate the stress of living with SM. Being unable to speak for much of the day, struggling to overcome anxiety in order to cope with daily life and meet new challenges, and coping with the unpredictability of other people's reactions create great strain. Children and young people need help to offload their stress both safely and appropriately.

When dealing with children's behaviour, it is important to recognise the three common reactions to stress:

FIGHT   lash out physically or verbally; look for an argument; steadfastly refuse to participate or comply.

FLIGHT   hide; cling to parent; immerse self in other 'more important' activities; seek permission to be excluded; deny there is a problem; drink alcohol or take drugs to unwind.

FREEZE   clam up; mind goes blank; look down and hope you won't be noticed; feel physically unable to move; muscular tension and clumsiness; use a flat, monotonous tone of voice.

Most of this manual addresses avoidance behaviour (flight) and the inability to speak (freeze) but, within this context, oppositional behaviour (fight) can also be expected. By following the treatment approaches described in this manual, you can expect difficult behaviours to subside, but this will not happen overnight.

It can be challenging to bear the brunt of pent-up emotions. Usually this occurs when children come home from school but, occasionally, they may be tipped over the edge at school, when they feel they are being treated unfairly. It will be hard to believe that a child has SM when they suddenly shout or swear at a member of staff, for example, but at this point, their fear of speaking has been outweighed by the fear of a threatened event. As various communication disorders demonstrate, swearing operates at an automatic level and is often the only language to be preserved. Aggressive behaviour and bad language cannot be tolerated so it is important to prevent outbursts, as far as possible, by ensuring that everyone takes reasonable steps to avoid setting off the child's panic alarm. It also helps to provide a calm place to unwind (where there are no violent computer games) before tackling homework or family chores, and a physical outlet for frustration after school such as trampolining, swing-ball or swimming.

Ironically, children who have SM often experience a 'meltdown' after doing incredibly *well*. This can seem like one step forward, two steps back but it is a natural, and usually fairly fleeting, reaction. The child is either exhausted after the extended period of intense emotion that accompanies doing something new for the first time – fear, doubt, determination, relief and elation – or fearful about the next step and future expectations.

When outbursts happen, they should be met with no more than short, calm reflection: 'I'm sorry you're so upset'; 'OK, you're feeling very angry right now'; 'You must be worn out'; rather than retaliation or attempts to reason or pacify. Time and a quiet, safe place are needed to defuse the situation and allow a highly sensitive child's reaction to run its course. Young children might have a den of blankets or soft toys they like to crawl into, while older children can be left on their own to listen to music, bash a pillow, write about or draw a picture of their feelings until they feel calmer. Let children come to you when they are ready, and see whether it helps to give them a choice: 'You can cry some more or we could go to the park'. Later, it will be important to acknowledge fully their frustration and take steps to deal with any specific triggers and underlying anxiety, while setting clear boundaries for what is acceptable and unacceptable behaviour.

Sometimes anxiety can be mistaken for passive aggression. It is impossible to sound enthusiastic when you are feeling tense or anxious. So, older children may unwittingly provoke others by speaking in a flat tone of voice which sounds uninterested, rude or confrontational. By rising to this, and getting annoyed, adults will escalate the child's stress level and push them into 'fight or flight'. However difficult it may feel at times, adults need to take a deep breath, stay calm and continue speaking in a gentle tone – and take time out if they feel they are about to lose their temper.

The fourth way to respond to stress is to **FACE** it and try to find a solution. However, this can also lead to inappropriate behaviour if children are trapped by their inability to speak. You need to look deeper than surface level to understand the reasons for apparently antisocial, disturbing or uncharacteristic behaviour in individuals who have SM. For example:

★ One student was so desperate to be noticed and have friends that she played tricks on her peers by moving their possessions between their school bags. When she was accused of stealing, her silence was taken as acquiescence.

★ Another student was afraid to use the school toilets because she dreaded running into a group of girls who had been teasing her. Her solution was to stop eating and drinking so that she could wait until she went home. Even though she was eating well every evening, staff members became far more concerned about her 'selective anorexia' than addressing her communication difficulties and the attitude of her peers.

★ A bright young man with a talent for languages started missing his German lessons and the teachers were convinced he wanted to drop this subject. It turned out that the last students to arrive at the German lesson always had to go into the next classroom to request a chair. Although this young person could answer factual questions and read aloud in class, he was as yet unable to initiate interactions or give lengthy explanations. By using the drawing in Figure 8.6 and changing the question 'Why don't you like German any more?' to 'What are you thinking when you say you don't want to do German?', he was able to complete the thought bubble. A chair was immediately reserved for him and he sailed through the rest of the course.

Of course, it is not just the children with SM who are stressed. Opportunities to combat stress through exercise, sports, yoga or massage, for example, should be a priority for *everyone* – staff members, families and the children themselves. This is about finding balance as well as recharging batteries. Everyone needs an all-absorbing hobby or out-of-school activity where, during that time at least, they can enjoy the moment and ignore their troubles.

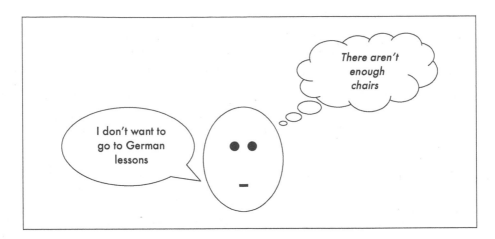

Figure 8.6: **What are you thinking?**

Two further reasons for inappropriate behaviour are the relief children feel when they are finally able to communicate, and the need to exercise some control over proceedings – control that most children gain through verbal expression. Children may become overexcited as they feel the burden of SM lifting. This may be regarded as natural exuberance and a degree of social immaturity, bearing in mind that they have missed out on such behaviour being checked in the past. It is not uncommon for the stronger personalities to express themselves non-verbally through cheekiness and deliberate game playing. In contrast with more general non-compliance, this behaviour is more evident with the people they cannot talk to freely and only occurs when they are feeling relaxed and 'safe'. Helene Cohen gives a moving and empathetic account of one such child's emerging self-confidence (in Sutton & Forrester, 2015).

Formulating an action plan

This chapter and the accompanying handouts have set out the rationale and guidance for ensuring that:

★ the child's anxiety is controlled and manageable

★ supportive environments are in place at home and in school

★ the child's fear of speaking is not strengthened or maintained.

The chapter concludes by considering the following online checklists to assist with identifying and implementing specific environmental modifications for individual children and young people, together with the personal action plan recommended at the beginning of this chapter.

a) Form 4 'Checklist of possible maintaining factors'

b) Form 10 'Reactions of family/friends/staff'

c) Form 12 'Environmental checklist for educational settings'

d) Form 13 'Environmental checklist for home setting'

Moving on to specific talking targets

There are several positive outcomes from ensuring that the home and school environments are as anxiety-free as possible. The child will:

★ be happy to go to school and separate from their parent

★ no longer stand isolated in the playground

Forms 12 and 13 list helpful targets to work *towards*; Forms 4 and 10 list potentially unhelpful behaviours that may need managing *differently*. Each maintaining factor identified on Form 4 is described in detail in Table 8.2 (page 134), which addresses specific maintaining factors and complements the general advice provided in this chapter and Chapter 9. It will also help practitioners and parents decide whether and why they need to be concerned.

It may not be possible, or necessary, to make all of the identified changes at once, so discussion is needed to agree the priorities (areas which are causing the child greatest distress), together with strategies, timescale and review date. Ideally, this will be done collaboratively at a meeting attended by parent(s) and staff members, but neither party should delay formulating and implementing an action plan while waiting for the other to come on board. Schools will probably prefer to use their existing additional needs documentation to record this plan. If not, they could use or adapt Form 14, 'Target sheet and action plan', which is also suitable for home use. There is a completed example of Form 14 on page 140.

Reviewing the action plan ... and sticking to it

Once agreed, we recommend that joint plans are reviewed every four to six weeks until all outstanding items on the checklists have been addressed. Personal plans can be reviewed and updated more often as each action point is achieved.

A word of warning: it may be easier to formulate a plan than stick to it, so regular reviews with mutual support and reminders are essential. The best-intentioned staff will be extremely busy; some people will be harder to influence than others; there will be new staff, and supply teachers to consider; and a strong lead will be necessary to ensure the plan is enforced. Professionals and specialists may be able to give telephone or email support between review dates to provide reassurance and quickly address any queries that arise. Remember, the child cannot enjoy school and make progress with their talking until all pressure is removed, however subtle that pressure may be, so time invested in getting it right at this stage will pay dividends.

Some parents may find the plan requires a complete turnaround in the way they handle their child's general avoidance behaviour; initially, the child may find this difficult and become more resistant. This is not easy for anyone, but please don't give up. Take a break to recharge batteries and find the strength to return to the plan the next day. Persistence will pay off and the child will, in turn, feel stronger and more secure with calm, consistent guidance.

Table 8.2: **Possible maintaining factors with alternative management strategies** ([N] = name of individual who has SM)

	Common responses to SM that may prevent or delay progress *(italics are the exceptions)*	How these behaviours could be maintaining SM	Alternative ways to manage SM as a backdrop to implementing an intervention programme
1	[N]'s anxiety about talking is ignored or dismissed	None is an issue on a one-off or very occasional basis but they should not be repeated with any frequency because they set [N] up to fail; make [N] feel extremely uncomfortable in the short-term; and lower [N]'s self-esteem in the longer term.	• Talk to [N] about SM (see 'the Pep Talk' on page 73). • Take [N]'s anxieties seriously and reassure [N] you will find a way through them together. • Talk to [N] in private if the presence of other people makes talking difficult. • Agree an alternative means of communication for people outside [N]'s comfort zone.
2	Adults or peers ask [N] questions and wait (unsuccessfully) for an answer		• If [N] cannot respond, keep [N] involved in conversation using commentary-style talk, rather than questions
3	[N] is given their turn to talk (eg at circle time or registration) but remains silent	In the absence of an explanation, [N] will find it increasingly difficult and scary to cope with their anxiety and the physical sensations it creates.	(page 122) and phrase occasional questions so that [N] can nod or shake their head in response. • Build rapport by focusing on enjoyable activities, rather than conversation.
4	[N] is asked why they don't talk, if they can talk or when they will talk (by adults or peers)		• Tell [N] you will not ask them a question in class unless they volunteer.
5	[N] is told 'I can't help you unless you speak'		• Ensure peers understand that the best way to help is to be friendly and *not* press [N] to talk.
6	[N] is encouraged, requested, pressed or offered rewards to speak, but without success	Expecting [N] to do something they cannot do is unfair and will raise [N]'s anxiety, making talking even harder. We need to watch out for situations which put pressure (however subtly) on [N] to speak, as disappointment or disapproval will be implied if [N] does not succeed.	• Wait for [N] to volunteer information about their progress. • Agree an intervention programme with realistic targets and strategies to ensure success. • Acknowledge [N]'s strengths and contributions; focus on what [N] *can* do, not what [N] can't do.
7	[N] is asked if they have succeeded in talking to others or what progress they are making with talking *(It is good to review progress together as part of a planned intervention programme; otherwise, questions like this make [N] feel judged and hurried)*		
8	Talking targets or expectations have been set for [N] (eg in a school report) but not achieved	Comparing [N] with people who are 'worse off' usually makes [N] feel criticised, weak or guilty, rather than more positive.	
9	[N] has been criticised, penalised, ignored, threatened or ridiculed for *not* talking	Any pressure to talk will raise [N]'s anxiety. These methods add humiliation, indignation, misery, fear or shame. [N] is even more anxious to avoid situations where they are expected to talk, in case the same thing happens again.	• Ensure this does not happen again. • Ensure that [N] receives an apology, either directly or indirectly. • Recognise that [N] is unable to speak in certain situations, so sanctions constitute discrimination. • Ensure that [N] is valued and included, whether they talk or not.

10	[N] hears adult(s) expressing concerns about their lack of speech *(It may very occasionally be necessary to talk directly to older disaffected students about the risks of not engaging with intervention, to secure their participation for a trial period, but most children need no additional motivation.)*	This will raise [N]'s anxiety about their future and the problems they are causing other people, creating extra pressure to speak.	• Ensure that any concerns or disagreements are discussed out of [N]'s hearing. • Reassure [N] that they will find it easier to talk in time. • Be positive about [N]'s achievements, efforts and potential. • Offer [N] solutions, rather than focus on their problems.
11	[N] talks when people insist, but not comfortably. *(Insisting on speech is not a problem if [N] talks freely at normal volume with relaxed facial expression and posture, or willingly as part of a small-steps programme to reduce anxiety around talking.)*	Sometimes [N]'s fear of talking is outweighed by fear of the consequences of *not* talking. If [N] speaks under duress to avoid eg disapproval, the unpleasant experience will strengthen [N]'s negative associations with talking.	• Don't force children to speak when they clearly feel uncomfortable. • Provide opportunities. rather than demands. to speak using commentary-style talk (see page 122). • Offer choices, both verbal and non-verbal, so that [N] has a say in how they contribute to activities.
12	[N]'s speech has been corrected, laughed at or criticised	[N] is likely to be distressed by incidents like these. They may be maintaining factors or initial triggers for SM and need to be discussed with [N] to ascertain their impact on [N]'s reluctance to speak, with reassurance and demonstration that any fears are unfounded.	• Ensure that any teasing/bullying/criticism stops and [N] is aware of the steps taken. • Ensure that different accents and cultures are valued and [N] is aware of this.
13	[N] or [N]'s peers have been told off too harshly for talking or making a noise *(No special rules should be made for N, and it is right to ask [N] not to talk if that is what is expected of the whole class. However, it is important to bear in mind [N]'s particular sensitivity to criticism and use a light touch, eg 'N, it's lovely to chat to our friends, but this is not the right time. Everyone can talk at lunch-time, OK?')*		• Ensure that [N] hears good examples of speech pronunciation, rather than being corrected and asked to repeat. • Ensure that [N] understands the reasons for reprimand(s) and knows adult(s) involved are no longer displeased. • Ask for an apology if [N] was told off inappropriately. • Let all of the children know the good times to talk and be noisy; lead by example to encourage exuberance at appropriate times. • Correct children's behaviour quietly and calmly.
14	Parents or siblings are not always comfortable speaking so they model silence (eg prefer other family members to do the talking; do not answer phone; avoid social situations)	If [N] sees that other people avoid or show dislike of speaking, [N]'s negative associations with communication will increase and they will be less likely to talk themselves.	• Be aware how easy it is to pass anxieties on to [N]; work as a family to keep communication a positive experience and make a game out of new challenges. • Set a good example by sharing personal anxieties, asking [N]'s advice, then setting and meeting a target. • It helps if immigrant parents learn the new language with [N], having fun and being relaxed about making mistakes in the process.

(Continued)

Table 8.2: *Continued* ([N] = name of individual who has SM)

	Common responses to SM that may prevent or delay progress *(italics are the exceptions)*	How these behaviours could be maintaining SM	Alternative ways to manage SM as a backdrop to implementing an intervention programme
15	Attention is drawn to the fact that [N] has spoken or made a sound *(It is good to praise [N] in the context of a small-steps programme you have set up together, or in private if [N] speaks openly about their SM. Be guided by [N]'s reaction: preschool children generally accept praise more than older, more anxious children.)*	Drawing attention to something that [N] feels very unsure about, especially in public, makes [N] feel uncomfortable and *less* likely to do it again. Praise can often backfire, as [N] senses how keen other people are for them to improve and worries that even more is expected now.	• Respond to what [N] *says* or *conveys*, rather than the fact that [N] spoke or made a sound. • Ensure that there is not a big reaction when [N] speaks. Tell peers that [N] *will* speak one day and, when this happens, they must carry on as if [N] has always spoken. • Give praise only in the context of agreed targets and in private. For example, put 'Well Done!' stickers in a book rather than on the child's jumper.
16	[N] has denied, or tried to cover up, speaking	[N] is terrified that if people outside their comfort zone know that [N] can talk, there will be increased expectation and pressure on [N] to talk to them. [N]'s priority is to keep their talking and non-talking worlds separate, rather than to talk more. Sharing recordings without permission also breaks trust and makes it difficult for [N] to believe future assurances.	• Ensure that everyone involved is on board and demonstrates to [N] that they understand SM. • Reassure [N] that people outside their comfort zone will be pleased but unsurprised to know that [N] can speak to others and will not expect [N] to speak to them until [N] is ready. • Explain to [N] why a recording was shared without their permission; apologise and assure [N] that it won't happen again. • Reassure [N] that any recordings are confidential and will either be deleted or only shared with their agreement.
17	[N] knows an audio or video recording of them talking was shared without their consent		
18	[N] does not want their sibling or twin to speak or vice versa	Trying to keep someone else quiet reflects your own fear of talking. Maintaining strength in numbers makes it easier to stay quiet and avoid anxiety.	• Talk to [N] and the sibling or twin at the same time about SM (see 'the Pep Talk' on page 73). • Provide reassurance that when one person speaks, there will be no pressure for the other to copy. No one expects them to go any faster than they can manage. • Get the children to work together on the intervention programme, as this usually results in the more anxious child following the less anxious child's lead.
19	[N] uses gesture, whispering, writing or pictures to communicate at school with no signs of progressing to speech with anyone *(Alternative modes of communication are necessary as part of a planned intervention to overcome SM.)*	[N] will not be anxious if their inability to talk is accepted and other forms of communication are made available. But the longer [N] avoids the need to speak, the more [N] will dread it.	• Help [N] work towards talking with a designated keyworker while using other forms of communication in the classroom. • Accept, but do not actively encourage, whispering by making it a target because it can be difficult to break the habit (see page 149).

20	Different arrangements are made so that [N] does not become stressed. *(It is good to make activities less stressful, so that [N] can participate with no or little anxiety, eg: a change of seating position from front to back of class, so [N] does not feel watched by others; a change of partner to a more sympathetic friend; arriving early to settle before the others arrive; doing only part of an activity; listening to music during exam.* *Always help [N] to work towards, rather than avoid, a challenge.)*	If [N] opts out of activities and social situations completely, or wants other people to stop doing things purely for their own reassurance, [N] will learn that the only way to cope with their anxiety is to eliminate it. [N] will become less and less resilient to even low levels of anxiety which are normal and to be expected. The danger is that [N] will become increasingly afraid of facing new challenges and make increasing demands to avoid anxiety.	• Acknowledge [N]'s anxiety and make activities more manageable, helping [N] to face their fear in tiny steps. • Aim for *participation* rather than talking. Talking will come as [N]'s anxiety decreases. • Help [N] to understand that a degree of anxiety is normal and goes away with familiarity and practice. • Acknowledge, commend and celebrate [N]'s courage in attempting new activities. • Recognise when [N]'s requests are based on 'What if?' thoughts (things that are highly unlikely to happen). Acknowledge [N]'s anxiety but stick to the plan; write it down ('This is what's going to happen') and help [N] ride through their anxiety in order to discover that their fear was unfounded. High fives all round!
21	Fun activities, treats or comfort (rather than reassurance) are provided when [N] pulls away from, or has been excused from, an activity *(It is good to have fun and provide enjoyable activities as a **distraction** for anxiety, to help [N] face their fear.* *If an activity was badly managed and [N] suffered unnecessary distress, it is right to **apologise** to [N] and assure them that steps will be taken to ensure this doesn't happen again.)*	When [N] receives hugs, extra attention or treats *instead of* participating in an activity, [N] gets the message that they were *right* to be afraid and pull away from a threatening experience. This strengthens their fear and increases the chances that [N] will opt out again.	• Try to follow desirable behaviour (eg being brave, kind, obedient, helpful) with hugs and attention, rather than undesirable behaviour (eg opting out). • Ensure that there is nothing for [N] to fear in the activity, other than unfamiliarity or uncertainty. There must be a good understanding of [N]'s SM and no pressure to speak. • If the activity is safe for [N], provide reassurance and coping strategies when [N] wants to opt out: eg suggest that they just watch for a while; explain that this is what 'worry' feels like when we get used to something new. Afterwards, give [N] a hug, extra attention or a treat for *staying or having a go.* • When [N] is excused from an activity that will be reattempted another time, provide an 'ordinary' rather than 'exciting' alternative. Don't oversympathise: calmly acknowledge that they found it scary and assure [N] this won't always be the case. If appropriate, reassure [N] that steps will be taken to make it easier next time and listen to [N]'s ideas.

(Continued)

Table 8.2: *Continued* ([N] = name of individual who has SM)

	Common responses to SM that may prevent or delay progress *(italics are the exceptions)*	How these behaviours could be maintaining SM	Alternative ways to manage SM as a backdrop to implementing an intervention programme
22	[N] uses gesture, whispering, writing or pictures to communicate with people they talk to comfortably at other times *(This is completely understandable when people outside [N]'s comfort zone are nearby.)*	If alternative forms of communication are successful, or gain more attention than talking, even when no one outside [N]'s comfort zone is listening, there is a risk that non-talking will become [N]'s default mode.	• It is helpful for people in [N]'s comfort zone to avoid responding to forms of communication other than talking when alone with N. If [N] uses gesture or whispers, etc, gently remind [N] that it's OK to talk now. • Avoid guessing what [N] wants (see page 172). • Ensure that talking is a relaxed, positive experience within the family.
23	[N] hears adults or peers warn others that [N] will not, cannot or may be unable to talk	This makes it very difficult for [N] to talk, even when relaxed, as [N] believes no one expects it. Talking would now draw unwanted attention to [N]. Once assigned a mute role, [N] is less likely to believe they can change.	• Ensure that [N] sees themselves as someone who hasn't spoken *yet*, rather than as a non-speaker. • Tell [N] that people know they will talk at some point and will not be surprised when it happens. • Explain to peers and adults that [N] will speak when ready. Until then, avoid asking [N] direct questions and chat to [N] without expecting an answer. • Advise strangers to let [N] talk in their own time.
24	Adults, siblings, friends or peers automatically speak for [N]	This can become a habit which reinforces [N]'s self-image as a non-speaker and denies [N] the opportunity to speak when they feel ready. 'Rescuing' the child by answering for them is a form of avoidance and the longer something is avoided, the harder it gets.	• **Parents** – See Handout 12 (online) which provides alternative strategies to rescuing. – Prepare doctors, opticians, etc in advance, as the child may need to respond by writing things down, pointing to a picture or answering the *parent*. – Ask older children how they would like to handle particular scenarios so that they can either prepare other people in advance or have a back-up plan (eg [N] could present a brief written explanation of SM). • **Teachers** – Ask the children *not* to answer for each other when asked a question and explain to [N] that you are happy for them to communicate non-verbally until they feel better about talking. – Accept and encourage messages through peers and expect [N] to confirm non-verbally that you have understood their peers correctly. – Encourage [N] to talk to their peers and give them space to do this until you can ask [N] questions through their pe ers (see 'Talking through other children' on page 182).

#	Concern	Explanation	Recommendations
25	There is little need for [N] to speak at home	It is vital to have experience of two-way conversation and humorous banter in at least one setting. Otherwise, [N] may find talking and general interaction more and more alien and become increasingly resigned to their non-speaking role.	• Beware of [N] spending increasingly more time alone, • Set up personal computers in a communal area, • Arrange for [N] to spend regular private time with the family members and friends they speak to freely, • Ensure that [N]'s voice is heard and that siblings do not automatically speak for [N].
26	[N] is becoming more withdrawn and talking less within their usual comfort zone (eg at home) *(This is normal behaviour for teenagers who are engaging in healthy social activity outside the home.)*	If [N] is feeling ignored or isolated they will be generally anxious or distressed and unable to concentrate on new learning or challenges to the best of their ability. If [N] is gradually withdrawing, it could be a sign that [N]'s SM is being handled inappropriately in one or more settings. Without help to put this right, [N] will feel increasingly pressurised and only be able to cope by opting out. There is a danger that [N] will feel there is no point discussing SM and become increasingly resistant to offers of intervention.	• Get involved in [N]'s interests and ask [N] to teach you new skills – show that you genuinely need [N]'s help. • Explain to peers and adults in private that [N] finds it hard to speak; is not being rude; needs their support. • No one should take [N]'s silence personally, make negative comments or push [N] to speak. • Lead by example to encourage inclusion: make a point of greeting and involving [N] in activities, playing on [N]'s strengths.
27	People have stopped speaking to [N]	The longer [N] lives with SM and the above maintaining factors, the more the cycle of fear and avoidance is reinforced and strengthened. Repeated unsuccessful attempts to intervene convince the young person nothing can be done, making it harder to engage them in intervention.	• Make time every day for shared meals and activities, including [N]'s friends when possible. • Involve [N] in using commentary-style talk (see page 122) if [N] is clearly uncomfortable with direct questions. • Reassure [N] that SM is temporary and focus on the essential foundation for speech – spending enjoyable time together on a regular basis through laughter, games, shared projects, physical challenges, favourite films, etc. Just 'hanging out' is vastly underrated!
28	It feels like there is no coordinated plan in place to help [N] overcome their fear of speaking		• Find out if anything has upset [N] in another setting and, if so, ensure this is addressed. • Ensure a consistent approach to managing SM across all settings. • Help parents and staff to change their approach where indicated, being mindful that they may feel hurt and criticised, having done so much to support [N]. They will also benefit from support and reassurance.

Form 14 TARGET SHEET AND ACTION PLAN (Completed example from initial planning meeting)

Name: _Shona Taylor_   Age: _8y 5m_   Planning meeting held on: _24.9.15_   at: _St. Ursula's School_

Desired long-term outcome(s): _"I want to have a good time at school and have friends to play with. I want my teacher to be pleased with me"_

What is happening now/ current situation	What we would like to see happening	Strategies needed to achieve this objective	Person(s) responsible for this action	Date to be achieved by
Shona looks anxious for much of the school day and is becoming increasingly resistant to going to school. Tearful in mornings and says she doesn't feel well.	For Shona to go to school happily, knowing everyone understands that she is not being naughty or difficult, and to appear relaxed at school.	Staff and parents will talk to Shona individually, going through points in Handout 1 (Pep Talk). SENCo to prepare a short talk for whole school staff meeting using Handouts 6 and 10a	Mr Blake (teacher), Miss Cook (teaching assistant) and parents. Mrs Piper (SENCo). All staff to read and follow advice.	9.10.15 9.10.15 9.10.15 onwards
Shona wet herself last term and is now afraid to drink until she gets home.	Shona may use the toilet without asking, to avoid accidents. She will resume normal drinking pattern.	TA will see Shona 3 x 10 mins a week to improve non-verbal commun and will explain the new toilet rule to Shona. Consider a toilet sign-out system for whole class, implement if practical and complete environmental checklist.	Miss Cook Mr Blake	2.11.15 2.11.15
Shona's Mum answers questions for Shona, to save her embarrassment.	Shona will start to answer questions with her Mum's support (mainly unexpected Qs from strangers).	Laura to follow WAIT – REPEAT/ REPHRASE – WAIT – MOVE ON sequence from Handout 12, and share experiences with other parents in local support group.	Laura Taylor SLT to notify Laura of date of next parent meeting	2.11.15 28.9.15
Certain relatives put a lot of pressure on Shona to talk and she no longer wants to visit them.	Relatives will recognise that pressure is not helping and be supportive so that Shona enjoys her visits again.	Laura to give relatives Handouts 2 and 5 and ask them not to ask Shona Qs (discuss commentary-style talk and being positive). First step is for Shona to talk comfortably in front of them, and no one must comment or act surprised when she does.	Laura Taylor	by October half-term (family party on 31.10.15)

The above actions were agreed by: _Parents, SENCo, class teacher and SLT_   Review date: _2.11.15_

★ participate comfortably in educational and social activities, knowing that they will not be pressurised to speak

★ move easily, rather than appearing to be stiff or frozen

★ transition easily from one activity to another

★ react to humour with mobile facial features rather than a fixed, frozen smile

★ be comfortable to communicate with relatives or staff either verbally, non-verbally or in writing

★ begin to talk to their parents or other talking partners in front of people who do not usually hear their voice.

The child will be ready to work on a talking programme when they:

★ seem comfortable in the target setting, as described above

★ have built rapport with at least one adult

★ have been reassured by the adult that it is fine if they talk and fine if they don't and (for children aged five years and above) that things will move at their pace.

Online resources for Chapter 8

The handouts, forms and appendices for this chapter are available at www.routledge.com/cw/speechmark for you to access, print and copy.

CHAPTER 9

FACING FEARS AT HOME AND IN THE COMMUNITY

Introduction

We believe that, for every child who has selective mutism (SM), helping them to face and overcome their fears about talking starts in the home environment. For most children, home is their comfort zone; the one place where they can be themselves and talk freely. This is precisely why parents are in the best position to support their child's generalisation of speech to other environments. For parents of children who are home-schooled, or whose children are more comfortable speaking in school than in the community, it may be a relief to find advice that does not revolve around the school setting. But we have found that even children whose main difficulty is talking at school do better when their school programme runs alongside home-based interventions.

★ This chapter therefore focuses on:

★ why parents are best placed to ease children out of their comfort zone

★ reducing avoidance of talking

★ strategies to help children talk to friends, family and practitioners

★ fostering friendships and socialisation

★ talking in public places and to strangers in community settings

★ additional considerations for adolescents

★ progressive mutism.

 In this chapter, 'parent' refers to not only parents and guardians but also any carer or professional who the child speaks to freely. We appreciate that there are some parents with whom the child is more withdrawn, and suggest that they are eased into the child's comfort zone in the same way as other adults.

You may think the handouts accompanying this chapter are rather prescriptive. This is not the intention; everyone has their own way of judging a child's anxiety level and readiness to move through the various stages. But the advice is very detailed for a good reason. Parents often say to us, 'What's your secret?'; 'He'll speak to you, but he won't speak to anyone else'; 'You've got the magic touch!'

We want to assure you that it is *not* magic! We follow the same procedure every time we meet children with their parents but in a relaxed way, so that it seems to come naturally.

We hope that, by taking you through our model of confident talking, and explaining exactly what we are doing, it will no longer be a secret. You will then have effective tools to share with other people. Of course, we are not the parents, so lack the emotional attachment which can make some of the strategies feel counterintuitive and therefore a little harsh. Please be reassured that, although our strategies may occasionally *surprise* children, they do not cause them distress. We know that they can be used by parents and professionals alike to good effect and, with practice, they will soon feel natural and comfortable.

Most of the strategies are very informal and introduced into everyday situations when other people are present and conversation feels difficult. Table 7.1 in Chapter 7 (page 108) is an overview of the progressions of confident talking which it may help to refer to while you read this chapter. It is also available online as Handout D2 in Appendix D.

Placing the child's comfort zone at the centre of intervention

First, consider again Binky, whose speaking habits are summarised in Chapter 4. Binky's parents reported that their six year old was a lively, chatty, fun-loving girl at home. The only concern they voiced initially was that she was not speaking at school. The four quadrants of the model of confident talking help to show the bigger picture (see Figure 9.1 opposite).

Binky had great difficulty speaking at school where her talking was limited to conversations with her mother and her best friend, Sara, when she perceived that no one else was listening. For example, they might talk next to the coat hooks if they arrived before anyone else, or at the edge of the playground. However, there were difficulties at home as well. Binky shouted and giggled inside the house and in the back garden, which had a high fence. But in the more open front garden, and on the pavement outside her house, she was much more restrained and aware of passersby. She spoke quietly and only nodded or shook her head to her mother when neighbours appeared. So it seemed there was a broader issue with talking in public.

Binky's parents confirmed that she would pull their heads down to whisper to them as soon as she noticed strangers standing close by in places such as shops or the park. She did this at home as well, when they had visitors. Her parents had put this down to shyness but they agreed that she was defintely not shy with people in her comfort zone.

On reflection, Binky's parents realised that, because she was at least speaking in other places, albeit by whispering, they had focused on school as being the main problem. But, in fact, her difficulties had been evident *before* she went to school. Her paternal grandparents, whom she saw infrequently because they lived abroad, had never heard her voice. Binky's parents agreed that if Binky could become more comfortable speaking to them in public, and to visitors at home, she would find talking in other settings much less daunting. Furthermore, only her parents could provide a bridge between the home setting and other environments and, although help was available to support Binky at school, this would not be extended to her outside activities such as ballet and Brownies.

Range of people

Binky only speaks to family members and her best friend Sara. Paternal grandparents have never heard her voice.

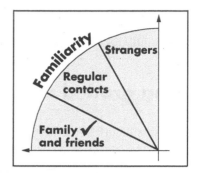

Talking in public places

Binky speaks very quietly in public and gestures or whispers in her parents' ear as soon as she knows she can be heard by anyone outside her comfort zone.

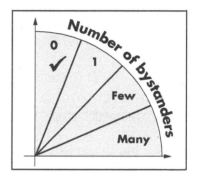

Group participation

Binky has plenty to say at family meals when only people in her comfort zone are present. No other talking in groups but Binky performs at larger gatherings in other ways (eg dancing; playing the recorder).

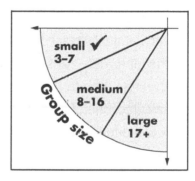

Social functioning

Binky interacts normally with her family and best friend, making comments, asking and answering questions, directing other people and negotiating. In school she initiates requests occasionally through Sara but usually requires adult prompting to make her needs known (responds non-verbally).

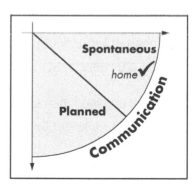

Figure 9.1: **Using the model of confident talking to consider speaking habits**

To summarise, by building support strategies for Binky into their everyday routines, Binky's parents could increase her tolerance to sharing her voice in a wide range of public places. This would, in turn, have a positive impact on her progress at school where Binky disliked being overheard.

Using graded exposure to help children overcome their fears

Graded exposure is the recommended approach for managing fears and phobias. By facing, rather than avoiding their fear, both adults and children can learn to overcome anxiety. The best results are obtained when the individual is exposed to *actual* rather than imaginary situations, while keeping their anxiety under control. In practice, this means:

★ finding a starting point with no, or minimal, anxiety

★ taking *very small* steps towards facing the feared object or event

★ repeating each step several times, in quick succession, until anxiety is no longer experienced.

In effect, the experience of achievement replaces the old, automatic fear reaction as a new positive memory is formed.

Helping children gradually face their fear of talking

Parents are ideally placed to carry out graded exposure. The child sees them every day in the settings that trigger anxiety. Most importantly, the child associates parents with positive feelings, rather than anxiety. From this starting point of low anxiety, parents are in a unique position to help children gradually face their fear of talking in ways that outsiders cannot. Bearing in mind that a large component of SM is the fear of being *overheard* (because this might lead to an expectation to talk), parents can help as follows.

1   Having educated adult friends and relatives about SM and the steps to take to build rapport with their child, parents can provide a bridge for their child between talking to them and crossing into the uncharted territory of talking to other adults for the first time. Similarly, parents can provide a bridge to facilitate conversation between the child and their friends.

2   Having engaged their child in conversation, parents can gradually move nearer to other people, helping the child to tolerate their voice being heard.

3   Having engaged their child in conversation, parents can help the child to tolerate the gradual approach of other people who will hear their voice.

4   By providing the comfort of positive associations and a safety net (the skills to move on conversations smoothly without embarrassment), parents can end their child's reliance on the avoidance strategies that replace talking and quickly become a habit. As part of this process, parents provide the support that children need to take advantage of daily opportunities to talk.

Points 1–3 are covered later in this chapter but, first, point 4 is considered – avoidance strategies.

Removing the need and opportunity for avoidance strategies

Most people cope with their phobias through avoidance because it removes all anxiety. Children who have SM are no different and will, of course, do all they can to avoid the need to speak in certain situations. Avoidance strategies such as whispering, gesturing and relying on other people to do the talking will certainly keep their anxiety under control. But unfortunately, as discussed in Chapter 2, avoidance *strengthens fear* and gives the child no opportunity to gain confidence through practice. It is the automatic response of good parenting to act as a cushion between a young, vulnerable child and an intrusive, or seemingly hostile, outside world, so it seems right to support the avoidance of talking.

However, as they develop, young children need to be weaned off this approach, so that they learn to fend for themselves and become independent. Naturally, no one wants children to feel unduly anxious, so the key to success is to adopt the stance of 'avoidance is not an option' while finding other ways to protect them from escalating anxiety.

Minimise anxiety

Following the advice in Chapter 8, to identify and address any maintaining factors, will go a long way towards reducing the child's overall anxiety. But when it comes to removing the need for avoidance strategies, the most important thing is to reassure the child that no one will mind if they *don't* talk. This is not the same as saying they don't *need* to talk! On the contrary, assure them that they will find it easy to talk in time. Meanwhile, it's not a big deal if they don't always manage it. Avoidance strategies will soon lose their value if everyone stays calm when the child doesn't speak, and parents smoothly move on the conversation without embarrassment, as described in the handouts for this chapter.

Lower expectations

The handouts also provide strategies to assist children so they can respond by nodding or shaking their head or saying just one word. By lowering adults' expectations, children are more likely to succeed and work up to a response of several words over the next few encounters. Build on this by telling the children that people will be very pleased with whatever they can manage: for example, a gesture such as a wave, smile or thumbs-up; a single word rather than a long answer; or a handwritten 'Thank you' in exchange for a present. Add the phrase 'just until you feel better about talking', to emphasise the temporary nature of their anxiety. It is also a good idea to practise a few simple answers in advance: for example, what they might say if someone asks them how school is ('OK'!) or which lesson they like best.

Children don't need rescuing

As explained in Chapter 8, it is important to ensure that children who have SM aren't repeatedly asked questions, especially by people who are keen to build rapport with them. But questions can't be ruled out completely and stepping in to answer for the child conveys the message that it is *essential to respond*. This completely contradicts the more important message that no one will mind if the child doesn't manage to talk. See Handout 12, 'Do I answer for my child?' (online) for what to do when someone asks your child a question. This is an excellent starting point for parents and it complements school intervention programmes well. The procedure starts by waiting five seconds, to give the child a chance to answer, followed by a set routine to move things on without answering the question for them. The only exception to this advice is when someone asks your child an unfair question which they cannot possibly answer: for example, 'You're very quiet, aren't you?' or 'So when are you going to talk to me?' In this event, move things on without waiting five seconds, as explained in Handout 4, 'What to say when …'.

> The five-second rule worked really well with my daughter, especially in public places when strangers approached her. She always replied – usually by the time I got to three!

Managing parental anxiety

You may experience a sense of panic as soon as your child is asked a question and, initially, have difficulty leaving that all-important five-second gap for your child to respond. Please be reassured that many other parents felt exactly the same way but found that this method worked and that it quickly got easier for them. Children and young people are often more fazed by their parent's anxious expression than by the question which they may or may not be able to answer. They will not become unduly anxious if their parent looks calm and relaxed. They will also benefit from the faith that parents show in them by *not* answering; and will be well supported by the alternative strategies that are recommended.

> The counting in my head really helped to distract my thoughts from waiting for Caitlin to reply. To make sure that I waited a full five seconds, I said 'seventy-one, seventy-two, seventy-three !'

In the handouts you will frequently see the reminder to 'smile'. There is a science behind this! The simple act of smiling – even a fake smile – sends a message to the brain that you are happy, which triggers the release of the feel-good hormone endorphin. Both you and your child feel better! So, if your anxiety rises at the thought of not answering, try to relax your shoulders, breathe slowly and *smile*, while you say one of the following sentences to yourself:

★ 'My child needs me to do this; they don't want to become dependent on me.'

★ 'This is worse for me than my child – they will survive a few seconds …'

★ 'We're working through this together; just as I helped him to be brave when he didn't want to …' (Think about a time when your child was afraid to do something but, with your support, they had a go and succeeded.)

Reducing reliance on gesture

Gesture is a valid form of communication which everyone uses and should, of course, be available to children. But the use of gesture should follow basic conversational principles – it is used as a quick, simple and clear alternative to speech. Imagine that your mouth is full of food and someone asks you a question. You would think nothing of nodding or shaking your head, or pointing to what the person wanted. But if this person needed a more detailed answer, or you wanted to ask them something, you would swallow the food and then speak to them. It is not normal, acceptable communication to expect the other person to guess what you were trying to say while you gestured. And it certainly would not be acceptable for you to get annoyed when they didn't do a very good job of it.

It's just the same with children who have SM. Of course, they can give a thumbs-up to show they feel OK, spread their fingers to indicate 'five', or nod or shake their head for 'yes' or 'no' when speaking is difficult. It's fine for them to point when offered a choice of items. These are very useful strategies to facilitate communication or when a quick response is needed. But it's not helpful to encourage an unnatural reliance on more complex gesture or the expectation that you will guess or interpret that gesture. If the child can't speak to you because other people are too close, move to where they *can* speak. Maybe the child needs to wait a moment while you finish what you're doing first, but that's OK. It's important to maintain talking as their primary mode of communication.

Reducing reliance on whispering

The situation is very similar with whispering. There are certain occasions when whispering is perfectly acceptable. But it's not something we generally encourage the rest of the time; it can appear rude and · socially unacceptable. However, there is also a physiological reason for ensuring that children who have SM do not get into the habit of whispering. Voice production requires the vocal cords to *vibrate* as air passes between them from the lungs. The voice will be very quiet if only a trickle of air passes through. But with a deeper breath, and a greater quantity of air, the voice will increase in volume. Whispering may be just as loud as a very quiet voice but it has one significant difference. When whispering, *the vocal cords do not move*. They are held taut in a frozen position, so that when air passes between them from the lungs, no sound is produced. For children who have SM, relaxing the vocal cords so that they vibrate is the final and hardest step required to produce a voice, so it's important to avoid the frozen position becoming a habitual 'default mode'.

Whispering is accepted, but not actively encouraged
Clearly *any* form of communication can be a huge step forward for a child who has SM, and this includes whispering. Whispering is acceptable in social situations when people outside the child's comfort zone are present, *as long as the whisper is 'public'* (not a private whisper in someone's ear). However, we recommend against actively *encouraging* whispering by lowering your head to invite a child to whisper in your ear, and to resist being pulled into this position. Handouts 13 and 14 provide alternative strategies. Essentially, move just far enough away from bystanders to a place where your child can talk to you face-to-face, even if this means asking the child to wait a moment until you are free to give them your undivided attention. Please note that none of this applies in situations where whispering is advisable: for example, during a concert or church service or in the cinema!

The model of confident talking: range of people

Children will find it easier to speak to family, friends and regular contacts outside their comfort zone when the stages of one-to-one interaction are observed, as shown in Table 9.1 (page 151). For example, children need to feel comfortable and relaxed and able to communicate *non-verbally* (stage 3)

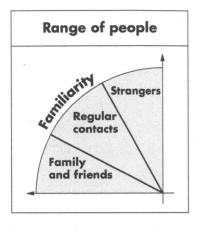

Range of people

Familiarity

Strangers

Regular contacts

Family and friends

before they will be able to talk freely. It is rather different with strangers with whom there is neither time nor need to build rapport. This is why young children generally find it easier to talk to people they know well. In contrast, most older children feel freed by the lack of personal history and find it easier to talk to strangers (see FAQ 18 in Chapter 1). This may well include practitioners (any therapist, psychologist or clinician working directly or indirectly with the child and family) whom they meet on a one-to-one basis.

For simplicity, we will refer to people the child has never spoken to before as 'new' people. The child may know them well but they are yet to enter the child's comfort zone.

Talking to friends, family and regular contacts

You could start by making a list of the most appropriate people to target and adding them to the top row of Progress chart 1 (online). This will remind you of the stages to guide each person through and let you see how far your child has come with each individual. However, this chart should not be shared with your child; they will see all of the challenges that lie ahead, rather than focusing on their achievements.

After the 'Pep -Talk' and maintaining factors have been addressed, there are several ways of helping children talk to new people:

(a) slowly does it …

(b) set up a talking bridge

(c) the Triangle Tactic

(d) the Sliding-in Technique

(e) desensitisation using voice recordings

(f) using a telephone or a webcam

(g) warm-up routines.

All of these methods are based on the stages outlined in Table 9.1, which shows how to progress from building rapport with a child, to facilitating speech. Figure 9.2 (page 153) is a handy reminder of the question sequence that is used during these stages, both for the new person being introduced to the child and for the parent who is trying to engage the child when another person is present. The most important point is to move *at the child's pace*, waiting until the child responds at one stage before proceeding to the next.

As well as the stages of direct interaction, Table 9.1 includes a bridging stage where the child talks to a parent in the new person's presence (see Figure 9.3 on page 153). This is optional – after all, parents are

Table 9.1: **Confident talking – establishing speech on a one-to-one basis through shared activity in natural settings**

Stage	Child's presentation	Target behaviours
0–3 (see Table 8.1, page 124)	Comfortable in adult's presence and beginning to communicate non-verbally	For the **adult** to: • talk mainly to parent, friend or sibling (if present) until child appears relaxed[1] • engage the child through shared activity rather than conversation • use commentary style[1] when talking to the child • ask occasional questions which can be answered by nodding, shaking the head or pointing, eg 'Is this the one you got for Christmas?'; 'So how do we turn it on – where's the switch?' For the **child** to: • sense that the adult is supportive and will not expect them to talk before they are ready • respond with facial expression and gesture (eg nods head).
Talking bridge[2, 3]	Tolerates voice being heard	For the **parent** to: • facilitate speech in the adult's presence by asking the child 'X or Y?' questions, eg 'Are the others still upstairs or outside?' • gradually include the adult, eg 'Shall we offer Aunty Pam one of your buns? Why don't you choose one for her?' For the **adult** to make this easier for the child by: • not watching the child closely • appearing to be occupied with other things • not reacting when the child talks to parent, friend or sibling. For the **child** to talk to their parent, friend or sibling in the adult's presence (voice is audible rather than whispered)[3]
4[2]	Talks to adult through parent, friend or sibling *in the adult's presence*	For the **adult** to ask occasional questions through the parent, eg 'Has Rory ever been to the zoo?'; 'This is delicious, can you ask Tilly what she put in the filling?' For the **parent** to: • repeat or rephrase the question and feed back the answer to the adult, eg 'Didn't you go to the zoo with your class? (Rory nods.) I thought so! Yes, Rory went last year' • continue to facilitate speech by asking the child 'X or Y?' questions, eg 'Was it Howlett's or Wildwood?' • redirect any questions initiated by the child, eg 'Rory wonders would you like to see his new pet?' For the **child** to answer a question repeated by the parent, friend or sibling or ask parent to convey a message to an adult, eg 'Does Aunty Pam want to see Fluffy?'
5	Uses voice with adult[4]	As the child relaxes further and becomes more involved in the shared activity, they respond directly to the adult's comments and jokes by laughing, or making sounds in the throat (often behind closed lips), to communicate surprise, disagreement, consent, etc.

(Continued)

Table 9.1: *Continued*

Stage	Child's presentation	Target behaviours
6	Uses single words to communicate with adult	For the **adult** to: • make deliberate mistakes, eg 'We start with four cards each' to provide the opportunity for the child to correct them, eg 'Seven!' • ask the child an occasional 'X or Y?' question about a shared activity, eg 'Is Fluffy a boy or girl?' If there is no response after five seconds, resume commentary-style talk[1] and move on, eg 'Maybe I can work it out if I have a good look!' • move on to factual questions once the child is responding easily to 'X or Y?' questions, eg 'How old is Fluffy?' (Questions starting Who/What/Which/How many/How old? are good for single-word answers.) • ask questions that show genuine interest or a need for information, rather than questions that test the child's knowledge. For the **child** to answer the adult using a single word.
7	Uses sentences to communicate with adult	For the **adult** to: • continue to ask occasional questions, wait five seconds and move on if there is no response (comments must outweigh questions) • give the child opportunities to make spontaneous comments by allowing five-second pauses after some comments, eg 'I can't make this fit'. Child: 'It doesn't go there!' For the **child** to: • respond to the adult's questions with a phrase or sentence • use sentences in a structured game[5] with the adult • begin to make spontaneous comments. For the **parent** (if present) to move away to a different activity or room, so the child does not become reliant on their involvement.

Notes

1 See page 122, Chapter 8.

2 These stages are only possible if someone the child talks to easily is present, such as a parent, friend or sibling. They can be bypassed on other occasions.

3 Children can also facilitate progress by trusting the adult to hear a recording of their voice, eg by leaving voice messages on the adult's phone or making the adult a Talking Greetings Card or Talking Photo Album (see 'Talking resources' in Appendix F).

4 This stage is often fleeting or bypassed and depends on the child's age, their relationship with the adult and the type of activity.

5 See Appendix A for activity ideas.

not always present. However, in our experience, as long as the new person shows no surprise when the child speaks, and does not suddenly switch their focus from the parent to the child, the child will soon start talking directly to them too. Therefore, it is always good to remind the other people present to give the child plenty of time to speak to their parents comfortably first, and to take this as the sign that the child's anxiety has dropped to a manageable level. At this point, it is safe for the new person to try a question because, if the child does not answer after five seconds, there is now a much better chance that they will answer when the parent repeats or rephrases the question.

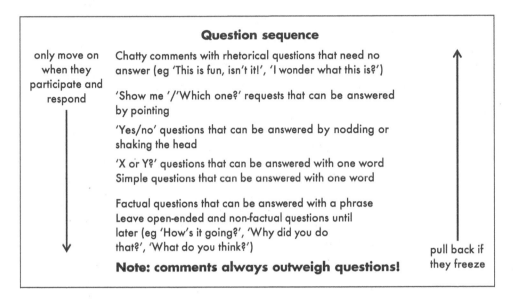

Question sequence

only move on when they participate and respond

Chatty comments with rhetorical questions that need no answer (eg 'This is fun, isn't it!', 'I wonder what this is?')

'Show me '/'Which one?' requests that can be answered by pointing

'Yes/no' questions that can be answered by nodding or shaking the head

'X or Y?' questions that can be answered with one word
Simple questions that can be answered with one word

Factual questions that can be answered with a phrase
Leave open-ended and non-factual questions until later (eg 'How's it going?', 'Why did you do that?', 'What do you think?')

Note: comments always outweigh questions!

pull back if they freeze

Figure 9.2: **Introducing questions to a person with selective mutism** (also in Handout D4, Appendix D)

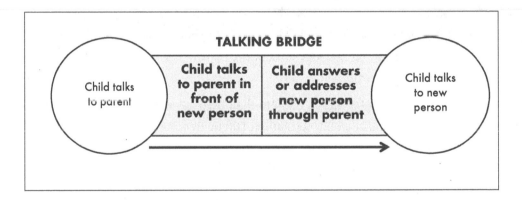

TALKING BRIDGE

Child talks to parent

Child talks to parent in front of new person

Child answers or addresses new person through parent

Child talks to new person

Figure 9.3: **Using a talking bridge to accelerate one-to-one interaction**

A word of warning here: none of the techniques described below will work to their best effect if the child is used to their parent talking for them in public, or if they are afraid of a surprised or overwhelming reaction from other people. The strategies in Handout 12, 'Do I answer for my child?', therefore take priority, along with priming friends and relatives to be calm when the child speaks.

Many children will also need help to attend social events in the first place – see 'Group participation' on page 167.

a) Slowly does it …

With sympathetic support, children can be gradually helped to speak to new people on a one-to-one basis during their normal routines and family social events. This may happen over one long session (eg a day at the beach or a family weekend) or over several shorter sessions (eg after-school club gatherings or music lessons). New adults will need some prior 'coaching': an email with the key points from Chapter 8 and the question sequence in Figure 9.2 can work well. Also, the child will need the usual reassurances that no one will mind if they don't talk. Other than this, no special planning is required, but if many people will be present, make sure that the child is given plenty of space and only approached by one new adult at a time.

b) Set up a talking bridge

The parent's bridging role can be an important part of the previous method's success on an ad hoc basis. But here, a parent and a new person set up dedicated sessions with the express purpose of gradually moving the child through the stages of one-to-one interaction. The new person (probably an adult) should be the only person present who the child does not talk to. There are no rules regarding how many sessions it takes, nor how long each session lasts, but if this is done in the environment where the child is most comfortable, most children will pass through several stages over two to three hours.

> My eight-year-old daughter was anxious about seeing so many relatives at her grandma's birthday party. But I kept reassuring her that she would be fine — no one was expecting her to talk if it was difficult and all that everyone wanted was for her to enjoy the day. (The relief on her face when I told her she didn't have to say 'Thank you' this time!)
>
> It worked! She enjoyed a big family event for the first time in years, helped as much as she could and spoke to a few people — in just a soft, quiet voice but she shocked herself that she had made this much progress!

Box 9.1: Fostering friendships

- Ask the teacher for advice about suitable classmates to invite round if your child has no suggestions, and introduce yourself to their parents.

- When inviting friends round, don't leave them to their own devices if your child is not talking to them yet. Also, remember that just being together can be awkward (eg during a meal or travelling in the car). Play games with them that your child enjoys, or get involved in something purposeful or physical (eg make pizza or jewellery, build a den, design a computerised kingdom, knock skittles over with giant water pistols, go bowling, make an obstacle course, train a puppy).

- Don't be fazed if your child does not talk the first time a friend comes round — other progress will be made instead. Use the Triangle Tactic to help them build rapport.

- Look for a club to suit your child's interests and talents rather than one you feel will be 'good' for them — drama isn't for everyone! Confidence grows from success and enjoyment, and activities such as computing, board games, Lego® and gymnastics all generate talk if there's a mutual interest.

- Help your child maintain friendships independently by supporting them to send a text or an instant message themselves, or to hand out a note or party invitations.

- Online friendships and gaming are a good start (taking the usual safety precautions), especially if communication progresses from messaging to speaking into a microphone, using a webcam or inviting a friend round for a shared session.

The sessions can start simply with the parent and the new person chatting together over a cup of tea, having agreed their 'double act' beforehand by going through Box 9.1 and Handout 13 'Easing in friends and relatives' (online). This handout is also useful for members of staff who can visit the child at home.

c) The Triangle Tactic

You may think that children should be less 'scary' than adults but this is certainly not always the case. Many children who have SM will also need structured support to make and talk to new friends. Box 9.1 gives some general tips for getting children together and, having achieved this, the Triangle Tactic will help to get conversation going. By staying until conversation is established, the parent provides two things: *support* for their child, as described in Handout 12 'Do I answer for my child?'; and *interest* for the new child. Without this, the danger is that the new child will get bored and wander off to amuse themselves, thinking there's no point talking to someone who doesn't reply. They may not want to return a second time.

As you can see in Figure 9.4, it may feel like two separate conversations for a while. The parent makes no attempt to persuade the two children to talk to each other, but involves them both in an activity and chats to them individually. Although the conversations are separate, the parent brings in the other child when they can: for example, 'I think Aadi's got one of those too, haven't you Aadi?'; 'Gosh that looks heavy. Peter, can you give Aadi a hand please?'

Following the usual question sequence (see Figure 9.2), the parent focuses on enabling their child to speak *in front of* their friend rather than directly to them, and then acts as a go-between. By redirecting comments in *both* directions, it is possible to make children feel as if they are talking to each other, well before they actually do. For example:

Parent:	So Peter, I hear you're into model making now?
New child:	Yeah, I've just got the Focke-Wulf 190A-8.
Parent:	Goodness! I've never heard of that. Have you, Aadi?
Child:	(nods)
Parent:	Aadi obviously knows a lot more about this than I do, Peter.
New child:	It's a German single-engine fighter aircraft.
Parent:	Wow! Aadi, do know which war it fought in?
Child:	(nods)
Parent:	World war one or two?
Child:	Two.
Parent:	Is that right, Peter?
New child:	Yeah, Aadi can see my collection if he wants.
Parent:	Would you like that, Aadi? You haven't got any model aircraft, have you?
Child:	I have!

It's a wonderful moment when the child who has SM eventually bypasses the parent and completes the triangle!

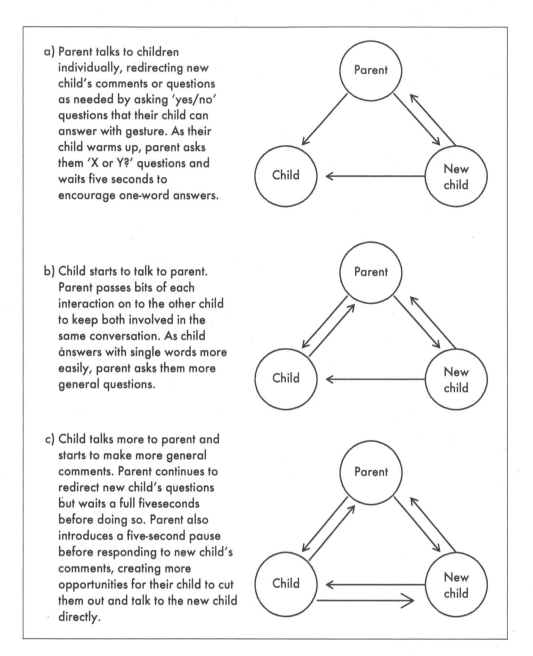

a) Parent talks to children individually, redirecting new child's comments or questions as needed by asking 'yes/no' questions that their child can answer with gesture. As their child warms up, parent asks them 'X or Y?' questions and waits five seconds to encourage one-word answers.

b) Child starts to talk to parent. Parent passes bits of each interaction on to the other child to keep both involved in the same conversation. As child answers with single words more easily, parent asks them more general questions.

c) Child talks more to parent and starts to make more general comments. Parent continues to redirect new child's questions but waits a full fiveseconds before doing so. Parent also introduces a five-second pause before responding to new child's comments, creating more opportunities for their child to cut them out and talk to the new child directly.

Figure 9.4: **The Triangle Tactic**

d) The Sliding-in Technique

This more formal method is described in Chapter 10 because it is normally used by members of school staff who have limited time for one-to-one sessions with the child. Based on classic exposure therapy, it gives them a way to fast-track progress with the minimum of 'warm-up' time. However, the Sliding-in Technique can also be used by families – see Sander's story in Chapter 14, and Maria's story in Chapter 15.

We recommend that practitioners ensure that parents are familiar with the technique, which enables children to gradually tolerate being overheard and spoken to. The new person literally slides in to the child's comfort zone. Parents should feel confident using it either as a fast-track method to introduce a new person or as a fall-back method when less formal approaches have not been successful. Some practitioners will demonstrate the technique first to slide themselves in as the new person and, second, to slide in a 'new' family member of the child or young person's choice. Finally, the child and their parent slide in other friends or family members without the practitioner being present.

e) Desensitisation using voice recordings

The whole family can get involved in recording and listening to silly noises, messages or songs for fun. Allowing someone to hear a recording of your voice is a powerful way to become desensitised to speaking for the first time, provided the listener reacts calmly and focuses on the message, rather than expecting face-to-face talking to follow immediately.

See 'Talking resources' in Appendix F for ideas such as photo albums, postcards and greeting cards which children can use to record messages or picture descriptions. Older children and young people can record voice messages on smartphones, tablets or laptops and send them to another person's device. Recordings can be played by the child themselves, as demonstrated in the BBC documentary *My Child Won't Speak* (see Appendix F 'Audio-visuals') or passed on and listened to without the child being present. Young children are often pleased to exchange voice messages with a familiar adult or use voice recordings in class, as described on page 187, seeing it as preferable to direct talking. Older children might need extra reassurance that the recording will only be heard by one person.

Using voice recordings as a step towards talking face-to-face is described next. If children resist making recordings because they hate the sound of their voice, see 'Desensitisation to the sound of your own voice' (page 159).

f) Using a telephone or a webcam

Talking can be made easier by putting some distance between the speaker and listener. In common with voice recordings, telephones and webcams introduce an extra step before face-to-face interaction, and offer a solution for people who the child does not see very often. Another advantage is that most of the work is done at home where the child or young person feels most comfortable.

Telephone

Chapter 10 outlines two telephone programmes which can be carried out with the child and the new adult in different locations for most of the steps. These may enable teachers to hear children read at home, for example, or allow geographically distant relatives to establish verbal communication after exchanging voice messages.

The two routes are summarised below; the details are in Appendix B (online).

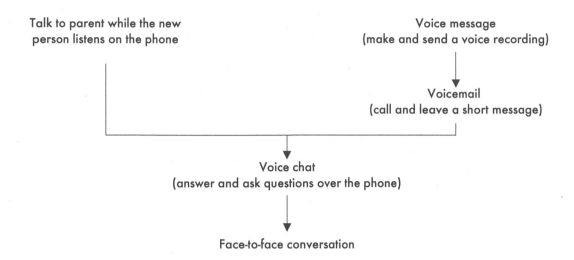

Chapter 10 also describes a telephone version of the Sliding-in Technique. This can work well for children who enjoy exchanging voice messages with school-based staff members, or talking to relatives on the phone, but are too anxious to talk face-to-face. Children can use walkie-talkies with their friends in the same way, starting at opposite ends of the garden, across the park, or upstairs and downstairs, and gradually approaching each other as they talk.

More informally, children may be able to join in a group 'Bye!' at the end of a phone call, take turns with their siblings to record the outgoing message on the home phone, or improvise with their friends using walkie-talkies or Talking Tubes (see 'Talking resources' in Appendix E online).

Webcam
Children and young people may be willing to move on to webcam chats after messaging or telephone contact. In our experience, they have always managed to talk to that person face-to-face after establishing audio-visual contact. One young man played games with his grandfather on a webcam to establish talking. First, they played a non-verbal guessing game where his Grandad drew a picture bit by bit and Nathan tried to guess what it was. Initially, he told his mother off-camera what he thought his grandfather had drawn. But, as he had to keep returning to the laptop to see the picture again, he soon didn't bother to move so far away when he spoke. It wasn't long before he was making general comments to his mother which his grandfather could hear. Nathan loved this special time with his Grandad and they progressed to other guessing games such as 'Colour I-Spy' and 'Animal Noises' (Appendix A online) until, one day, Nathan simply didn't bother to go off-camera to speak.

Older children usually prefer to establish verbal communication *off*-camera by telephone or Skype, before progressing to live webcam or FaceTime conversations. Another useful stepping-stone is to record and send video messages on Skype or a smartphone.

g) Warm-up routines
Once children have used a small-steps programme and know that it works, they are usually very good at working out their own condensed version to break the ice quickly with more new people. All of these

routines operate on the principle of starting with a low-risk activity in which the child or young person does not have to worry about the actual words they are going to say.

For example:

★ Becky invented her own ball game to replace the Sliding-in Technique counting sequence. She and the visiting friend (and initially her mother) would throw a ball to each other, counting aloud – one … two … three – to see whether they could get to 20 without dropping it.

★ Having read to his teacher over the phone, Richard would read a short passage to visiting relatives and then answer questions about it.

★ Janis would leave a couple of voicemails on a new person's mobile phone and then share photographs with them when they met. After several appreciative comments from the new person, she could answer simple questions about the pictures. Sentences soon followed.

All of these routines seem too simple but they succeeded because each person had already worked through a much slower, gradual, step-by-step approach with other people. Also, they had learned that it was possible to speak without anxiety if they did things at their own pace. With a sympathetic audience who fully understood the situation, they now needed to get out just a few words before their anxiety subsided and talking became easier.

Parents can introduce similar warm-up routines and ice-breakers when they have visitors, with non-taxing games or activities that their children know well. Friends and relatives may also like to see 'Talking through toys, puppets or animals' in Chapter 10 (page 182).

Desensitisation to the sound of your own voice

Most children regard voice recordings as a helpful stepping-stone towards speaking face-to-face. Although they may initially be nervous about the new person hearing their voice, their anxiety centres on where this might *lead*, rather than the sound they are making. However, it is not uncommon for children to state that they don't want to speak because they don't like the sound of their voice.

Try not to get too side-tracked by this. In the majority of cases, these are children who have never been given an adequate explanation for their SM. They know they hate talking and are bright enough to realise that there must be a reason for this. Not liking the sound of their voice seems like a reasonable explanation, particularly as: (1) their anxiety is clearly linked to the act of speaking; (2) *no one* likes the sound of their own voice! Not on first hearing, at any rate. But, as with other things, with exposure we get used to it.

To avoid children developing an aversion to their voice, and to address this when it happens, use as many of the following suggestions as feel appropriate.

a) Have fun playing with toys that have an instant record and play-back facility, such as Repeating Parrot (see 'Talking resources' in Appendix F).

b) Encourage the use of voice messaging within the family, as an addition to regular text messaging.

c) Reframe 'I hate my voice' and 'My voice sounds horrible' to 'You didn't like hearing the recording because your voice sounded so different from how it sounds in your head when you talk' and 'Your voice sounds different to you from how it sounds to other people. Other people hear a nice voice'. When the child disagrees, stick to the same message: 'I know your voice sounds strange to you, but it sounds lovely to other people'.

d) Reassure the child that you did not like your voice either when you first heard it, but now you have got used to it.

e) Give the scientific explanation: we hear voice recordings via sound waves travelling through the air, which is how other people hear our voices, and we hear our own voices via vibrations that travel through the bones in our head and fill the spaces in our head. The latter sounds much more rich and resonant (compare how voices sound in the open air with how they sound echoing in a cave), so it is a shock for *everyone* to hear their recorded voice.

f) Give the psychological explanation, as outlined above and in 'The influence of SM on thinking and reasoning' in Chapter 2 (page 33).

g) Use techniques such as the Sliding-in Technique and the reading route (Chapter 10) which do not require voice recordings!

Talking to practitioners

Unlike teachers, practitioners can decide whether they will provide support through parents and teaching staff and remain a relative stranger to the child; or whether they will have direct contact with the child. The reasons for direct contact include:

★ facilitating further assessment

★ addressing an additional difficulty such as a communication or learning difficulty or social anxiety

★ acting as a keyworker in the short term (see page 196, Chapter 10)

★ helping a young person to understand their difficulties and transition into a new setting with the added boost of having spoken to someone new.

When working directly with the child, there are ideas for facilitating communication at the initial meeting in Chapter 5. If further meetings are needed to work towards talking, for young children we suggest informal methods. See 'Slowly does it …' and 'Set up a talking bridge' in 'Talking to friends, family and regular contacts' (page 150), and 'The informal Sliding-in Technique' (page 180), all of which can be used in a variety of settings. For children aged 5 or 6 years and above, use more formal small-steps programmes (see Chapter 10, page 188).

Talking to strangers – family support

It is impossible to lead an independent life without talking to strangers. Children need sensible advice about when it is *safe* to talk to strangers, rather than blanket warnings *not* to talk to strangers. Growing up being able to talk to strangers, albeit briefly with a parent present, is the best possible preparation that children with SM can have for coping in new environments where they don't know anyone.

We suggest following the steps below.

1   Use Handout 12 'Do I answer for my child?' to help children cope with unexpected questions from shop assistants, receptionists, and so on.

2   Prepare adults such as doctors and opticians in advance, following the guidance in Chapter 6 (page 100).

3   Increase children's tolerance of talking *near* strangers, as a first step towards talking *to* strangers. This is covered in the next main section, 'Talking in public places'.

4   Remind children that, in most situations, strangers are far too busy to start a conversation. If they do, it is OK to smile and say nothing – the stranger will know they have overstepped the mark.

5   Use role-play games with younger children, and rehearsal with older children, to prepare them for shopping, ordering food or drink, changing library books, answering the phone, etc. Cashiers and servers in supermarkets and fast-food chains tend to have a predictable greeting and patter!

6   Once children are making good progress and talking to more of their regular contacts, it is time to hold back when talking to safe strangers on their behalf. This will feel difficult at first because your child has needed your support for so long. However, often it is only habit getting in the way of your child discovering their potential. Choose your moments and try the sequence below in situations where it won't be the end of the world if you don't step in.

    ★   Gently make your position clear. For example, you are too busy to stop what you are doing when the ice-cream van comes round, or too settled at the table to return to the counter to ask for ketchup.

    ★   Remind your child how well they are doing with other people, and how little the child needs to say.

    ★   If they hesitate, calmly say, 'It's OK, you don't have to go if you don't want to'. Make no attempt to persuade them to go and don't watch them. In this way, there is no pressure, and it is entirely the child's decision.

Safe strangers

(Check against your local school or neighbourhood watch policy)

- People working in a public place and doing their job

    e.g. people wearing a uniform who are trained to help; people working behind a counter, in a shop or school, or on public transport.

- People who talk to you when you are with your parent or teacher.

★ If they miss out on this occasion, it is hard not to feel horribly guilty but keep it light and calmly say, 'It's OK, you can try another time. I know you're going to get really good at this'.

After this gentle nudge, expect to be pleasantly surprised!

7 Help older children prepare for secondary school, college or work placements by focusing on talking to strangers, as recommended in Chapter 11, 'Making a fresh start' (page 247). This can be done informally with parents, as discussed in this section, or with more formal assignments, as discussed below. In both cases, it will first be important for the young person to:

★ understand the *reason* for their fear – a phobia that causes an imagined rather than actual threat

★ recognise that gradually facing fears is the only way to banish them

★ believe that, by talking to strangers, they will be challenging their phobia. This will help them to leave it behind when they join a new community circle or transition to a new educational setting.

> 'My 14-year-old home-schooled son was initially very angry when I talked to him about phobias and explained to him that the only 'cure' for SM was for him to face his fear. He stormed off and nothing more was said. But that weekend we went shopping and he suddenly disappeared. I was about to panic when he reappeared clutching something – he'd collected his weekly magazine for the first time in his life. I was amazed but he calmly said 'You said if I made myself do things they'd stop being scary'. He is now back at a very supportive school and talking more every day.'

Talking to strangers – working on assignments

Practitioners and educational mentors may consider individual sessions, group work or summer schools for older children and teenagers with SM, focusing on assignments in community settings which involve talking to strangers. See the further notes on group work on page 165.

Establishing an incentive

Tackling children's long-standing fears about approaching and speaking to strangers will need considerable motivation. Therefore, it will be important to link assignments to a personal goal or an area of life that the young person would like to improve, as identified during the assessment or subsequent meetings. For example, if a young person has identified going to college as their priority, a follow-up session could involve considering various components such as the interview, travel, using the college library and canteen, meeting fellow students, participating in discussions and asking for help. Sequencing them in the order they will be encountered, or ranking them in order of importance, will provide a focus for practical support and assignment setting.

Form 15 'Talking to strangers' (online) may also help. It builds on items 4–7 of Form 8b. It also provides a baseline and accompanying notes to use in preparation for individualised target setting. This could be preceded by asking young people to rank the areas of 'Going out with friends and family', 'Shopping independently' and 'Travelling independently' in order of their personal priority.

Identifying underlying anxieties

Section 1 of Form 15, 'General independence', needs further comment. These items are rarely identified as priority areas because they do not represent end goals, but they are fundamental to an overall sense of freedom. Therefore, we incorporate them as steps towards personal goals, where appropriate, and monitor the remaining items to see whether progress in other areas has a positive impact. Persistent difficulties here may underpin a dependency on other people and resistance to going out unaccompanied. They could also be a symptom of social anxiety disorder (see Chapter 13). It will be important to help individuals recognise what is at the root of their anxiety, so that they can be helped to identify more useful thinking patterns and practical coping strategies.

For example:

★ Are they in constant dread of being seen, approached and spoken to by other people?

★ Could they cope if they missed a bus or got separated from their friends?

★ Do they worry excessively about their safety or what other people are thinking or saying about them?

★ Are their anxieties directly related to their inability to talk? If so, there is even more reason to work on assignments with strangers.

★ Are there issues that go beyond the act of talking which might be more appropriately addressed at a cognitive level?

Clearly, these are complex issues which practitioners can only be expected to explore and address within the context of their particular area of expertise. Suggestions are included in Chapter 10 under 'Additional considerations for adolescents and young adults' (page 214).

Choosing appropriate settings

When choosing settings for assignments, there will inevitably be an overlap with the next part of the model of confident talking: 'Talking in public places'. Therefore, it is important to consider the location and time of day because children will initially prefer there to be few bystanders and little chance of being observed by people they know. Each assignment can be broken down into several smaller steps to reflect their increasing tolerance to being overheard. For example, ordering a drink in a fast-food restaurant could be broken down as follows.

★ Talk to mentor sitting at a side table.

★ Tell mentor what I want to drink in the queue.

★ Tell server what I want when it's quiet (better chance I'll be heard first time).

★ Tell server what I want when it's busy (I'll have to repeat if necessary but that's OK, the server is used to that).

Preparing for the assignment

Rehearsal is always useful and children can run through verbal exchanges before actual assignments, with their mentor taking the role of server, shop assistant or stranger on the street. Similarly, they can practise face-to-face or telephone exchanges with strangers who have been briefed, such as the mentor's work colleagues, before going out into the real world.

Older children can also prepare by making themselves comfortable, breathing slowly in and out, closing their eyes and *visualising* themselves succeeding in their assignment. The more they 'see' and 'hear' themselves run through the routine, the more familiar the activity will feel when the time comes.

Imposing a time limit always adds to the pressure, so build in extra time for some slow breathing to calm the nerves and use phrases like 'It's OK to go up whenever you're ready', or 'I'm joining the queue now, follow me as soon as you're ready', rather than 'OK, go!' Breathing is covered in more detail in Chapter 10 under 'Additional considerations for adolescents and young adults (page 214)'.

Talking to strangers – using the phone

In this age of electronic text-based communication, it has become increasingly unnecessary for young people to use the telephone to speak to anyone other than close friends and family. Many households have personal mobiles, rather than a shared landline. Yet care should still be taken to ensure that young people don't develop an intense dislike or fear of using the phone, in addition to their SM.

Many jobs rely on a good telephone manner or the ability to quickly resolve a problem with a phone call rather than an email. Just as confidence has a ripple effect, fear breeds fear – it is difficult for an individual to feel in control and free from SM when they continue to avoid a specific aspect of communication. In addition, the telephone provides a rich source of practice in talking to strangers, combined with complete control. You can end the call at any time, blaming it on the signal or battery, without losing face!

We therefore make the following suggestions.

★ Look at Form 15 in conjunction with 'Telephone programmes' in Appendix B. The 'robot route' uses telephone services with automated voice recognition as a starting point for talking to strangers, without the 'warm-up' time you get with other people.

★ Consider the possibility that adults close to the child are modelling telephone avoidance and conveying anxiety about saying the wrong thing, sounding stupid or bothering other people. These messages usually reflect personal insecurities and what we think of *ourselves*, rather than what other people are thinking. It is OK to make a mistake, stumble over a word, repeat ourselves more clearly or ring at an inconvenient time. All of this is good and normal and not what people remember after the call. Tell children that if we are polite, patient and helpful, we will always make a good impression!

★ Encourage children to answer the phone at home, either informally, to help parents out, or as an assignment, as shown in Box 9.2 (overleaf). The child is learning two things: that they are capable of

dealing with unplanned encounters with strangers; and that they can extract themselves from *any* conversation if they need to. Terminating a phone conversation is a skill which can give confidence in using 'get-out' phrases such as 'Sorry, I need to go' or
'Excuse me' in face-to-face encounters. Having an escape route is the first step to not needing one!

Box 9.2: Example of telephone homework

Read through the notes below to remind yourself of the strategies we agreed. Answer the phone as much as you can, even if you don't recognise the number, and keep a record of how you are doing. The more you answer the phone, the less anxiety you will feel.

What will happen when I answer the phone

1 I will say '**Hello**'. Then, if it's for me …

   That's easy!

2 If it's a sales call …

   I will say '**No thank you**' as soon as I can and **hang up**.

3 If they ask for Mum or think I am her …

   I will say something like '**She's out – can you call back after 4 pm?**'

   or '**She's not here, do you want her to call you when she gets back?**'

   or '**I'll just get her.**' (It's good to interrupt as soon as possible!)

Every time you answer the phone, make a note of what happened, and how much anxiety you felt on a scale from 0 to 10, as shown in the example below.

Date	What happened	Anxiety
4.1.16	It was for Mum, I interrupted and said 'I'll go and get her'	6
4.1.16	I could see it was a sales call, I felt worse the longer I left it and hung up without saying anything	7
5.1.16	Sales call – I said 'No thank you' straightaway and felt much better.	4

Group work

We have used paired and group sessions to develop understanding, maintenance and management of anxiety in general and SM specifically; to share experiences and coping strategies; and to tackle assignments, as discussed in this chapter.

Working in pairs or groups is not always possible but we recommend it, particularly for older children and teenagers. In our experience, children can be spurred on by seeing other group members rise to a challenge. To this end, speech and language therapists may be able to team up with their local dysfluency service because the issues of anxiety and avoidance in SM are very similar for young people who stammer.

The young people we have worked with report that one of the things they find most helpful is to know that they are not alone. Meeting others within the same school or locality shows them how much more common SM is than people realise. When asked whether they prefer individual or group sessions, they opt for both in our experience, saying that it helps to come to a group session, confident that they can already speak to the facilitator with whom they have built rapport on a one-to-one basis.

The model of confident talking: talking in public places

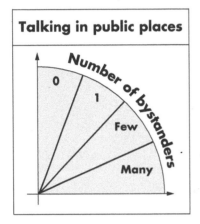

Some children who have SM speak happily to their parents in public places until someone linked to their school appears. Others rarely speak in public and withdraw when a visitor arrives in the home. No two children are the same but they will all benefit from help to increase their tolerance of talking in front of general *bystanders*; that is, people who are not part of the child's group or activity but yet might still hear or see the child speak.

The issue for the child is not usually the actual number of bystanders, but rather:

★ the number that the child is *aware of* and their proximity

★ whether they perceive the bystander to be listening or not

★ the possibility of bystanders approaching

★ fear of reaction or disclosure – will the bystander be surprised, or tell someone what they have witnessed, thus raising the expectation that the child will talk to others?

Handout 14 'Talking in public places' sets out strategies for parents to help children talk to them more in public, with reduced reliance on avoidance strategies. It is aimed primarily at community settings outside the home, but the same strategies can be applied at larger family gatherings where the onus is on general mingling rather than group activities.

> 'We just had a very successful family birthday party where we coached everyone beforehand on how not to ask Ted questions or put any pressure on him. He was very quiet and withdrawn for the first hour but, when he realised others were leaving us to our corner of the garden, he played and talked to us, even when there were a few people around.
>
> By the end, he was leaving us and helping himself to food which I thought I'd never see!'

Children may enjoy the challenge of the Walkabout Technique on page 205. It is often used in schools to encourage continued talking when walking from point A to point B. Equally, it can be made into a game on the way to school or the shops, for example.

Progress chart 2 'Talking in public with increasing numbers of bystanders' (online) can be used to keep a record by adding the places your child most frequently attends in the first column. For simplicity, the progression used (zero–one–few–many) refers to the number of people who are close enough to hear or see the child talking. However, the actual situations chosen to practise tolerance of bystanders must depend on the individual child, so that settings associated with highest anxiety are left until last. Generally, it is easiest for children to talk to people in their comfort zone when any bystanders are complete strangers with no interest in the conversation. Table 9.2 gives some examples of the progression in practice.

Table 9.2: **Talking in public places – community settings**

	Number of bystanders who may hear or see the child speak			
	0	**1**	**Few**	**Many**
EXAMPLES OF PUBLIC PLACES	Park or beach – people in distance Empty aisle in supermarket Standing round the corner out of sight Deserted street on way to school	Home with visitor present A friend's house or car with their parent Empty reception area apart from receptionist Taxi Private music lesson	Café/restaurant when quiet Shops/changing rooms Supermarket/cinema queue Library Park Street Clinic waiting room	Café/restaurant when busy On the bus/train Playgroup, dancing class, gymnastics, youth club Accident and emergency department (A&E) Church service Wedding reception

The model of confident talking: group participation

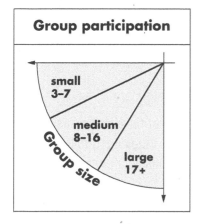

Group participation

small 3–7

medium 8–16

large 17+

Group size

This quadrant of the model is mainly covered in Chapter 10 and refers to times when children are *part of a group activity* such as a class discussion or roll-call; or *addressing a group*, such as speaking in a play or saying their lines at an enrolment ceremony.

Families will find that they are already helping their child to cope better in group situations by following the advice in Chapter 8 and the earlier sections in this chapter. A good practical method is to start with a non-verbal option (for example, a party game forfeit could be to count to 10 backwards or stand on one leg for 10 seconds) or to ask the children to speak in unison. It may also be worth checking whether organisational policy is being followed. For example, the UK Scout Association states that children must not be made to feel self-conscious or worry about forgetting words: young children should not be required to say their investiture Promise alone, and older children would usually repeat the words line by line. Box 9.3 gives additional tips to help children face social events.

Box 9.3: Helping children who have SM to face and cope with social events

- Educate adults in advance and ask them to involve the child in a friendly way without expecting them to talk straightaway. (Don't ask questions; instead, make chatty comments and allow the child to speak in their own time.)

- Reassure the child that no one will insist they say 'Hello', 'Thank you', 'Goodbye', etc and that it's fine if they talk and fine if they don't.

Family occasions

- Involve the child beforehand with a job that plays to their strengths, such as making a notice or baking biscuits. Make sure this is manageable and not an overwhelming challenge for them!

- Arrive early, before it gets crowded, and get the child involved with helping in some way so that they are occupied from the start.

- Ensure that the child is seated where they don't feel 'trapped', eg near a door.

- Arrange fun activities that don't require taking turns and being the centre of attention. Physical activity is good for relaxing the body, having fun and taking the focus off talking.

- Allow the child to take something like a book, favourite toy or tablet computer, so that they can retreat a little when they need to, and join in again as they feel more comfortable. Find a quiet corner where they can spend short breaks.

- Encourage the child to take something they are proud of, such as a possession, game or family pet, to show people by way of conversation or interaction.

Clubs and organised activities

- Go on your own beforehand to do a trial run. You can then describe to your child the format, facilities, etc in advance.

- Ask a receptive adult to 'Meet and Greet' and oversee the child's involvement, so that they are not left to fend for themselves; someone to find them a job to do, ensure they have somewhere to sit, assign them to a group, etc.

- If available, take a friend or sibling for support.

- Arrive early, before it gets busy, and make sure the child knows where the toilets are.

- Build in an escape route: arrange for the child to just watch or only stay a short time on the first visit (they can always stay longer if they want to) or be outside half an hour early if they need to leave. (Don't go in – it's enough for the child to know you are there and the leader has your phone number if there any problems.)

The model of confident talking: social functioning

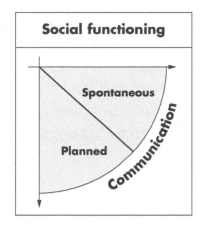

This quadrant of the model is covered in Chapter 10 because most children's speech is less animated and spontaneous in educational settings where there are more people around. However, the progression applies to all settings.

Social functioning concerns *how* the child uses their speech. It is not enough to be able to speak when prompted by questions or instructions. We need to use language effectively to meet our needs and express our opinions; to say *what* we want, *when* we want – within reason, of course! The progression moves from 'low-risk' communication, where the talking is planned, structured and factual, to 'high-risk' communication, which is spontaneous, child-initiated and possibly personal. It is the unpredictable outcome of these exchanges that make them high risk.

Appendix A (online) provides guidance for supporting the progression from planned to spontaneous activities.

Additional considerations for adolescents

The strategies described in this chapter are equally suitable for older children and teenagers when used with age-appropriate activities and conversation topics. We routinely use the question progression in Figure 9.2 with young people who say we come over as 'understanding' and 'not pushy' – they are not aware of being 'therapised' (thank you Maria for that lovely word!). So parents can either introduce the informal strategies without explanation, or let older children know exactly what they are doing, as described in Handout 12 'Do I answer for my child?'. The strategies are methodical and sensitive; they gradually increase expectation at a pace to suit the individual. They should also appeal to a young person's logic in the context of phobia and anxiety management.

But what about young people who seem increasingly withdrawn, perhaps giving up on their ideas of going to college, who spend most of their time at home, unable to face the outside world, let alone their fears of talking? The future is a very scary place for them and they have no idea how to approach it; they prefer to avoid thinking about it altogether.

We hope that reading this manual will give you confidence that your teenager *can* be helped. However, without an open channel of communication, it is difficult to know where to start. Teenagers do not respond well to being told what to do. They need to find their own motivations, hopes and dreams, and anxious teenagers seem even more resistant. Every suggestion parents make somehow conveys that they are disappointed in their child and wish they were different. But simply being patient and giving them their space is not enough to turn things around; they need reassurance, gentle guidance and connection with the outside world to believe there is a way forward, without feeling pushed. They need to know that their parents see a whole person, rather than their difficulties, and are interested in what they know, feel, like and dislike.

There are no quick fixes here but don't give up and they won't either. Let them know that you are there for them, fully and unconditionally. You know it will take time, but you have faith that they will work out what they want to do and you are ready and willing to provide whatever support they need. Acknowledge that this is a difficult and scary time but you will find a way through it together. It will be OK. Enjoy their company without feeling offended if they don't say much. Try to let only a very small part of your total conversation be about their SM and future plans, even if that is often all that is on your mind. Keep them as involved in family life as possible. Ask them for their help and do things as a team, rather than giving them jobs to do. Get everyone in the family to choose an activity day with only one rule: everyone has to join in, whether they think they will enjoy it or not!

Do the little things together and the big decisions can wait. For example, if a school, college or work placement has broken down, there will be a reason. Don't let your son or daughter think it was their fault (see Chapter 8, 'Maintaining factors', and Chapter 11, 'Transitions'). Tell them you understand SM much better now and know that it can be different another time. Be positive about a gap year (or two …). This is the time to learn to drive (always a massive confidence boost, even if it takes several attempts to pass), sign up to a photography course, do voluntary work or learn to cook. Colleges welcome mature students and they have to support students with extreme social anxiety (check out the Equal Opportunities policy on the college website), so that place will wait until your son or daughter is ready to take it. Somewhere out there are people who want to help, given the right information. And other parents to support you and share the journey.

Chapter 10 also includes a section for adolescents and young adults.

Progressive mutism

There are few things more distressing than when a child who has SM stops talking to family members when they previously had no difficulty, and becomes silent at home. The following advice is for the people to whom the child used to speak freely.

Try to identify the reason

First, we suggest reading through FAQ 14 in Chapter 1, to think about when speech stopped, and to see if any of the scenarios fit the preceding events. This may provide clues to the practical steps to take, in addition to the progression of treatment described in this manual.

For example, the child may need:

★ private time with their parent(s) away from other household residents to rebuild rapport before following Handout 13, 'Easing in friends and relatives'

★ help to deal with a trauma such as a house fire or burglary

★ an apology and adjustment for a misunderstanding or unfair treatment.

The child will need calm reassurance that it is not surprising that they stopped talking, given their specific circumstances (it is distressing and confusing for them too), plus assurance that things will be different now. You are there to help and it is safe for them to start talking at home again whenever they feel ready.

Convey confidence that the child can and will talk, without any pressure to talk

This sounds like a tricky balance! It is so important not to panic about the future because any anxiety will be conveyed to the child and increase their negative association with communication. It is impossible to *make* children talk, so all you can do is provide an environment where they feel relaxed, happy, safe and confident, and *need* to talk.

Maintain a relaxed, calm and smiling exterior yourself, being careful not to convey disappointment or hurt that the child is not talking to you. Talk to the child in commentary style (see page 122), bringing as much fun and laughter into your interactions as possible, to convey that you enjoy the child's company, whether they talk or not. However, you still provide the *opportunity* to talk; statements and rhetorical questions, followed by a pause, are far more likely to evoke a verbal response than asking direct questions, especially when you say something that the child feels driven to correct (see Tables 9.1 and 10.2 on pages 151 and 183 for ideas).

Supporting younger children

All or some of the following strategies may be helpful, depending on individual children's needs and the pattern of communication within the family.

Revise the child's internal rule system

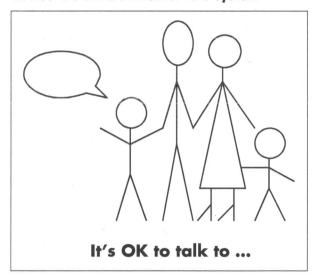

It's OK to talk to ...

Children with rigid rule systems (point (a) in FAQ 14; see Chapter 1, page 15) can be presented with a new rule to say to themselves: 'It's OK to talk to [names of immediate family and pets]. I like it when no one else can hear.' Note that 'It's OK to ...' is not the same as parents or other adults saying 'I want you to ...', 'You need to ... ' or 'Go on, you can do it'; all of which constitute pressure and raise anxiety. Display the 'It's OK to talk to ...' image where the child will see it often (eg on their bedroom wall) so there's no need to mention it again. Later, they can add further rules, such as, 'It's OK to let my teacher hear my voice'.

Encourage general vocalisation

Build in games and activities where the emphasis is on laughter, making sounds or physical exertion, rather than talking. For example, blow bubbles with lots of 'oohs' and 'ahs'; have a pillow fight or tug-of-war; make 'brum brum' and 'beep beep' noises while you play with toy cars; or accompany their turn on the swing or slide with 'whoosh!' and 'whee!'

Avoid the common 'talking traps'

This may be the hardest thing to do but it is very important in turning things around. Handout 14, 'Talking in public places', explains these traps, and how it is possible to inadvertently encourage silence by giving lots of attention to the use of non-verbal communication. To guess what the child wants, and to allow gestures such as pointing to become the main means of communication, effectively normalises silence and makes the act of speaking less and less familiar to the child as time goes on.

This is *not* a recommendation to make children go without something unless they speak. Life will go on as normal and your child will be provided with all they need. However, there are many non-essential things and it is important for the child to see that you have faith in their ability to talk again. After one attempt to understand what the child is trying to communicate, calmly say that you are sorry, but you don't know what they mean, and move the conversation on by continuing with what you are doing or by changing the subject. You can say 'Don't worry, you can let me know later' or 'It's OK to tell me if you want' or 'I know it feels difficult at the moment but soon you'll be able to explain and help me out'. You can even suggest that the child asks their favourite toy to tell you (see Chapter 10 'Talking through toys, puppets or animals', page 182), but don't get into a lengthy discussion about it or wait for the child to speak there and then. When the child *does* speak, suppress your relief, which may overwhelm them; simply make it a positive interaction by responding to what they have said.

Supporting older children

The situation is rather different with older children who have lived with SM for years and gradually shut down as they become increasingly despondent. It may not only be talking that has stopped within the family. Changes may be needed to increase interaction in general, as a foundation for talking. See Table 8.2 on page 134 for some ideas, particularly items 1–8 and 25–27. Some young people start to re-engage with their parents after a specialist in SM has spoken to them about their difficulties and convinced them that they can be helped, or an outsider shows a special interest and involves them in a practical project where they rebuild their sense of value and purpose.

Providing reassurance

The basic reassurances are still needed:

★ you understand what they have been through

★ you are there to support them

★ you will find a way through together

★ you are ready to listen when they feel like talking again

★ you know this needs to be in their own time.

The last point is probably the most important. Young people are sometimes afraid to start speaking again because they fear that everything will move too fast for them – if they speak to one person, it might be assumed that they can speak to everyone. In addition, you will need to say that you won't be offended if they talk to other people and understand why this might be easier for them. For example, they might want to talk to someone outside the family who is less emotionally attached, but feel guilty or anxious about this. They won't want to risk being overheard if they think this will upset you or lead to pressure to talk in other situations.

Written communication

We do not normally recommend alternative modes of communication for close family members. However, a written form such as email correspondence may be the best option for a young person who has long-standing, progressive mutism. It should be regarded as a valuable stepping-stone towards recovering verbal communication and may be helpful in sharing your new-found understanding of SM.

Responding to a request for help

It is possible that a young person will ask for, or agree to, their parent's help to speak to them again, especially when SM is better understood. However, after such a long period of silence, the young person may experience the typical SM 'freeze' when attempting conversation. Questioning will tend to trigger anxiety so will have to be avoided until later. First, you need to establish *voice*. Do not try to find meaningful or interesting topics. The most important thing is for the young person to get used to their parent hearing their voice again. The less they have to think about *what* they are saying, the better it is. Use the reading route (page 197) or the progression in Box 9.4. The young person should try to breathe slowly and evenly and should not force the voice (allow it to gradually get louder as anxiety decreases).

Once the young person is answering simple questions in practice sessions, without feeling anxious, start to introduce 'X or Y?' questions into general conversation (eg 'Shall we have custard or ice-cream?').

Box 9.4: Progression to re-establish speech with a talking partner such as a parent

Repeat each step below several times until it feels comfortable. Take a break whenever you need to.

1   Start with just one word. Say 'two' after partner says 'One …'

2   Say two words by counting up to four, taking it in turns. Partner starts by saying 'One …'

3   Increase to counting up to 10, taking it in turns.

4   Try two numbers each. Partner starts by saying 'One, two …'

5   Take it in turns to say an item from a familiar sequence, such as the days of the week, months of the year or letters of the alphabet. Try saying two or three items each.

6   Move on to sentence completion, where the partner starts a sentence and you say the last word. See Appendix A, Stage 6 (online) for 'Finish the sentence – numbers' and 'Finish the sentence – automatic phrases'.

7   This leads into simple questions. For example, 'One and one make …' ('two') becomes 'How many thumbs have I got?' ('two').

8   Practise phrases and sentences using activities from Appendix A, Stages 7 and 8, or personal interests and areas of expertise.

Practising alone

Finally, here are a few words for young people who desperately want to talk again but are not ready to approach other people. It takes courage but, if people close to you are doing things that are making it difficult for you to talk to them (see Form 10 online), take the time to explain this to them in an email. Talking aloud to yourself is also a good way to prepare for working with an understanding adult. See 'Breathing' (page 217) and 'Voice production' (page 219) in Chapter 10 to understand how your voice works, and 'Lone talking' and 'Shaping' programmes in Appendix B for small steps. Don't be surprised if hearing your voice after so long makes you panic at first. You are recalling the times that you were expected to talk to people who triggered your fear reflex. This feeling will subside as you tell yourself that there is no pressure, you are going to set the pace. One step at a time, one day at a time.

If you cannot achieve voice – even when on your own with no chance of being overheard – other possibilities may need to be explored, taking into account your medical history and significant life events (for example, see 'Psychogenic voice disorder' on page 56). Meanwhile, it is fine to work through the programmes in Appendix B, using a very gentle whisper to avoid vocal strain.

Online resources for Chapter 9

All of the forms, handouts and appendices accompanying this chapter are available at www.routledge.com /cw/speechmark for you to access, print and copy.

FACING FEARS IN EDUCATIONAL SETTINGS

Introduction

This chapter considers how staff and practitioners working in and alongside educational settings can help children and young people who have selective mutism (SM) to overcome their fear of talking. Working within the framework of the model of confident talking, the methods are less formal in early years settings than for older children.

This chapter focuses on:

★ an overview of exposure therapy

★ general points about intervention for all ages

★ early years settings

  – informal strategies

★ school and college settings

  – informal strategies for everyday management

  – general principles of small-steps programmes

  – talking to the keyworker

  – generalising to other adults and children

  – involving the child's classmates

  – working towards spontaneous speech

★ additional considerations for adolescents and young adults

★ letting go.

A quick guide to exposure therapy

Flooding

In this method of phobia management, which dates back to the 1960s, the individual was confronted with the source of their fear and unable to escape. The theory was that, after a while, they would learn that there was no real danger and their fear response would be extinguished. However, the combination of a sudden escalation of anxiety and no control simply made the exposure sessions a terrifying experience. We know now that exposure must be gradual, and at the individual's pace, so that they experience only manageable levels of anxiety.

Systematic desensitisation

This method was less invasive because individuals *imagined* their fears. The fear was broken down into a hierarchy of situations – for example, being in a room with a plastic spider, a tiny real spider, a larger spider, and so on – and the individual imagined each situation once they were in a very relaxed state. When they could think about the least anxiety-provoking situation calmly, the next level was introduced. In time, individuals could endure the *actual* situations with less anxiety.

This approach also had its limitations. It was designed for adults and relied on a skilled therapist, a good therapeutic relationship and the individual's ability to learn deep relaxation before the process of visualising fears could begin. But it clearly demonstrated the value of the small-steps approach and the role of imagination in desensitisation.

Desensitisation is often used in SM work to precede other more direct methods. The individual does not actually speak to a new person; instead, he or she imagines what it would be like by allowing the new person to hear a recording of their voice. By experiencing this event without negative consequences, the thought of actually speaking to the new person starts to become less threatening.

Graded exposure

This direct approach is effective in overcoming fears, phobias and specific anxieties in all age groups. It is a key element of cognitive behavioural therapy (CBT) for phobias and obsessive compulsive disorder (OCD). There are two main approaches – shaping and stimulus fading – both involving *real* situations and exposing the individual to their fear in tiny increments. When the individual has mastered their anxiety at one level, the next increment is introduced.

Shaping

The individual's behaviour is gradually 'shaped' into the desired behaviour. The individual starts by doing something manageable and is then encouraged to do a little bit more each time. This method has one particular limitation in SM intervention. When consciously working towards talking – for example: gesture a word; mouth a word silently; whisper a word; say a word – the leap from no voice to voice is too great. Many children who have SM cannot lower their anxiety sufficiently to produce voice, even for a single sound. However, as a general approach to target setting, the practice of making only one small change at a time works well. Therefore, we mainly use an *informal* shaping approach where there is no expectation to attempt the next level – only an opportunity to do so.

Stimulus fading

The individual's reaction to a stimulus or 'trigger' is gradually faded until the stimulus no longer has the same effect. What makes this so useful in SM intervention is that the *stimulus* gradually changes, rather than the individual's behaviour. Individuals are encouraged to talk in a comfortable situation and *while they are talking* a new person very gradually approaches and joins in. This is the basis of the Sliding-in Technique (see pages 180 and 196).

General points about intervention for all ages

Applying exposure therapy to SM

In practice, a combination of desensitisation, stimulus fading and shaping is used, depending on individual circumstances. As discussed in Chapter 9, parents are ideally placed to support the child in graded exposure work, but members of staff will need access to a variety of techniques they can use with and without parental involvement. In all cases, patience is key! If the child gives even the tiniest indication of relaxation or improvement in response to your planned activity, keep it up! For example, a 'frozen' child might pick up a toy or a snack, look at it briefly and then put it down. Don't be disappointed. This is a step forward; before actually taking or eating the item, the child has to be sure that their action will not result in increased attention or unwanted comments.

Using the model of confident talking

Figure 2.5 (page 47) shows the model of confident talking and Table 7.1 (page 108) gives an overview of the progressions of confident talking within this model. Tables 8.1 and 9.1 (pages 124 and 151) expand the stages of one-to-one interaction, with guidance on how staff members can build rapport and facilitate communication, with and without parents present. It will help to refer to them as you read this chapter and consider each quadrant of the model of confident talking.

The most important point for school staff to bear in mind is that the child should be helped to speak to *one person at a time* and that this will only gradually generalise to talking in the classroom and speaking spontaneously. Don't assume that having spoken once, or in a 'safe' structured activity, the child is 'over it'. At this point, some children do indeed feel a great release and improve rapidly, especially on a one-to-one basis, but most meet the description of 'low profile' rather than 'high profile' SM (see Handout 3, 'Quiet child or selective mutism?' online). Springing questions on them, or expecting an answer when other people are present, can set them back, so take things gently and regard talking to a new person as the *first*, rather than the final, step in their programme.

Choice of activity

Different activities carry a different level of 'risk' for children who have SM and any other child who is anxious about making a mistake or has not yet mastered the language required. When establishing and generalising speech, it is very important to minimise anxiety by initially choosing low-risk activities with known content and fixed duration. Only move towards high-risk activities as the child gains confidence and is speaking more freely.

Table 10.1 summarises low- and high-risk activities, and will help staff members make sense of apparent incongruities in the child's behaviour. For example, it explains why saying a line in a play in front of the whole school, or carrying out a survey by reading out questions from a clipboard, are far easier than joining in classroom discussion or answering an unexpected question.

Table 10.1: **Summary of low- and high-risk activities**

Low-risk activities* (content is explicit and manageable)	High-risk activities (content or outcome is unknown)
Speaking or singing in unison	Speaking alone under time pressure
Continuing a rote sequence such as counting, days of the week, months of the year, letters of the alphabet	Activities involving ambiguous content or unfamiliar subject matter (child may need more information or be unsure whether their answer is acceptable)
Reading aloud (if the child is a competent reader)	Reading aloud (if the child is a poor or beginner reader)
Planned or rehearsed activities with known content and time for preparation	Conversation (unplanned content and duration)
Activities requiring only single words or phrases with factual content and no risk of error or rejection	Questions involving reasoning or explanations which require longer answers.
Adult-led activities (no need for child to get the listener's attention at a suitable moment)	Child-initiated interaction
Structured activities with a familiar format and a fixed end-point.	Content based on personal opinion or contributions which may therefore need further explanation or justification
* Provided they do not draw unwanted attention and an increased expectation to talk	

Preparing to help the child face their fear of talking

Before using the techniques described in this chapter, try to ensure that:

★ All members of staff involved understand the nature of SM, the importance of environmental modifications (Chapter 8), and the need for a coordinated team approach.

★ All staff members are familiar with the stages of one-to-one interaction, have realistic expectations of the child and are aware of the best way to communicate with the child at each stage. The most important point is moving at the child's pace, waiting until the child responds at each stage before proceeding to the next one. See Appendix D (online) for useful handouts.

★ A designated adult has spoken to the child to share their understanding of SM and the setting's willingness to provide support (Handout 1 online). The child is aware that there is no rush and they will be able to talk as and when they feel ready.

Programme planning and monitoring

★ For simplicity, people the child has never spoken to before are referred to as 'new' people. The child may know them well but they are yet to enter the child's comfort zone.

★ The term 'talking partner' denotes anyone with whom the child uses sentences *without any signs of anxiety*), provided no one else is in earshot. Initially, these sentences may be limited to responses and structured activities but, in time, the child should be able to converse with talking partners spontaneously and to initiate comments or requests. Always remember that children may not wish to discuss some subjects, and may be unable to talk in many places for fear of being overheard by other people.

★ The term 'keyworker' describes an adult who has been designated to support the child on a regular basis and to carry out a programme designed to facilitate confident talking. The keyworker will work towards becoming a talking partner and then help the child to generalise to other people and places, gradually building their confidence to both respond to and take the lead in conversations.

★ The child's education plan, targets and review meetings will be coordinated by a designated person, perhaps the special needs coordinator or a practitioner from outside the school. Parents may need support to select appropriate targets and strategies from Chapter 9, as part of a coordinated intervention plan.

★ The term 'practitioners' includes any therapist, psychologist or clinician working in school directly or indirectly with the child. Many children will not have (or need) a practitioner; much will depend on the educational setting's experience of SM and local resources.

★ Unless specified, 'children' in school settings means both children and young people.

★ The online resources for this chapter include the following selection of Progress charts. (Of course, staff members can devise their own record-keeping documents.)

   a) Overall progress charts to show at a glance how far the child has come, and what remains to be done. These are designed for staff and parents.

   b) Records of individual sessions to document the child's response and inform further planning. These are designed for the child's keyworker.

In addition, recording systems such as target sheets are created during individual sessions to show the children their short-term targets and achievements. See Appendix C (online) for examples.

Early years settings

Staff in early years settings will focus on two quadrants of the model of confident talking – 'range of people' and 'group participation'. Parents are best placed to work on 'talking in public places'. After talking to people in preschool settings, one-to-one and in groups, followed by a carefully planned transition to primary school at about five years old (see Chapter 11), most young children seem to complete the generalisation process without further intervention.

The practitioner's role in early years settings is more likely to be around support and advice for parents and staff, than direct intervention.

The model of confident talking: range of people

Talking to staff

The programme coordinator could use Chart 1 to record progress, writing down the staff in the child's setting in the top row. This will show how far the child can communicate with each adult. While everyone should be able to help the child relax and participate in general activities, only one person should take the lead in building rapport on a one-to-one basis at any one time. Otherwise there is a danger of several people 'having a go' and overwhelming the child.

Range of people

Six ways to help children talk to playgroup or nursery staff are described below. They are not mutually exclusive; several may be useful for any one child.

a) Taking the pressure off

b) Talking through the parent

c) The informal Sliding-in Technique

d) Shaping (from gesture to sounds to talking)

e) Talking through other children

f) Talking through toys, puppets or animals

a) Taking the pressure off

When SM is recognised early, sometimes all that is needed is to remove the need to talk and show the child you enjoy being with them, whether they talk or not. You gain their trust by being positive about their efforts and achievements, holding back on questions, and conveying no disapproval. This approach requires time with the child on a one-to-one basis, either at nursery or through one or more home visits. Box 10.1 (page 181) describes how to prepare for a home visit, ways to interact with the child and some suitable activities.

b) Talking through the parent

Parents can provide a useful talking bridge, as explained in Chapter 9 (page 154). This technique can be used very informally when parents visit the preschool setting or during a home visit, as shown in Table 9.1 (page 151). If a child does not speak spontaneously, subsequent home visits can gradually help them speak to a member of staff, as described on Handout 13 'Easing in friends and relatives'.

c) The informal Sliding-in Technique

Another way to take advantage of a parent's reassuring presence is to work with them in the preschool setting. It is always a good idea to encourage parental attendance, as suggested on Handouts 9 and 10a.

> When Emma was three years old she was so lucky to have an amazing teacher at her nursery class. As soon as the teacher heard about Emma's difficulty talking she invited us round to her house for tea, putting no pressure on her to speak and letting her have a lovely time exploring her garden. She then joined us for an afternoon at the beach with her own children a couple of weeks before term started. This made all the difference between me having the confidence to send Emma to nursery and keeping her at home.

Box 10.1: Home visits for younger children

Home visits are a good way to break down the barrier between home and school because most children who have SM are comfortable talking with close family members at home. The following strategies often lead to some talking, either directly to or in front of the visitor.

- Prepare for the initial visit by explaining to the parent that:
    - it will be a very informal and relaxed visit
    - it may be helpful to occupy the child with a favourite activity before you arrive, so that you can show interest while you chat to the parent to begin with
    - it works best to talk to the child as they would do normally but don't try to get the child to talk to you, or be embarrassed if they don't talk.

- Suggest that the parent tells the child in advance that:
    - you are coming round to play and get to know them
    - they may talk if they want to but you won't mind if they don't.

- If appropriate, say that you know they have been a bit unhappy or worried about playgroup, nursery or school and you want to help make things better. During the visit ensure that there is no pressure on the child to talk:
    - give them the opportunity by talking in commentary style (see page 122) but don't ask them questions other than through their parent (see page 180)
    - if the child seems very anxious, find an excuse to pull back for a while and allow the child time to relax with their parent
    - don't show surprise or praise the child when they talk – just enjoy it!

- Helpful activities include:
    - showing the 'visitor' their toys or pet
    - listening while you read them a story
    - playing games which can include siblings
    - spending time in the garden to relax the child further by providing a less enclosed space and allowing more physical play.

As well as involving the parent in activities as part of the main group, it is important to allow the parent and child enough space to play on their own because the child will find it easier to speak at these times. If available, somewhere like the home corner, book area or even the staff kitchen can be useful to provide a little more privacy. Once the child is able to talk to the parent on this basis, an agreed member of staff can gradually approach until the child can tolerate their presence, as described on Handout 15. This informal version of the Sliding-in Technique can also be carried out in the child's home. It is recommended for children aged five and under.

d) Shaping (from gesture to sounds to talking)

Shaping is very successful with young children aged 3 to 5 years and is a useful way to help children talk to staff members because it doesn't need a parent to be present. After initial rapport building with a designated adult (see Table 8.1, page 124), the child works through a progression of informal activities which facilitate a gradual increase in communication from gesture to sounds to speech. These activities are presented as an opportunity to *play* with the adult, rather than a time to talk. They are done in a quiet area without interruptions, on a one-to-one basis.

Table 10.2 opposite shows how the adult can move the child forward, alongside the target behaviours which indicate the child's readiness to move on to the next stage. If there is another child at the setting who the child with SM talks to, it may be advantageous to include them in some of the games to act as a 'go-between' (see the next section, 'Talking through other children').

> Davey was too nervous to talk to his Mum around other people at playgroup but he was happy to go with me and nod and shake his head. We set them up with a small table in the kitchen and, once he was talking to Mum, we warned him that I would need to pop in very quickly while he was playing. I smiled and waved at him as I went in but didn't look at them after that.
>
> The first time, Davey was quiet but, by the third time, he carried on talking to his Mum as usual. I was really pleased but remembered not to comment. Later on, I said it looked like a lovely game, and maybe next time I could watch a bit longer to learn how to play it.
>
> We progressed from me watching from the other side of the room to me joining them at the table. I couldn't believe it when I asked if I could join in and Davey gave me a toy dinosaur and said 'You have that one!'
>
> (An early years member of staff tries out the informal Sliding-in Technique)

Aim to organise a play session three or four times a week, lasting 10 to 20 minutes, and invite the child to choose or bring their own games to play. There is no formal target setting; the designated adult simply keeps a record of progress, perhaps using Progress chart 1 for an overall summary and Progress chart 3 for a daily record. As the child talks to the adult, other children or adults can be included in the sessions.

e) Talking through other children

If the child has friends in the preschool setting who they talk to easily in other settings, these friends can be used as a bridge to talking to a new adult (see Table 10.3 on page 185). Some young children who have SM will start speaking spontaneously to the new adult when they reach Stage 4, in which case the rest of the progression can be abandoned.

f) Talking through toys, puppets or animals

Encourage children to bring a pet or favourite toy they talk to in other settings. Invite the child who has SM to involve them in various activities, eg 'Show Fluffy what to do' or 'You can put Teddy to bed and read him a story'. Given space away from the watchful eyes of adults, some children will begin to talk to their companion and gradually allow an adult to join in their play. It helps if the adult addresses the toy or pet initially, rather than the child. When the child talks comfortably to their toy or pet in front of the adult, the adult can ask the toy or pet simple questions to see if the child answers, eg 'Fluffy, would you like fish or chicken for dinner?'

Table 10.2: **Confident talking – establishing speech with young children on a one-to-one basis using informal shaping activities**

Stage	Child's presentation	Target behaviours
3	Uses non-verbal communication	For the adult to create the *opportunity* for the child to talk, rather than the demand or expectation. See Table 8.1 (page 124).
Talking bridge (runs *alongside* Stage 5)	Tolerates voice being heard	For the adult to: • tell the child that talking often feels a bit difficult to start with, so they might like to try songs and story-time noises with the other children instead • encourage the child to bring in toys or animals which they talk to at home. Ask the toy or animal questions, rather than the child, and talk *for* the toy or animal, showing no surprise if the child joins in and talks too • encourage the parents to have fun with the child at home using, eg, a Talking Tin or Talking Photo Album to record their voices (see Appendix F 'Talking resources'). For the child to do one or more of the following: • sing, chant or make noises in unison with other children (animal noises, sound of wind, fireworks, siren, etc) • talk to a favourite toy or pet in the preschool setting • play a voice recording made at home.
5	Produces sound and voice	For the adult to create the opportunity for the child to say a sound or repeated phrase by *pausing for several seconds* before carrying on (the adult *does not ask* or encourage the child to copy): • read the child a story with accompanying sounds, eg 'The little mouse said 'Eek!' The little mouse said _____' If no response, the adult says 'Eek!' and carries on • read stories with repeated phrases such as 'Oh no!' to see if the child joins in the chanted phrase or continues after a pause • make noises during pretend play, eg 'Shhhh' (rock the baby doll), 'brmm!' (toy car), 'psss!' (open a fizzy drink) • introduce a toy which can only speak in sounds, eg 'He's trying to say fork. This is a "f-or-k"'. This is a "f_____"' • include the child in early phonics work by saying 'The tap says_____' rather than 'What sound does the tap make?' If there is no response, the adult says 't' and carries on. For the child to do two or more of the following: • laugh audibly • make audible sounds using musical instruments, straws and body parts (eg clapping, tapping, blowing, sucking) • make animal or transport noises (eg hiss like a snake, meow, squeak, roar, engine sounds, horn or siren) • hum, eg play a kazoo, or join in an action song by humming the rhythm • say letter sounds, eg *d* for 'drum', *t* for 'tap' • join in with familiar songs, rhymes, or repeated phrases with an adult.
6	Uses single words to communicate with adult	For the adult to: • ask occasional 'X or Y?' questions during shared activities, eg 'Who do you want to be now? Superman or Batman?', 'Shall we make pizza or a cake?' These should be *genuine* questions, rather than questions that test the child's knowledge, such as 'Is that a horse or a cow?' • read a familiar book and encourage sentence completion by pausing, eg 'Bobo's hiding, he's in the _____?' If there is no response after 5 seconds, the adult finishes the sentence and carries on

(Continued)

Table 10.2: *Continued*

Stage	Child's presentation	Target behaviours
		• make deliberate mistakes, eg 'This one goes in the bedroom!' and wait several seconds. If there is no response, continue with an 'X or Y?' question, eg 'Oh no it doesn't! Let's see, does it go in the kitchen or the bathroom?' For the child to respond with single words in one-to-one fun activities such as book sharing, pretend play, games and crafts.
7	Uses sentences to communicate with adult	For the adult to: • read a familiar book and pause for several seconds mid-sentence to encourage the child to continue • use 'I wonder' statements during play and wait several seconds before continuing, eg 'I wonder where this goes?' • 'lose' things and see whether the child says where they are, eg 'Oh dear, where did I put my glasses? I can't see them …' • encourage the child to talk to their toys, eg 'Teddy doesn't know how to get dressed, does he? Can you tell him what to do?' If there is no response, start it off, eg 'Teddy, put your vest on' • gradually ask questions starting 'Who / What / Which / Where', etc. For the child to respond with phrases or sentences.
8	Connected speech or conversation	For the adult to: • encourage the child to help a new child or a friend who's not sure what to do • ask the child to bring a favourite book (one they know off by heart and love to 'read' to parents) and see whether they can 'read' it to the adult • ask the child to bring in a collection of objects from home (ideally belonging to various family members) and go through them, telling the adult about each object • make the child 'teacher' or 'mummy' and become a 'child' who has to be told what to do. The adult keeps getting it wrong, eg sits on the floor instead of the chair. For the child to: • begin to make spontaneous comments • talk freely during free play or a creative activity (this may be more of a running commentary than directed to the adult, but the child is not fazed when the adult asks a question) • string a few sentences together, eg tell a story or give the adult instructions in a structured game or activity.
Note: see Appendix A (online) for games and activities to adapt to an age-appropriate level.		

Table 10.3: **Confident talking – establishing speech on a one-to-one basis through friends the child talks to easily**

Stage	Child's presentation	Target behaviours
3	Happy to communicate non-verbally to adult and talks to friends out of sight or earshot	For the adult to: • discourage friends from answering for the child by saying, eg 'It's OK Richard, Jimi can tell me by nodding or shaking his head (or pointing)' • give the child space to spend time with friend(s) they talk to at home, away from the adult's gaze • make it 'safe' to talk, eg 'It's OK, you don't need to talk to the grown-ups yet, I know it feels difficult at the moment. You can just talk to Richard, like you do at home'; 'You two can tell each other what you want to build while I go and sort out the drinks'; 'Jimi, can you look for Richard outside and tell him I've found his robot?' • demonstrate that it's fine to use friend(s) as a go-between, eg 'Jimi, tell Richard if you get stuck and he'll let me know'; 'Richard, can you ask Jimi what he wants to drink and then come and tell me?' • engage the child and their friend(s) in turn-taking games where the child does not need to speak (see Appendix A, Stage 3). For the child to: • build rapport with a designated adult (Table 8.1, page 124) • talk to friend(s) at the setting, even if they are away from the main group.
Talking bridge	Tolerates voice being heard	For the adult to continue as above but in closer proximity to the child. The adult ensures the child's comfort by: • not watching the child closely • appearing to be occupied with other things • not reacting when the child talks to friend(s). For the child to talk to friend(s) in the adult's presence (voice is audible rather than whispered).
4	Talks to adult through friend in the adult's presence	For the adult to facilitate talk through a friend *when both children are present* and ensure their comfort by keeping other observers or listeners to a minimum: • ask occasional questions through a friend, eg 'Your turn now, Jimi! Richard, can you ask Jimi if he wants the bike or the scooter?' • ask the child to talk to a friend in a structured turn-taking game (see Appendix A, Stage 4), eg 'We take it in turns to pick a card and tell the person next to us which picture to find to make a pair. I'll tell Jimi; Jimi, you can tell Richard; and Richard, you tell me'. For the child to answer a question repeated by a friend or participate in a turn-taking game, addressing their friend rather than the adult.
5	Uses voice with adult (This stage is optional: it may be fleeting or bypassed)	For the adult to maintain focus on fun and validation of the child's contributions, without directly referring to the fact that the child has spoken in their presence. For the child to interact directly with the adult by laughing audibly or making sounds in their throat (often behind closed lips), eg makes a sound and shakes their head to indicate 'No, not that one!'
6	Uses single words to communicate with adult	For the adult to: • reverse direction of turn-taking games so the child addresses the adult rather than their friend • ask the child occasional questions during play with their friend (see Table 9.1 for progression and examples) • play games without the friend's support (see Appendix A, Stage 6). For the child to address and/or answer the adult using a single word.
7	Uses sentences to communicate with adult	As for Table 9.1.

Adults may also introduce a toy or puppet and speak for them, using a different voice – the funnier the better! Speaking for this toy, the adult can address the child directly or talk to the child's toy or puppet. It may feel much 'safer' for the child to answer this new character, who comes without any associations of expectation to interact. Once the child is talking to the new character, the adult can gradually use their normal voice too, to create a three-way conversation as described under (e) 'Talking through other children' on page 182.

Some children use a toy to express themselves, referring to themselves in the third person, eg 'Faye wants a biscuit', despite using 'I' correctly at home. This shows that the child wants to communicate but is not ready for direct and unrestricted conversation. In addition to accepting this interim step and responding via the toy (eg 'See if Faye would like one of these'), the adult should take the opportunity to reassure the child, again through their toy. For example, 'Please tell Faye it's OK if she wants to ask me for a biscuit herself. I know she's not ready to talk a lot and that's fine. She only needs to talk when she feels happy about it.'

Talking to children

There are six ways to help children talk to a new child.

1   **Play dates.** Staff can give parents ideas of who to invite home or to the park with their child, to provide a more comfortable setting for the child who has SM to develop their talking (see Chapter 9, 'Talking to children').

2   **Choice of play materials.** Playing with walkie-talkies or Talking Tubes (see Appendix F 'Talking resources') may enable the child who has SM to communicate with others by putting a helpful distance between them. Similarly, using masks and puppets detracts attention from the child and may make it easier for them to speak.

3   **Providing private spaces.** Children can often chat more easily to another child if they are out of sight of others, eg in or behind a tent, book corner, screen or bookcase, home corner or fort made of large cardboard boxes or four sides of crenellated cardboard. This might be possible in the playground too, in a tunnel or under climbing apparatus, or simply in a den against the fence under some material or coats.

4   **Involving other children in jobs.** Jobs and errands such as washing hands or paint brushes, tidying the book corner or taking the register to the office are good informal activities which children can do in pairs. Involve parents where possible as these informal and sometimes brief times may enable a child who has SM to talk in front of or to another child.

5   **Involving other children in games.** Once the child is comfortable talking to parents or a staff member in a corner of the classroom or playground, another child can be invited to join in.

6   **The Triangle Tactic.** This is a very informal way of helping the child talk to a new friend. The technique is used when an adult can speak to two children individually, but the children don't yet speak to each other. See page 155 and Figure 9.4 (page 156) for details, substituting the adult who the child talks to in the early years setting for 'parent'.

Talking to strangers

This area is more appropriately covered by parents – see Chapter 9, page 161.

The model of confident talking: group participation

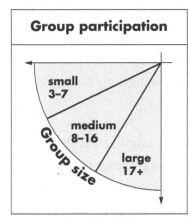

Having gradually increased the number of adults and peers who the child can talk to, they may be used to talking in small groups of three (parent, adult and child; or adult and two children) but be daunted by larger groups. This can be facilitated in the following ways.

a)   Parents or staff can gradually include one extra child at a time in games and activities with the child, and vary the group participants. Once children have talked with at least half of the class, they will be much more inclined to join in whole-class activities.

b)   Roll-call can be managed by self-registration, a wave or talking in unison (see Handouts 9 and 10a which were discussed in Chapter 8).

c)   Circle time can be managed by providing advance warning of the turn-taking activity and giving the child a non-verbal way to participate. For example, the child 'tells' their news by bringing in a clue and the other children guess what they have done while the child nods or shakes their head. Even better, the child records their contribution at home and plays it during circle time (see Appendix F 'Voice-recording devices' for suitable products).

d)   Encourage the child to bring in a toy containing a message they have recorded using a mini-recorder and play this individually to the other children and adults. Alternatively, they could use the toy in a puppet show so that everyone hears their voice (see Appendix F 'Voice-recording devices').

e)   Ask groups of children to speak in unison whenever possible to balance out individual turn-taking activities which are difficult for children who have SM. Make it 'safe' for children to speak or sing in unison by saying, 'I know that talking on your own is a bit too scary at the moment, but it's OK to sing or join in with the others if you want to'. Try not to watch the child too closely to see whether they join in. When they think that their voice will be drowned out by the others, and no one is looking, they will test the water! And, although you will be thrilled when they do, praise the *whole* group for their wonderful singing, farmyard noises, nursery rhymes, etc, rather than just the individual child

f)   When reading stories to groups of children, engage the child who has SM with actions and objects, rather than asking questions. Again, get the group talking in unison as much as possible; books with repeating lines are ideal for this. (Search the internet for 'books with repeating lines' or 'repetitive texts' for inspiration!) Rebecca Bergman's *Stories for Talking* (2008) sets out clearly differentiated language levels so that children who do not yet talk can get as involved as the chatty ones by focusing on comprehension tasks initially (see Appendix F 'Talking resources').

School settings

The advice given in 'Early years settings' may be all that some five to six year olds need; and home visits (page 179) are useful at any age for initial introductions and for students who are home-schooled or planning a return to educational settings.

This section describes:

1   The formal approach of structured small-steps programmes which many school-aged children need to address persistent levels of anxiety, particularly when their difficulties have been poorly understood in the past.

2   Informal approaches which may be enough to help children work through their difficulties, particularly when SM is caught early and handled sympathetically from the start, and when students are making an actively managed fresh start (see page 247). In other cases, they provide a useful stop-gap while putting small-steps programmes in place, and should continue as an agreed part of the overall programme.

Small-steps programmes – general principles for effective implementation

The techniques to establish and generalise speech are based on the behavioural principles of graded exposure. So, first, it is vital to ensure that the psychology and organisation of successful small-steps behavioural programmes are understood and observed. If the guidance in this section is followed, children who have SM can be expected to make good progress. If problems arise, please see Chapter 12 'Troubleshooting: why isn't it working?

Finding a keyworker

First, find a suitable person to take the role of keyworker – someone to take the main responsibility for establishing and generalising the child's talking in school, by working through targets on a regular basis. Keyworkers may be experienced professionals or willing volunteers, but some people are better suited than others, as Box 10.2 indicates. Although the task may be daunting at first, the best understanding of SM undoubtedly comes through experience as a keyworker. School staff who have successfully taken on the role frequently report that few teaching experiences have been as rewarding.

Sometimes a keyworker cannot be provided and a parent has to take the role. This is not ideal because it is a formal role which benefits from a degree of detachment which does not always feel comfortable for child or parent. Yet it can be done, particularly when children are younger and generally more amenable to parent visits to their school. Success relies on a good working relationship with the school because parents will need the same flexibility and influence as a school-based keyworker.

Length and frequency of sessions

Structured small-steps programme sessions to establish talking should generally be 10 to 15 minutes long and take place a *minimum* of three times a week to keep up the momentum. Positive learning requires frequent repetition and reinforcement. If infrequent, the targets achieved can be wasted because of the need to backtrack completely each session to get to where you were before. Older children and young people can tolerate and benefit from longer sessions to tackle specific targets, but they still need to meet more than once a week if building on previous targets.

Box 10.2: What makes a good keyworker?

A good keyworker is someone who:

✓ Has a good understanding of the principles underlying the development and treatment of selective mutism.

✓ Has a relaxed temperament and the ability to convey a calm, positive attitude even when they feel anxious, frustrated or disappointed (all of which are bound to occur at some point).

✓ Is able to make mistakes, have fun and and laugh at themselves.

✓ Is liked and trusted by the child.

✓ Makes the child feel that this respect is mutual.

✗ Does not take it personally when the child does not speak or cooperate, but empathises with the child's anxiety, and considers ways of reducing the anxiety another time.

✗ Does not get too emotionally involved or possessive.

✓ Asks for help whenever needed.

✓ Celebrates the child's success, even if this means letting go.

Fixed times for the sessions give the child greater control over their anxiety and facilitate risk taking as the end is always in sight. Set a timer or show the finish time on a clock.

Linking the work to the child's priorities

Perserverance and success are likely to be greater if programmes incorporate and work towards the child's interests and priorities. See Chapter 5 for how these can be elicited during assessment and examples of how they were used in the treatment programme.

Getting children to sort, rank or rate people or situations during the programme can also be important, to help you plan what should be done next. This also reassures the child that you are taking their preferences and perspective into account. For examples of sorting, ranking and rating activities, see Figures 5.6 and 5.7 (pages 89 and 91).

Fully involving the child while providing a clear lead

Good communication with the child is important for good progress but too much detail can be overwhelming. While it is important to give an overview of the programme (eg 'We can gradually help you talk to one person at a time'), it is best to then focus on just one goal at a time, such as talking to the keyworker or reading with a small group of peers. Tell the child exactly what is involved at each step, planning targets around their interests and priorities whenever possible (see above).

Note, however, that when working with anxious individuals, it is counterproductive to expect them to set their own targets: contemplating situations they have previously avoided creates too much anxiety for them to think clearly about what is and isn't possible. Children need to feel confident that the keyworker knows how to help, and this is best demonstrated through clear guidance, that is: 'You're ready for this now', rather than 'What do you think we should do next?'

However, having steered children in a certain direction, it is good to offer *choices* as appropriate. For example, say 'You're ready to have a friend join in now – is there someone you'd like to choose?' or 'Would you like it to be [X] or [Y]?' Let them select from the register or photos if necessary.

Setting suitable targets

A successful programme has only one target (or small step) to work on at a time, whether this is set by the keyworker within a session or given to a child for homework. Once this is achieved another is added, so the child is never looking too far ahead at one time.

Small-step progressions are created by changing only one variable at a time, for example:

★ the choice of person present

★ the proximity or seating position of the person present

★ the number of people present, either as part of the task or hovering in the background

★ the direction of turn taking (is the child addressing a familiar or new person?)

★ the extent of physical involvement (articulatory effort, eye contact, gesture, movement or touch)

★ the length of the task (keep it short and specific rather than open-ended, eg 'read five words' or 'read for one minute', rather than 'read to me')

★ the nature and 'risk level' of the task itself (see Table 10.4 at the end of this section for the categorisation of activities into low, medium and high risk).

There is no requirement to achieve a set number of targets within a session; the child simply continues until time runs out or they need a break. There are specific examples of small-steps programme targets in Appendix C.

Starting each session with a 'warm-up'

If a specific target is achieved in a session through a series of small steps, children cannot be expected to start the next session at the same point. We recommend backtracking and repeating two steps before moving forward. The confidence gained saves time in the long run.

When children are working on a new goal, such as talking to a different person or in a different place, it is not possible to backtrack and repeat targets. The warm-up is then provided by running through the chosen activity beforehand either with the keyworker alone or in the usual setting, so that the child is prepared for what is coming up.

Once children can speak spontaneously, they will not need warm-up activities to speak to that person again – even after a break of several weeks or months.

Keeping a record of achievements

Children will be encouraged by keeping a clear record of what they have *achieved*, rather than a daunting 'To Do' list to work through. Younger children can mark each target achieved with a tick, star or sticker, while older children might add an index card to a personalised storage box. The only time children are presented with several targets at once is when they are familiar with a technique and repeating it to generalise to other people. A computer print-out might then be used to remind them of the plan. There are examples of children's recording systems in Appendix C.

Note that the use of attractive stickers to record progress is not the same as a reward system. Stickers simply add to the fun and help to make the sessions more enjoyable.

Using rewards as incentives

When a child reaches a target, that success will be its own reward if the rationale of the programme has been explained and the child is clear about the benefits. And if the child has a good relationship with their keyworker, just spending time together will be enjoyable and validating. It should, therefore, not be necessary to provide external motivation through rewards. Indeed, introducing rewards can add an unnecessary *pressure*, and emphasise how much the adult wants the child to succeed. However, it is good to reward hard work and effort, rather than talking itself. We recommend using rewards to celebrate achievement, rather than to increase motivation or appeal to a child to behave in a certain way. For example:

★ 'You've been working so hard, I thought we'd have a treat today!'

★ 'I had such good fun with you yesterday, this is to say "thank you".'

★ 'You're doing so well, how shall we celebrate when you've filled another sticker chart?'

Introducing the right person at the right time

Care must be taken to introduce new people at the appropriate time. For example, if the child has little rapport with a particular member of staff, or sees them as an authority figure, or is afraid to fail or wants to succeed almost too much, their anxiety level may be too high to allow any techniques to be successful initially. They will gain more confidence if they are first helped to speak to a less 'threatening' adult or child. Similarly, the child may have strong associations of failure with their current teacher, having tried to speak and failed on many occasions. In this case, it may be better to develop their communication with a classroom support worker in the first instance, and work towards generalising speech to a different teacher in the next year group.

Checking the child's anxiety during the session

Use quick checks to monitor the child's level of anxiety or relaxation during sessions. For example, use an anxiety rating system, such as a numbered scale, or a set of 'happy to glum' faces or raising one to five fingers (see Figure 8.3, page 126). This is vital feedback about how the child is managing and indicates to them that you are factoring this in to your programme planning. Once adults have a greater insight into each child's set of anxiety triggers, they will be in a better position to modify their interactions with the child and plan appropriate support.

Ensuring that the child uses an audible voice

A whispered voice is only ever set as a target for voiceless sounds such as 's' and 't' in a shaping programme. The child must use an audible voice to achieve talking targets, however quiet that may be. Occasional reminders to 'use your brave voice' or 'switch your voice on' may be necessary but, generally, the programmes are set up to ensure anxiety is low enough to permit voice. Volume then usually increases naturally as short manageable tasks are achieved, anxiety dissipates, and the child relaxes and breathes more deeply. If necessary, activities involving silly noises and humming can help, likewise blindfold or barrier games in which the keyworker can't lip-read and says 'Pardon?' when unable to hear.

Coping with unachieved targets

Children should *never* be allowed to feel that they have failed – only that their anxiety was too great to allow them to succeed. The keyworker's job is to make the steps towards a challenging target smaller, so it is easier for the child to manage. This can either be done immediately, with a shorter or simpler task, or by ending the session early with a very casual 'Let's stop there. I can see it's difficult. It's OK, we'll try again next time'. An experienced keyworker will use both of these options to the child's advantage, but less experienced keyworkers are advised to opt for early termination. This provides breathing space and planning time. It also means the child will feel disappointed that the session is over (assuming they have a good relationship with their keyworker), rather than relieved that the pressure is off.

Sometimes it is impossible to make a target any smaller and 'all' that is stopping the child succeeding is their panic associated with uncharted territory. Extra strength and determination are needed to push through the fear barrier. This is when the experience of ending a session early can help, to create the drive that is needed to reattempt and achieve the target, thus ensuring that the session continues.

For this reason it is vital that programme sessions are not filled with unchallenging fun activities when targets get too difficult. Many children will naturally attempt less and less when they know that their time with the keyworker is secure, whether they achieve their targets or not.

In our experience, a session has never been terminated more than twice after the same target, and children have succeeded on the third attempt. However, we must emphasise that this is done only when it is certain that the target cannot be made any smaller. Even when terminating a session early, ensure that the child finishes 'on a high', with a focus on something they have done well (for example, completed the warm-up activities at breakneck speed!).

Table 10.4: **Classification of activities by level of risk (anxiety load)**

Risk	Single-word activities	Sentence-level activities
Low	*Rote speech:* counting; days of the week; months of the year; letters of the alphabet (spoken on a turn-taking basis, each person says one item at a time, initially, and then two or more items at a time). *Factual speech:* answer questions with 'yes' or 'no' (eg 'Can babies fly?'); answer 'X or Y?' questions (eg 'Is grass green or purple?').	*Rote speech:* counting; days of the week; months of the year; letters of the alphabet (recited initially on a turn-taking basis, each person saying several items at a time, in sequence. Later, the child recites the sequence alone.). Sing or talk in unison; say repetitive 'catch lines' in stories or rhymes. Rehearsed speech (eg lines in a play). *Factual speech:* simple sentence completion or word pairs (eg 'fish and chips'). *Reading aloud:* familiar material (for confident readers); take part in reading a play. *Structured turn-taking:* play games such as 'Battleships' or 'Guess Who?'.
Medium low	*Factual speech:* name simple pictures (eg play 'Pairs'); complete stock phrases or sentences with a single word (eg 'You sit on a _____?', 'hot and _____?', 'table and _____?'). *Reading aloud:* simple single words; answer questions by finding answers in the text (confident readers); play 'Word Dominoes'.	*Factual speech:* provide a definition or describe a picture so that others can identify the word; answer questions which require a simple phrase or sentence. *Semi-structured turn-taking:* play simple request games (eg 'Fish', 'Happy Families'). *Reading aloud:* pair up cards to make a sentence, rhyme or question/answer; read a sentence and supply the missing word; read out and solve crossword puzzle clues. *Personal information:* provide details such as full name, age, date of birth, address, telephone number, school, name of teacher.
Medium high	*Factual speech:* answer easy questions without a picture reference (eg 'How old are you?'); give an item from a category (eg colours, food, animals). *Reading aloud:* identify the missing word in a sentence: order words to make a sentence (for confident readers). *Likes and dislikes:* give favourite item from a category (eg colour, drink, car, recording artist); repeat with least favourite or 'worst ever' item.	*Semi-structured turn-taking:* play games requiring questions and reasoning (eg 'Hedbanz', 'Twenty Questions'); give directions to complete an activity; follow directions and seek clarification when unclear what to do. *Social routines:* say 'Thank you', 'Yes, it is', 'No, I haven't', 'I'm not sure', 'No, I don't know', etc, rather than nod, shake head, shrug or say a simple 'Yes' or 'No'. *Connected speech:* give detailed instructions on 'How to ...' (eg make a sandwich, catch a fish, fly a kite, get ready for bed, add sound to a PowerPoint presentation). *Unplanned speech:* answer unexpected questions.
High	*Thinking skills:* eg play 'Word Strings', riddles. *Guessing games:* eg 'I-Spy', 'Hangman'. *Reading aloud:* difficult words (for underconfident readers); sound out and blend words. *Initiation:* call out, eg 'Snap!', 'Bingo!', 'Stop!' *Social routines:* say 'bye', 'hi' or 'hello', 'please'.	*Conversation:* initiate contact or requests; ask for help; correct mistakes; negotiate. *Verbal reasoning:* inference and deduction; alternative solutions; explanations. *Personal contributions:* tell jokes; share opinions, fears, frustrations, wishes. *Unstructured turn-taking:* play games such as 'Don't Say It!', 'Give Us a Clue', 'Sussed!'. *Connected speech:* talk for 30 seconds about a favourite film, television programme or hobby, or on a topic such as 'My Family'.
Notes		

⚠️

- When devising a programme to elicit and develop speech, start in the top left-hand box and progress *across* and *down*, never diagonally.
- Select one or more activities from each box according to age, ability and interests – there is no need to complete them all.
- Including an extra person, background audience or time pressure will add to the anxiety load.
- Leave high-risk activities until last and return to easier activities when introducing another person or change of location.

See Appendix A (online) for details about individual, group and whole-class activities.

The model of confident talking: range of people

The hope is that children who have SM will eventually talk to *everyone* in their school setting but, realistically, it will be important to identify and focus initially on key staff and a few classmates. Progress chart 1 (online) can be used to record overall progress, having entered their names in the top row (see the example on page 233). This chart is for staff information only and should not be shared with the child, as explained in Chapter 9 (page 150). Parents may also like to keep a separate record for contacts outside school.

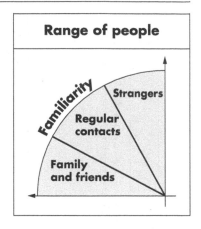

Informal strategies

In addition to the small-steps programmes which follow, there are three informal strategies that all members of staff need to be aware of and use with caution, as detailed below.

a)   Using parents or friends as go-betweens

b)   Graded questioning

c)   The Triangle Tactic

These strategies must be used at private moments with the child, and not in front of the whole class. For example: in a parent–teacher consultation meeting; in a group discussion in a corner of the library; or in a one-to-one interaction on the sidelines of the sports field. The first strategy may allow children to feel sufficiently comfortable to speak to others in the staff member's presence. This step, if handled appropriately, often leads to direct communication. The second strategy involves establishing good rapport with the child, carefully monitoring their anxiety level, and gradually introducing a series of question prompts as their anxiety decreases. Once the child can speak to a particular member of staff, the third strategy can be used to help them talk to another adult or peer.

Success depends on the child knowing that their difficulty talking is understood, and believing that, for as long as they need, they may communicate in other ways when this is more comfortable; for example by speaking through other people or writing. If they are afraid that speaking to one individual will bring an immediate expectation to talk to other people in other situations, there is a strong chance that they will remain silent.

The effects of these informal strategies are not necessarily seen immediately: patience and consistency are required. They are particularly effective during extended periods of one-to-one interaction. For example:

★   A teacher picked up a young child who had SM from home and accompanied her to school each day until she was settled. Within months, the child was talking freely at school.

★   A classroom assistant built rapport with a girl aged 10 during the summer holidays in the local park, initially with the girl's mother present. Their relaxed conversation assisted a gradual generalisation to other people when the child returned to school.

★ Work experience with the school groundsman enabled a teenager to speak at school for the first time.

★ A college student was taken under the librarian's wing and developed an interest in archiving alongside building his confidence in talking.

a) Using parents or friends as go-betweens

This approach is detailed in Table 9.1, Stages 0–4 (page 151), and earlier in this chapter, 'Talking through other children' (page 182).

Having asked a question through a parent or a friend who the child talks to, it is always best to avert eye contact; for example, say to the parent 'Perhaps you could ask Peter now which subject he prefers?', then look down and appear to be busy with notes. Make sure that parents are also aware of the strategy and simply ask their child the question, rather than telling their child to reply to you. Once children are comfortable talking in front of you, the next strategy has even more chance of success.

b) Graded questioning

Staff members who see the child regularly should slowly and gradually build rapport as part of their everyday interactions and systematically change their questioning style, as indicated in Table 9.1 (page 151) and Figure 9.2 (page 153). Although this strategy can be used by any staff member, it is important not to overwhelm the child with too much attention. The progression must move at the child's pace, only going up a level as the child responds at each stage, with relaxed body language and steady voice.

For example, once a child talks comfortably to their friends in your presence, or responds good-humouredly to rhetorical questions such as 'OK, shall we just say that art is not my best subject?!', you can try asking 'X or Y?' questions such as 'So is the answer nearer 20 or 200?' *It is extremely important to do this out of earshot of other people.* After all, the child has been assured that they will not be picked out to answer questions in class at this stage, unless they volunteer. In the initial stages at least, *ask questions that the child can answer easily.*

After asking a question, look away and slowly count to five. If the child answers, carry on calmly as if talking was the most natural thing in the world. If they don't answer, move the conversation on without any hint of displeasure or disappointment; for example, say 'Once you've decided, the answer goes here'. Either way, return to commentary-style talk for a while (page 122) and make sure the child is completely relaxed before trying again. If you are confident that the child is on the verge of speaking, repeat the original question once more and count to five again, to give them another chance to respond, eg 'What do you reckon – 20 or 200?'

 It is important to monitor the child's reaction to being asked questions. If there are signs of increased anxiety or avoidance (eg no eye contact or missed lessons), the strategy should be ended while the overall plan is reviewed and alternatives are considered.

c) The Triangle Tactic

The Triangle Tactic can help children to speak to each other for the first time without the need for a formal session outside the classroom. It needs to be managed carefully with a peer who the child with

SM feels comfortable with, in places away from public scrutiny, such as a corner of the library or the school playing field.

The Triangle Tactic also has the following advantages.

★ It helps to break the habit of other children speaking for the child.

★ It promotes generalisation after children have spoken to each other in structured activities (see page 201).

★ It is a good way to facilitate group discussion in general, with children, teenagers and adults alike.

See page 155 and Figure 9.4 (page 156) for details (the facilitating adult takes the parent role).

Talking to the keyworker using a small-steps programme

If children who have SM have not spoken after a few sessions of rapport building, or during the first few weeks of term at a new school, *it is not wise to wait and hope for the breakthrough which may never come.* A small-steps programme using a specific technique will fast track progress and enable them to talk to a keyworker who can then help them to generalise their talking to other people, as discussed in 'Generalising to other adults and children' (page 200) and 'Group participation' (page 202).

Practitioners may train staff in educational settings to use the following techniques, or they may use a technique themselves to enter the child's comfort zone before handing over to a school-based keyworker, or supporting a student through the transition to a new setting.

a) The Sliding-in Technique

b) The reading route

c) Lone talking

d) Telephone programmes

e) Shaping (moving from non-verbal communication to sounds to talking)

The choice of technique depends on the availability and commitment of staff and parents, access to a restricted area and the child's age and anxiety level. With children up to about 15 years old we don't normally provide a choice. Instead, we introduce the method that seems most viable, explaining how it can help them speak without anxiety and when we are going to start. But, as children get older, once they understand they are dealing with a phobia of talking, we would explain the various choices and help them weigh up the pros and cons.

a) The Sliding-in Technique

The Sliding-in Technique was first documented in 2001 in the first edition of this manual. It remains our usual method of choice when children persistently freeze, whisper or produce a very unnatural voice when trying to speak. This is because, for most children, it creates least anxiety (see 'Graded exposure' at the start of this chapter, page 176). It relies on a parent, or other talking partner from the child's comfort zone, being available to work regularly with a keyworker and on the child being comfortable to work with their parent. This isn't always the case; older children, for example, might be embarrassed about their parent coming in to the school. An alternative is to carry out the technique at home, or over the telephone, as explained below.

Wherever the Sliding-in Technique is used, it is important to find a quiet room which is free from interruptions (put a 'Do Not Disturb' sign on the door if necessary). Another consideration is the time of day: if the room is on a busy corridor, where other students can be heard passing by, the child will be too aware of their presence to relax. The child's classroom can be used if no other children are around, before or after the main school day, for example.

It may take a total of 1 to 2 hours of target-setting time to help the child reach Stage 7 with the new person (use of sentences in a structured situation), so allow up to six 30-minute clinic or home-based sessions, or six to ten 10–15-minute sessions at school, over two to three weeks. Subsequent sessions may be needed to move towards spontaneous speech, as described later in this chapter. Experienced or confident keyworkers can 'slide' themselves in successfully in a single extended session. We favour this for older children (about 9 years upwards) who fully understand the rationale and have good rapport with the new adult. The single session can also work well for younger children who are in an environment where they feel comfortable and display little body tension. (See Appendix C, Example 1, in which a six-year-old boy spoke to two people for the first time within 30 minutes.)

 If it is impossible to find a room free from interruptions, consider using the building when it is empty for a single session (for example, during school holidays). This may also be easier for parents who have difficulty taking repeated time off work.

There are detailed instructions for the Sliding-in Technique on Handout 16 (online), along with Progress charts 3 and 4 to keep session notes and a record of overall progress. *The process is not complete until the parent or other talking partner 'slides out'*, ensuring that the child can talk independently to the new person.

b) The reading route

Reading aloud is usually the least daunting of verbal activities because the child does not have to worry about saying the wrong thing or being expected to enter the unpredictable and personal world of conversation. It is a method which can be used with or without a parent or other talking partner. It is also an excellent starting point for children who are competent readers and able to read aloud when on their own with a keyworker, *using a natural-sounding, albeit quiet voice*. As such, it represents a fairly quick route to establishing conversation, suitable for many older children or young people and children with 'low profile' SM. Once again, success depends on the child knowing that their difficulties are understood, and trusting that by reading aloud they will not suddenly be expected to speak any more than they feel comfortable with.

Young children may approach this route through reading groups, where children read the same text in unison and join in as best they can, following the text with their finger and saying whichever words they can manage. Alternatively, they may be happy to read aloud to a parent initially, with their teacher or keyworker listening in, either at school or on the telephone (see 'Telephone programmes' below).

Older children may be asked to read aloud after completing Form 8a or 8b, having rated reading aloud as less anxiety provoking than other activities. Some students may be relieved to be given a one-to-one reading assignment to replace a class presentation, while others will be willing to give reading a go after a period of rapport building and an explanation of their difficulties. Introduce the task by saying that you understand that certain things, like being asked unexpected questions, can be very difficult, but that reading aloud is usually easier because they won't need to find their own words to express themselves. Give them a short passage to read aloud, indicating where they should stop. It helps to sit beside them, rather than opposite, so that the child does not feel they are being scrutinised while they read.

Reading aloud represents a 'voice' target (Stage 5) in the stages of one-to-one interaction because it does not involve actual communication. Activities can be moved towards true communication in a few sessions, as described on Handout 18, starting with a familiar paragraph or piece of work which the child has looked at in advance. If the voice is whispered or strained, the child may start by reading aloud in an adjacent room (see 'Lone talking' below).

> Ty's first assignment was to prepare instructions to embed a moving image in my PowerPoint presentation. He did a great job and I followed his written commands while he watched, giving non-verbal feedback.
>
> His second assignment was to prepare instructions to install some freeware and to read them out so that I could concentrate on the laptop screen. This was the first time he spoke during our sessions.
>
> For his third assignment, I rang him for similar instructions which led to a more natural two-way exchange as I asked questions and tried to find the right part of the screen. After that, Ty spoke easily during our sessions.

c) Lone talking

Lone talking is an option when a talking partner is not available and the child cannot read aloud in the same room as the keyworker or practitioner. This method starts with counting or reading aloud in a normal speaking voice when alone, in a place where the child feels confident they will not be overheard. There are full details and suggested targets in Appendix B. Younger children could read aloud to a therapy dog or a much-loved pet.

In essence, once the child can tolerate the possibility of being overheard, steps 1 to 3 on Handout 18, 'The reading route', are carried out with the child in an adjacent room, with the door slightly open. Step 3 is then repeated while the adult slowly enters the room and joins the child. Steps 4 and 5 complete the process.

d) Telephone programmes

★ The remote talking route

This method helps children get used to talking to their parent, or another suitable talking partner, while a chosen person listens in on the phone. It has been used successfully by teachers to hear children read at home, for example, before transferring to the school setting. See Appendix B (online) for details.

★ The voicemail route

This method does not rely on an additional talking partner's involvement and progresses from telephone messages to face-to-face interaction as follows:

– text message, email or written word

– voice message (making and sending a voice recording)

– voicemail (calling and leaving a short message)

– telephone conversation

– face-to-face conversation.

Voicemail is closer to actual communication than voice messaging because it is 'live' and therefore more anxiety provoking. It relies on the recipient not inadvertently answering their phone, so texting may be useful to send advance warning. See Appendix B for details.

★ The Sliding-in Technique using telephone handsets

This works in the same way as the Sliding-in Technique – continuous talking using a low-risk turn-taking activity (counting) while the new person gradually approaches – but it can be done without a talking partner. It is also an alternative to lone talking for children who cannot talk in an adjacent room or when a private area cannot be found within a school. Younger children may benefit from a parent's support, but the main requirement is good rapport between the child or young person and new adult. See Handout 17 (online) for the details. By the end of the activity, the child will be able to count with the new adult in the same room. They can then continue with the standard Sliding-in Technique (Handout 16) or the reading route (Handout 18).

> Felix (aged 9) communicated well with me non-verbally, but stopped talking whenever I went into his house. He had told his Mum that he wanted to talk to me, so we started the Sliding-in Technique from my car at the end of his road. He and his Mum counted alternately to 20 and then his Mum rang me and switched their phone to loudspeaker. They repeated this with me listening. I then started 'one', his Mum said 'two', Felix said 'three', and so on, up to 10. We repeated this as I gradually approached his front door. I told Felix my starting point each time and he marked his progress with stickers on a map we had drawn. Soon I was in their hallway and, for the first time, Felix was using his voice, knowing I was in his house.

e) Shaping (moving from non-verbal communication to sounds to talking)

Although the gradual shaping approach from gesture to sounds to speech works well on an informal basis with children up to the age of five or six (page 183), we do not usually recommend it for small steps programmes with older, more anxious individuals. It takes much longer than the above approaches to build up to a single word. However, it may be useful if parents are not available and the child cannot read or talk aloud when on their own. Young people with long-standing SM may opt for shaping because the starting point of a single sound may be all that they can contemplate.

Desensitisation is an important part of shaping programmes. Children record themselves and become accustomed to the keyworker or the practitioner hearing their voice. For this reason it is possible to manage an entire shaping programme by email in the initial stages. The young person records sounds, syllables and words on their laptop, smartphone or tablet and emails the files to their keyworker. This requires great trust and the keyworker may need to assure the young person that they will delete the recording as soon as they have listened to it. This provides a useful alternative to face-to-face meetings when regular sessions or travel is difficult. For full details of the shaping approach, see Appendix B, with examples of targets in Appendix C.

Generalising to other adults and children

Once speech has been established to sentence level (Stage 7), the reading route, telephone targets or the Sliding-in Technique may be used or repeated to introduce other key adults and children. Ideally, a school-based keyworker will lead this generalisation process as the child's talking partner, but parents could take this role if a member of staff is not available.

The use of frequent stickers or ticks to acknowledge progress is quickly faded out during the generalisation phase. While it may help to repeat the same small steps and tangible acknowledgement with a key adult such as the child's teacher, this is neither necessary nor advisable with peers – not unless they *all* get a sticker at the end of the session. The child is familiar with the technique, so the generalisation target is to include a new person in an activity. Progress is acknowledged at the *end* of the session on a one-to-one basis.

After the child has spoken to each new person, it is very important for the keyworker to leave for part of the session, if only to get on with some work on the other side of the room, or to step outside for a few minutes. The child then completes an activity with the new person on their own. It is also useful to set a talking activity where the child and the new person start *without* the keyworker. This is particularly important if the parent is acting as a keyworker; otherwise the child may only speak when the parent is in the school building. Whenever possible, time should now be set aside outside the designated sessions to allow a further opportunity for the child to talk to the new person on a one-to-one basis in a low-risk activity. For example, to read aloud to a teacher, or play a game with a peer (see Table 10.4, page 193, for low-risk activities).

Although sessions with the child are still away from the main class at this stage, the time taken to talk to each new person decreases with the child's growing confidence and it will not be long before the programme moves into the classroom (see 'Group participation' on page 202).

Short cuts

Once a small-step technique has been used two or three times in succession, new people can be introduced more informally in fewer steps.

The steps are reduced to:

a)   a warm-up activity without the new person

b)   the new person joins in

c)   a low-risk activity

d)   a follow-up activity

e)   an activity repeated without the supporting adult.

There are some examples of these 'short cuts' in Chapter 9 (page 158), 'Warm-up routines'. Example 7 in Appendix C shows how the telephone was used to help a child quickly generalise to members of staff he rarely had contact with.

Children can be asked how they would like to start short-cut procedures or to select from various options. For example, new people can take a starting position across the other side of the room, rather than outside the room, or sit in a turn-taking circle facing *outwards* for a few rounds of rote sequences, before turning round to face the child. Rote sequences can be swapped for another low-risk activity such as reading aloud or a favourite game.

> Carrie, aged 14, was determined to talk to the school counsellor without the support of her keyworker. She wrote a short explanation of her difficulties with a proposal that the counsellor should leave the room and slowly enter after one minute.
>
> Once alone, Carrie started to read aloud and continued as the counsellor entered the room. The counsellor was then able to ask some simple questions about the passage she had read, before Carrie went on to discuss her difficulties in making friends. Carrie knew that she would be able to talk freely, once she had crossed the barrier of allowing the counsellor to hear her voice for the first time.

The Triangle Tactic

This informal strategy helps to ensure that children continue to talk to each other outside the designated sessions. Don't forget that the organised activities provided clear speaking roles and an agreed turn-taking sequence. Success in these structured activities does not guarantee that the children will manage spontaneous general conversation. It may even feel strange or awkward at first, after what may be several years of silence and minimal social interaction. Once children have spoken to each other in a formal session, it therefore helps if adults who both children speak to individually try to find quieter moments to chat to both children and support them in talking to each other.

See page 155 and Figure 9.4 (page 156) for details (the facilitating adult takes the parent role).

Talking to strangers

Children who are receiving help from education staff or practitioners, in preparation for transition to another school or college, will do better to focus on talking to strangers in public places *outside* the school (see Chapter 9, page 162).

 When setting specific targets for the child, focus on *either* talking in school *or* talking in the community, but *not* both at the same time. This does not include the parent targets which make it easier for children to talk to strangers. These are discussed in Chapter 9 under 'Removing the need and opportunity for avoidance strategies' (page 147) and 'Talking to strangers – family support' (page 161).

The model of confident talking: group participation

Talking in the classroom requires two aspects of generalisation: the ability to talk as part of a large group; and the courage to talk to your neighbour or teacher while being watched or overheard by several bystanders. Small-steps programmes will therefore need to cover this area of generalisation in tandem with the next area, talking in public places.

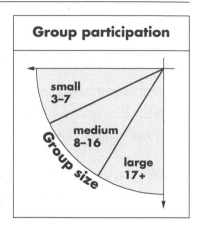

Talking in the classroom is more likely when:

★ there is a general understanding and expectation that the child will speak when they are ready

★ the child has experience of talking in smaller groups of five to seven people, including the keyworker and the teacher

★ at least half of the class members have heard the child's voice (not necessary with a 'Fresh start', page 247). This could be in a small group session, by a voice recording or by passing or working nearby when the child is talking to the keyworker

★ the child has spoken to the teacher when alone, with the keyworker outside the classroom or with a small group of peers

★ the child is not concerned about the reaction of their peers (see the next section 'Talking in public places').

Increasing group size

By now, the child will have practised talking in groups of three when speaking to a new adult or peer with the keyworker. Group size must be gradually increased to ease the child into whole-class activities, as described below and under (c) and (e) on pages 204 and 205. Ideally, this will be done outside the classroom initially, to keep the child's anxiety level as low as possible. If this cannot be factored into lesson time, it may mean holding sessions for a fixed period at break times or during activities such as whole-school assembly at the SENCo's discretion. The emphasis is on quickly enabling peers to hear the child's voice in single-word and sentence-activities, and with careful planning, most peers only need to join the group once or twice to achieve this. Peers will have noticed how little their classmate says, so they won't be surprised to hear that you have arranged some activities to help the child get used to talking in small groups before they speak in class. They will appreciate that you have chosen them to participate because of their thoughtful nature.

Section A of Progress chart 5 (online) provides an overall record of achievement and paves the way for transferring speech to the classroom.

a) Short cuts

Aim to increase the group size to four to six children by adding a new child to each activity.

Use the short cuts described in 'Generalising to other adults and children' (page 200).

b) The Talking Circle (extended Sliding-in Technique)

Once the child is familiar with the Sliding-in Technique, and confident that it can be relied on, more than one person can be introduced at a time. Two or three extra chairs are placed in a circle and the child and the keyworker start counting alternately. After an agreed signal, a new person enters the room, slowly takes their place in the circle and joins in the counting. (For example, the keyworker could open the door to let each new person in, while maintaining their turn in the counting sequence.) This is repeated until everyone waiting outside has joined the circle and the keyworker ends the counting.

> Kelly's form tutor played a board game with her and a friend in the lunch hour, while four girls she had spoken in front of on a school trip waited at the other end of the room. The games involved throwing a dice and picking up a word-challenge card to match the colour landed on. Some games involved asking each person their favourite animal, television programme, etc, to practise talking to each person in the group.
>
> After each complete round, one of the waiting girls came over to join in. After this, Kelly began talking to them in class, starting in lessons where background music obscured their voices.

Activities then move from single words to sentences, moving round the circle in different directions. Finally, the keyworker slides out, leaving the child talking unsupported in a structured activity with the new people. This process can soon be speeded up even further by seating new people in the circle on chairs facing outwards, rather than starting with them outside the room; one at a time they stand, turn their chair around and join in the counting.

The Talking Circle technique can be used to slide in several new peers or teachers in the same session, as shown in Appendix B, Example 5.

c) Low-risk activities

As the child talks to more children, use the small groups to rehearse activities that can be transferred to the classroom, starting with low-risk activities involving rote language, number sequences or reading aloud. For example, the child could:

★ practise reading alone to the keyworker, then in a small group and with the whole class, before finally reading aloud in their class assembly

★ reply to a group roll-call before answering the register in class

★ take it in turns with peers to take the register (with the teacher's approval!)

★ practise a turn-taking activity such as counting up in fives, before it is done as a whole-class activity.

See Appendix A (online) for more ideas (stage 5 includes reading activities which can be incorporated in the classroom). Also see 'Talking in the classroom' on page 209.

The model of confident talking: talking in public places

When children start talking to individuals at school, initially it will be very hard for them to do this in the presence of bystanders; that is, people who are not part of their group or activity, yet might hear or see them speak. There is a dread that the bystander will expect the child to talk to them too and become offended or annoyed if they don't.

Talking in public places

Supporting the child to talk in public places

You can help through coordinated planning, reassurance, and gradual exposure to places around the school where the child will be overheard. Progress chart 2 (online) might be useful for both planning and recording progress. It also provides a central record for 'sightings' from other staff as the child speaks spontaneously to their friends or adults around the school.

a) Parental involvement

Liaise with parents who can help children increase their tolerance of talking in public outside the school, as explained in Chapter 9.

b) Reassurance

Reassure the child, as part of their Pep Talk or ongoing support, that it is 'safe' to talk to their family and friends around the school: all staff understand (make sure they do!) and know that the child is working hard at getting used to talking to other people; they will also be pleased to see that the child is relaxed and talking; and they won't comment or expect the child to talk in class before the child feels ready.

Follow up your reassurances by allowing children and their friends to use outside spaces to work and play in as much as possible; this provides a welcome break from the perceived scrutiny of the classroom. Encourage school trips, residential stays and work experience for the same reason. They often represent a breakthrough for the child, in terms of both general confidence and being able to talk more openly.

c) Change the location of planned activities

Extend the child's talking programme to include activities in public places within the school such as their classroom, the dining room, the corridor and the playground. Start by repeating activities in the new setting with no bystanders. Then gradually increase the likelihood of the child being overheard by other people, using Table 10.5 for ideas. As always, keyworkers should introduce tasks confidently. For example: 'Today you're ready to start working in other places around the school', but it is wise to let the child retain some control by inviting them to select the activity.

When children are used to counting in sequence as a turn-taking activity, use counting as a way to do a quick head count or roll-call when moving around the school or leaving the school premises. Initially in small groups, and ultimately as a whole-class exercise, children can call out their number on the class register, rather than responding to their name, or be given a number to remember and call out later when getting on the school bus, etc.

Table 10.5: **Talking in public places – educational settings**

	Number of bystanders who may hear or see the child speak			
	Zero	**One**	**Few**	**Many**
Examples of public places	Empty classroom at lunch-time, after school or in school holidays Private work room with window shut and a 'Do not disturb' sign on the door Behind the bike shed Round the corner, out of sight	Private work room with another child or member of staff working at a different table Empty reception area (just the receptionist present) Empty dining room with member of staff laying tables	Private work room with window or door left open Library Toilets Corner of playground/ car park/ playing field Reception area Corridor or area just outside the classroom during lesson-time	Classroom, eg circle time, roll-call, classroom discussion Playground Canteen Assembly hall Corridor at break time Changing rooms After-school club

d) The Walkabout Technique

Once the child can talk in small groups, they can try the Walkabout Technique. Initially, this is done on a one-to-one basis, then as a small group activity, starting with talking to the keyworker in a 'safe' area where no one else can hear. The challenge is to continue talking while walking to another safe area or back to the original spot; for example, walking down a corridor from one room to another, or circling the playground at lunch-time.

Focus on flow rather than content by choosing a simple turn-taking activity to begin with, such as counting aloud, reciting the alphabet, alphabet strings (eg banan**a**–**a**ppl**e**–**e**lephan**t** ...) or 'I went to market'. The choice of activity is important, particularly for older students who don't want to feel foolish. However, the rationale behind the walkabout is more important than the activity itself. In reality, people may *see* the student talking but they are unlikely to overhear them because it is a private 'chat'. The activity enables the student to discover that they can be seen to talk without reprisal, and ensures that people who see them won't be surprised when they talk later in class. This is why the walkabout is also an excellent activity when visiting a new school or college campus for the first time.

> Once Raj had spoken in three different places – the resource room, his empty classroom and the preschool nursery – we made a map of his school and he stuck smiley faces in those areas.
>
> He loved adding more stickers as he talked around the school, and always got an extra one if there were other people nearby!

e) Informal strategies

Once the child is talking freely to the keyworker in private, the keyworker can start to talk to the child *outside the structure of planned sessions*, when moving around the school building. This must be introduced very gradually to avoid a sudden increase in anxiety. Initially, it will involve occasional 'X or Y?'

questions such as 'Is it Danny or Lee who can't come this afternoon?' Handout 14, 'Talking in public places' (online) gives more detailed advice that supports the child to eventually respond to the keyworker in the classroom in front of their peers.

The keyworker can also get other children or adults working at a separate table during designated sessions, so that the child who has SM gradually becomes used to being overheard during structured activities with the keyworker. Choose the children carefully, one at a time initially, and tell them in private that they must not comment when they hear their classmate speak for the first time. Divide your attention between both tables until it feels natural to come together for a shared activity.

Talking to the child about reactions from other people

Talking in a classroom of peers *who do not expect the child to speak* requires more than practice talking in large groups. Many children will also need to address their fear of an unfavourable reaction when they *do* speak. This is not normally an issue for younger children but, after an extended period with the same peer group, it can bring progress to a standstill.

As the child makes progress talking to individuals outside the classroom, it will be important to ascertain their feelings about speaking in class for the first time. Most children who have SM learn to hang back to avoid unwanted comments and questions, so this represents a radical change in their behaviour. The keyworker or parent should ask the child:

★   whether they have thought about the time when they will be ready to talk in class

★   what it will feel like

★   what they think the other children might say when they start to talk.

If the child does not answer, they will probably feel ambivalent at best, which is a concern. Forms 9 and 10 (online) can be used in full or part with older children to get a clearer picture of the issues to address.

The next step is to discuss how to allay any concerns. There are essentially two options:

★   to take a risk – after all, talking may cause some surprise the first time but it will soon become old news

★   to take control and let the child's classmates know what to do.

Ultimately, it is the child's and the family's choice but, if the child seems unconvinced by the first argument, for the speediest results, we recommend the second option, as discussed in the next section.

This does not apply when 'Making a fresh start' (Chapter 11, page 247). The child's new peer group could regard them as being on the quiet side but they are probably more concerned about establishing their own role within the classroom. Talking in class still represents a major challenge, of course, because the child has never done it before. They may need help to be convinced that their peers have no reason to be surprised and that it is better to take the plunge sooner, rather than later. We recommend the article in *Finding Our Voices*, issue 4, 'What if you suddenly talk and people make a big deal about it?' (see Appendix F 'Other websites').

Involving the child's classmates

It is important to ensure that, when the child finally speaks, the reaction of their classmates does not set them back, as shown by Robbie's story (page 297). The essential message that child, peers and staff alike should embrace is it is only a matter of time before the child speaks and, when it happens, no one should be surprised. There is no need for cheering or comments; they should simply carry on talking as if the child has always spoken. There are three ways to convey this message, as follows.

a) Talk openly about SM like any other childhood fear

Respond to other children's natural curiosity by talking about the child's SM openly and supportively in class as it crops up (see Chapter 8, 'Dealing with unhelpful comments', page 122).

Time can also be set aside to talk to the class, at an age-appropriate level, about lack of confidence and how 'I can't' turns into 'I can' with small steps and lots of practice. Ask the children to share which skills they are working on (eg swimming, diving, reading, cooking, talking) and agree that, rather than 'I can't', it is 'I can't *yet*, but I will!'

b) Enlist support through a class discussion

With the family's agreement and the child's knowledge, read a book to younger children such as *My Friend Daniel Doesn't Talk* (Longo, 2006) which is aimed at four to eight year olds. Alternatively, simply chat with the class about how to be a good friend and best support the child, as described on page 31 of *Can I Tell You About Selective Mutism?* (Johnson & Wintgens, 2012).

For example, Maria, aged seven, was relieved when this was suggested as a solution to the pressure she was experiencing from her peers, and chose to be present. The chat took place before Maria's group programme and she talks about the positive effect in Chapter 15 (pages 312 and 324). As a result, the class became involved in a carefully planned team effort and Maria was proud to receive the praise that children with less control of the situation often recoil from.

c) Enlist support through a personal message

For older children of nine upwards, it can be very effective to present a personal message to their peers. This can be seen in a class of 10-year-old children in the BBC documentary *My Child Won't Speak* (see Appendix F 'Audio-visuals'), which uses a script from the first edition of this manual. The script in Box 10.3 can be used as a starting point for a letter, inviting the child to keep, change or delete the words. Working on this together will usefully pinpoint exactly how the child would like their peers to behave towards them. The letter can then be read out by an adult or, even better, recorded by the child as an audio or a video message. The child might like to play this to a favourite teacher, support staff member or small group of peers first, perhaps choosing to be absent in the first instance. Being brave enough to allow the class to hear your voice in this way takes a tremendous leap of faith, but we have never known there to be a poor outcome. Peers have always been interested and supportive, and it has enabled the child to take the next brave step of speaking in the classroom.

Box 10.3: 'My Story' script

As you know, my name is _____ and I am ____ years old. When I was very young, I developed a fear of speaking in public. It started when I first went to playschool. It was such a shock to be on my own with complete strangers that I panicked and couldn't speak to anyone. After that, I dreaded going back. Every time I met a new person I'd just freeze again and my words wouldn't come out. It was a horrid feeling but there was nothing I could do to stop it. I was fine with my family – talking's never been a problem at home! It was just when I went out that I couldn't talk.

Over the years, my anxiety got worse – I knew my words would end up getting stuck, so I avoided talking as much as possible. I tried to get out of things like parties and it must have looked like I didn't want any friends. But I was just scared that people would talk to me and I wouldn't be able to answer. I really wanted to talk but, each time I tried, I'd get the same anxiety I felt all those years ago in playschool.

This anxiety has a name. It's called selective mutism and the way to deal with it is to very gradually get used to talking a tiny bit at a time until the anxiety goes and you feel comfortable with the situation. I know it works because in the last ____ months I have started speaking to several people for the first time. It's much harder though with people who know me. I feel they will be shocked if I talk and this makes it very hard to feel relaxed.

Now you know how I feel, I have something to ask you. I really want to get over this, but I need your help. I am going to keep practising until I can talk more, but please don't make a big thing of it when I do. It will help me if you don't stare or comment when I speak. Just treat me the same as anyone else and carry on like I've always been talking. It may take a bit of time and it will be easier for me if you do most of the talking to start with. If I don't say much at first, please don't give up. Just treat me like one of your friends and it will get easier and easier for me.

Thank you for listening and thank you for trying to understand.

Older students might like to make a PowerPoint presentation to educate both staff and peers with the option of adding a soundtrack. There is further inspiration on YouTube where many young people have written or spoken out about their SM.

Noah (12) could speak in a small room with some adults and two or three children but was terrified of talking in class. This fear dated back to reception class when he finally spoke a word and everyone clapped him. He was then taken round the whole school, from class to class, so that everyone could congratulate him – he had never forgotten this. After gentle persuasion, Noah recorded his letter to his class in his own voice. He asked for it to be played in his absence and his teacher said the children listened very carefully and asked lots of interesting questions. They talked about their own fears also.

Noah seemed to shed a great burden immediately. His whole class had heard his voice and the world hadn't ended! He felt reassured that other children at least partly understood his situation. Perhaps he needed some time to check for 'fall-out' but, less than three weeks later, Noah spoke in the classroom – not the whisper he had occasionally managed before, but in his usual audible voice.

d) Is it necessary to involve peers?

Some children do talk a little in class, if only to one or two friends or to answer the register, and there is not the same need to prepare their peers for when they might speak. However, the same children often resist individual or group work because they do not want their peers to find out about their difficulty talking. It is important to address this anxiety. Calmly tell the child that their classmates know already; they see that the child does not talk much in class. They don't comment because it's not a big deal to them – they are happy if the child speaks and happy if they don't. All children have got things they need to work at and, just as the child who has SM would be happy to help a friend practise catching a ball, there are lots of children happy to help with talking.

Talking in the classroom

Progress chart 5 (online) gives an overview of programme planning in the generalisation phase, and indicates when children have made sufficient progress to start talking in the classroom. It can also be adapted to support pupils making a 'Fresh start' (page 247). For them, sections A and B won't be relevant but sections C–E provide guidance for ensuring appropriate reassurance and a gradual easing in to class activities through 'low-risk' activities.

For example, pupils could first be asked to participate non-verbally by keeping score, holding up work or advancing the slides in a PowerPoint presentation. Talking would be confined to times when they *volunteered* an answer or had the opportunity to contribute to one-to-one or small-group discussions at the side of the class. Low-risk verbal activities would then be introduced with prior warning, such as rote sequences (eg each pupil to respond to roll-call by saying their number on the register; numeracy practice), answering in unison, reading aloud and rehearsed lines. Class presentations are a good way forward, as pupils can read aloud from prepared text, perhaps from their seat at first and then facing the class (see Appendix A, Stage 5 'Reading aloud' for further ideas). Only very gradually would pupils be chosen to answer general questions, ideally after priming the whole class what to do or say when they are not sure of the answer. For example, to emulate a popular television show, pupils could be allowed to nominate a friend, ask the 'audience' or request '50:50' (for a choice of two possible answers). Or explain that it is fine to say 'I don't know' or 'I'm not sure' but encourage pupils to take a guess by welcoming all answers as 'good thinking' and a valuable contribution that other people can work on.

It is absolutely right to keep nudging students forward using low-risk activities but take care to maintain the small-steps approach of changing only one thing at a time. It is a big leap, for example, from chatting to a few friends informally in the classroom to presenting to the whole class. If in doubt, ensure that the student or parents have the opportunity to suggest an easier step in preparation for a new assignment. Students often hide their true feelings at school for fear of making a scene and it cannot be assumed that their lack of opposition is the same as tacit agreement.

 A word of warning: some teachers have sprung surprises on students without a gradual easing-in, and have been delighted to get a verbal response in front of the whole class. However, it tends to be a short-lived success. Faced with the fear of looking stupid in front of their peers, it is possible for students to summon all their strength and speak out. Unfortunately, the shock can lead them to drop out of further classes, or develop severe anxiety symptoms such as nausea and vomiting, which inhibit further progress.

Spontaneous contributions to classroom discussion represent the final step for most children who have SM and cannot be forced; just as there will be other quiet children in the class who tend to listen rather than volunteer information. See Sander's story in Chapter 14 (page 306) for an excellent example of a sensitively handled transition. By focusing on low-risk activities in the classroom, Sander was able to take the next step when the time was right for him, and he became a regular contributor to classroom discussion. Children who do not take this step and respond only when spoken to, or when they perceive that speaking is the only way to avert an even more stressful situation (low profile SM), will need continued support, as covered in the next section.

The model of confident talking: social functioning

It is one thing for children who have SM to be able to speak when the exchange is planned or prompted, but quite another for them to say what they want, *when* they want. Until they have the freedom to communicate spontaneously in this way, their speech will have limited social purpose or function. If not achieved this is the most disabling impact of SM, leading to increasing mental health issues and a sense of lost identity if not resolved (see Chapter 15, where adults describe the effects of SM on their lives).

Table 10.6 overleaf breaks down the areas considered under **social functioning** and the shift towards spontaneous speech. Essentially, this is looking at a progression from low-risk verbal activities – where the emphasis is simply on managing to speak – to high-risk activities which have social value but cause greater anxiety. This is mostly because of the individual's lack of control over other people's behaviour and the resulting uncertainty about the outcome.

Progress chart 6 (online) complements Table 10.6. It highlights the importance of ensuring that children are helped to move beyond the vulnerable, low profile stage of SM, where they simply speak when spoken to. It may be used to consider aspects of social functioning which can be incorporated into planned activities and role play; to monitor the emergence of spontaneous language to meet the child's academic and social needs; and to alert colleagues to areas of ongoing concern. All staff members need to be realistic about what can be achieved in the time they have with each child. But they should never lose sight of the big picture and recommendations for ongoing work to continue the journey towards fully effective social functioning.

Planned activities

Once the child is working well with structured activities at Stages 6 and 7 (single words and sentences), the keyworker needs to progress their programme in two directions *in tandem*:

1) generalise to new people and new settings while repeating the *same* activities

2) work towards a higher level of social functioning by introducing *new*, higher-risk activities, on a one-to-one basis. This will include Stage 8 activities.

So, for example, the child and the keyworker could start their session with a warm-up activity followed by a familiar low-risk game with a new child, and finish with a less structured or connected speech activity on a

Table 10.6: **Confident talking – working towards effective social functioning**

Social functioning Working towards spontaneous conversation to meet the child's needs			
LOW RISK ——————————————————————➤ HIGH RISK			
PLANNED		**SPONTANEOUS**	
Prompted	Child-initiated	Prompted	Child-initiated
Factual content	Emotive content	Factual content	Emotive content
Structured	Unstructured	Structured	Unstructured
Within a small-steps programme, activities gradually move from:			

Planned Taking place within a designated programme session or rehearsed with known content and fixed end-point	➤	**Spontaneous** Taking place as part of everyday routine, ie involving other people and/or time pressure, or introduced without prior warning
Prompted Child responds to a question, cue or prompt	➤	**Child-initiated** Child initiates the interaction by asking a question, giving an instruction or gaining someone's attention
Factual content Child's contribution will not be challenged and is known to be correct. No other answers are possible	➤	**Emotive content** Child's contribution may be challenged or require clarification. Content involves personal information or opinion, explanation or doubt (eg more than one answer)

Structured Agreed turn-taking sequence; set language; clear rules for activity and task completion; no initiation required other than taking turn.	➤	**Semi-structured** Structured turn taking, but some turns may take longer than others; language may vary; rules are in place but unpredictable duration; some initiation may be required, eg to cue next person, stake a claim (eg 'Snap!', 'Bingo!'), correct other people or give/seek clarification.	➤	**Unstructured** Talking is not in fixed turn-taking sequence and may require 'calling out'; language generated by participants; activity itself may be structured but interaction follows usual conversational and social rules and may involve negotiation or improvisation; initiation required for balanced participation.

Note: see Appendix A for activities which are coded into these categories at each stage of interaction.

one-to-one basis. In time, the riskier activities can be repeated in group work, helping the child to feel more comfortable about speaking in class and in other unplanned situations.

Working towards spontaneous speech

Most children start speaking spontaneously to keyworkers or practitioners they see frequently when:

★ they have established good rapport and worked towards communicating in sentences (Stage 7) without feeling pressurised

★ they do not feel inhibited by their parent's presence (they may be used to parents answering for them, or concerned about 'disloyalty' to family members they do not yet speak to)

★ they have a *reason* to talk; for example, something they are interested in and want to share

★ they are sure no one else can overhear

★ the keyworker primarily shares, rather than seeks, information.

For other children, the move towards spontaneous speech can be facilitated after Stage 7, as follows.

a) Ease into conversation

Respond to any spontaneous comments in a calm, friendly way, rather than with exuberant praise or reaching for a sticker. This is a special moment and your interest in *what* the child is saying is all – and everything – they need.

Gradually introduce unplanned questions at the end of sessions that have gone well. See Figure 9.2 (page 153), 'Introducing questions to a person with selective mutism'.

b) Follow a progression from low- to high-risk activities

Work from sentences to connected speech (Stage 8) and from structured to semi-structured and unstructured activities. See Appendix A (online) for activity suggestions, and Tables 10.4 and 10.6 in this chapter for guidance on the appropriate progression. You will probably have many more creative ideas to slot into this framework.

c) Increase the child's comfort with initiating interaction

Help the child to feel at ease with initiating exchanges by losing the habit of prompting the child in turn-taking games; eg 'It's Sammy's turn now', 'Your go!'. Look at the child, smile, look away and *wait*. If necessary, cue with eye contact and a slight nod of your head, but try to fade this out over time, so that the child learns they do not need to wait for approval before they act.

When the child can ask questions and give instructions in structured activities, set them tasks which require them to initiate interaction without a prompt. For example: delivering messages; fact finding and reporting back to you; being responsible for time keeping; giving you a reminder at the end of the session. In particular, set targets where the precise timing is up to the child, for example:

★ Put up your hand in class today and answer a question.

★ Choose two colours for the glove puppet you are making and tell your teacher what you would like before next Tuesday.

★ Phone me some time after school and recommend a good television programme to watch this evening.

★ Ask [N] where he got his trainers from before I next see you.

This type of target will probably pose the greatest challenge for children who have lived with SM for several years. The fear that their efforts will be laughed at, or rejected, can be very strong. Older children may need help to initiate contact by email or text before they are comfortable with verbal tasks.

d) Rehearse greetings

Play the 'Quick-fire Greetings' game (see Appendix A, Stage 7) in three consecutive sessions. After the third one, say that, from now on, you would like the child to do their best to respond after you say 'Bye' at the end of your sessions. If they succeed, this may be acknowledged at the beginning of the *next* session, so that the actual exchange is enjoyed at a purely social level. Having said that, a smile and a thumbs-up never go amiss! We do not set 'Hi' as a target, believing that children enjoy their sessions more if their first word is spoken in their own time, but we do find that, after the 'Bye' target, spontaneous farewells and other ritualistic social language begin to emerge.

e) Practise contradiction

Build assertiveness by giving specific practice at contradicting and correcting other people, such as:

★ Make deliberate mistakes during an activity, eg 'Now we put the pastry case into the jam' and continue to play dumb until the child corrects you.

★ Read out sentences to which the child says either 'silly' or 'sensible'. If silly, the child has to reword it: eg 'The king sat on his crown and put his throne on his head'.

★ Do some sums which the child has to mark with a tick or a cross. If wrong, the child tells you the correct answer.

★ Read out a passage after priming the child that it has a certain number of deliberate mistakes. The child must stop you and correct each one they spot.

f) Develop self-help skills

Build self-help skills by giving specific practice at seeking clarification, such as:

★ Read out deliberately vague or overcomplicated instructions for drawing a picture or making an object. The child must ask for more information (eg 'What does perpendicular mean?') in order to complete the task.

★ Adopt a whole-class approach to encourage children to say when they don't understand and ask appropriate questions at the appropriate time. (See *Active Listening for Active Learning* by Johnson & Player, 2009, in Appendix F 'Therapy resources').

g) Support conversation

Use glove puppets, cardboard cut-outs, computer avatars or simple illustrations of social situations to engage in and rehearse appropriate dialogue for scenarios such as a friend staying over, getting first-aid for another child, reporting bullying, or returning an incorrect or unwanted item. Many children find role play much easier when providing a character's voice or imagining what other people might be saying.

Include targets which involve longer interactions with other children, for example:

★ Show [N] around the school and answer all of their questions.

★ Walk around the playground with [N], taking it in turns to ask and answer a question.

★ Explain the rules of this game to [N and N] and make sure that they are playing it properly.

★ Read your poem or story or give your presentation to your tutor group and answer their questions afterwards.

h) Group work

Explore the options for ongoing group work for social and conversational skills, self-esteem and assertiveness. Various structured programmes are available or children could meet more informally for a lunchtime session with a facilitating adult. This could include eating and talking together, sharing and teaching each other games, and problem-solving activities.

Ultimately, it is practice, practice, practice that makes something which initially seemed impossible feel entirely manageable. The support of other students who don't necessarily have SM but lack confidence in expressing themselves can help to both validate and re-evaluate personal feelings and perceptions.

Additional considerations for adolescents and young adults

As children transition into adolescence, it is somewhat ironic that they experience a spurt in thinking skills and abstract reasoning, at exactly the same time as hormonal changes trigger acute self-consciousness and irrationality. It is a very self-centred time: they are thinking *too much* about how other people see them; while unable to think *enough* about the effect their behaviour is having on other people. But, equally, it is a time of great conflict: their desperation for greater independence exists alongside a fear of self-sufficiency and the continued need for emotional support.

Parents bear the brunt of their adolescent children's frustration, insecurity and dismissive behaviour and very often feel that whatever they say is rejected. This is, therefore, a time when outside professionals and mentors have a particularly important role to play. Their rational explanations, alternative points of view and approval are more likely to be taken on board, partly because they come from an unbiased source (unlike the parents' words of wisdom), and partly because respectful adolescent young people (all credit to their upbringing) can control their impulsive tendencies for long enough to listen and reflect. This is also when the thoughtful young adults they are going to become first appear!

There is little in this manual that does *not* apply to adolescents and young adults. This section covers additional interventions that are particularly appropriate for this age group, including those with a coexisting diagnosis such as high-functioning autism. We suggest considering any interventions that seem to meet a particular need, in conjunction with the booklet for teenagers and adults 'When the words won't come out' (online), which contains the main messages we want to convey to young people.

Body language, eye contact and posture

Body tension and averted eye gaze may have become such a habitual part of being around other people that, even when they can speak, the young person finds it hard to change these physical aspects of communication. They may not appreciate the messages they are unconsciously conveying to other people, or that what they do to avoid drawing attention to themselves actually makes them stand out. They also do not realise the direct link between a relaxed physical state and a general sense of well-being.

The following strategies aim to increase self-awareness and help the young person adopt a more natural posture.

Blending in

Help individuals to understand that the best way to blend in is to look the same as everyone else and encourage them to observe photographs, their peers or the general public to work out the appropriate posture to emulate. They may believe that hanging their heads and avoiding eye contact is a way to avoid being asked questions when, in fact, it was their teachers' or relatives' awareness of their difficulties that reduced questioning. Without this awareness, the same stance usually invites a question to keep them involved or to ask whether they are feeling OK.

In most situations, it is easier to think about keeping your back straight and chin up than to focus on eye contact. An upright posture conveys the message 'I am OK' and does not draw attention. It is also essential to a relaxed breathing pattern, as discussed below.

Eye contact

It is possible to work on eye contact using the activities marked 👁 in Appendix A. These aim to make eye contact necessary and comfortable. If young people are using sentences but struggling to make eye contact, even after these activities, introduce some of the following rules.

★ No eye contact makes you look bored or uninterested and, therefore, appears rude.

★ It is polite to look at someone while they are speaking, as it shows you are listening. Older individuals with high-functioning autism spectrum disorder can explain that they don't mean to appear rude, but they listen better if they look away so they can concentrate on the words.

★ A tiny bit of eye contact is all that is needed and is better than too much! If you look at someone continuously as you speak to them, you will appear aggressive or intimidating.

★ It is fine to look away while you speak – everyone does this while they think about what they are saying. But keep your chin up – literally! If you let your head hang down, you will look ill or depressed.

★ When speaking to someone, always look at them as you finish speaking. This lets them know that you have finished and it is their turn.

★ When speaking to someone, the objective is intermittent eye contact otherwise it looks like you are talking to yourself. When it doesn't come naturally, try out the following and use the one that feels easier:

  (a) establish eye contact but lower your gaze for a few seconds occasionally

  (b) look away but make eye contact for two seconds now and again.

★ If you are in a group and looking at different people as they take turns to speak, move your whole head, not just your eyes, to avoid looking shifty!

Relaxation

Overall body tension impairs breathing and contributes to a general feeling of being constricted or trapped. However, trying to get young people to relax in front of you usually makes them acutely self-conscious, so we recommend a more indirect approach. Encourage the release of muscular tension through physical activity whenever possible. Sports are not for everyone but is there a wall or a cupboard that needs demolishing at home or a bonfire to build? Young people should compare how their bodies feel when they are relaxed and engaged in enjoyable pursuits with the tightness they experience when feeling anxious; and practise a conscious release of tension whenever possible.

Working within any physical limitations they may have, ask young people to check their bodies for tension when they are alone by making the following simple movements which you can demonstrate in both a free and a constricted fashion.

★ Lift your arms above your head and drop (not *lower*) them to your sides.

★ Lift your shoulders up as far as possible and drop (not *lower*) them back into place.

★ Stand up and swing your arms loosely in front of your body and behind, as you swivel your waist from side to side.

★ Do the same movement (swivelling from the waist) while you are sitting down, with your back straight and hands in your lap. We say 'Wiggle your shoulders' for this, but it is only possible with a relaxed, upright spine. Aim for this loose, upright position, with the shoulders back rather than hunched forwards. Note that the instruction 'Shoulders back' tends to result in tension rather than free movement.

Aim for a relaxed upper body posture during sessions by lifting the chin slightly and dropping and wiggling shoulders into place; this opens up the chest and ribcage to allow unrestricted breathing.

It is also important to check the lips and jaw for tension and relax the face, keeping the upper and lower teeth apart with lips barely touching. Gentle blowing may help to unclench the jaw.

Breathing

Staying alive aside, breathing is important to SM management for anxiety control and voice production.

Using steady, controlled breathing to reduce heart rate and anxiety

By breathing slowly in and out, the heart rate can be reduced, which automatically reduces anxiety. We recommend five slow breaths in and five slow breaths out whenever a moment of calm is needed. This is particularly helpful when working on assignments (see page 162). But first demonstrate good posture, as described above, because it is only when the ribcage can move freely that the lungs can draw in enough air to permit slow breathing.

Show young people how a hunched position traps the ribs, so they can't swing out and draw air in. When this happens, people compensate by taking short, rapid breaths which fill only the top of their lungs – this is called 'shallow breathing', which *creates* a feeling of anxiety. The faster they breathe, the more they will get a sensation of breathlessness caused by an excess of carbon dioxide in their blood. Slow, deep breaths balance out the oxygen to carbon dioxide ratio and restore a sense of calm.

Using steady, controlled breathing to produce and maintain voice

Understanding the mechanism of voice production is extremely helpful when experiencing any kind of disruption to speech output. By appreciating the physical effect of their anxiety, young people who have SM can begin to override their emotional response to a situation, and learn to consciously control their vocal mechanism. For example, many individuals hold their breath just as they try to talk, which makes speech physically impossible, as Figure 10.1 shows.

Being able to visualise voice production is helpful so, in addition to using simple diagrams like Figure 10.1, you could accompany the written explanation with gesture, as follows.

1   Place your hands on your ribcage and swing them outwards and inwards to show the lungs working like bellows, with the ribs drawing air in and out. Use a small constricted movement for a quiet voice; a bigger movement for a full relaxed breath and louder voice.

2   Demonstrate vibration of the vocal cords by placing your outstretched hands alongside each other, palms down and a few centimetres apart; then rapidly and repeatedly move them together and apart.

3   Now clench your fists to show how anxiety causes the vocal cords to tighten and contract, holding them apart. In this frozen position, the vocal cords can no longer vibrate and, at best, you can whisper. To demonstrate the link between exhalation, whispering and talking audibly, first gently breathe out with airflow only, no voice: 'hhhhhha'. Towards the end of your breath, move the lips together and apart to demonstrate a whispered 'pah-pah' (your lips are moving but not your vocal cords, so keep your fists clenched).

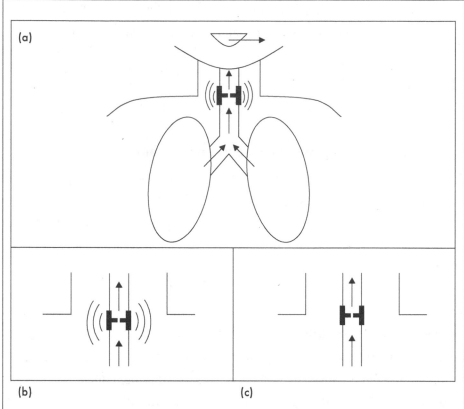

a) Air passes from the lungs, through the windpipe and out of the mouth, passing through the larynx (voice box) on the way. It is only possible to activate the voice box and speak as you breathe out.

b) If the vocal cords are relaxed, they vibrate against each other as the air passes between them to create voice. A small amount of air produces a quiet voice; more air makes the voice louder. Extra volume comes naturally when you breathe deeply, fill your lungs (inhale) and have plenty of air to release through the voice box as you breathe out (exhale).

c) If the vocal cords are stiff and tense they cannot move together and vibrate, so no sound is produced. All you can produce is a whisper, which is your outward breath, shaped into different sounds by the articulatory movements of your lips and tongue.

Figure 10.1: **The mechanics of voice production**

Repeat, adding voice: 'hhhhh**ah**-p**ah**-p**ah**', and vibrate your hands together from their relaxed position each time you say '**ah**' (Figure 10.1b).

By concentrating on breathing while preparing to speak, and specifically focusing on the outward breath as a run-up to their first word, individuals can help to prevent their throat 'seizing up'. A safe time to practise this is when leaving voice messages because there is always the option to end the call! (See Appendix B 'Voicemail' and 'Robot routes', and Example 8 in Appendix C.)

> I used to think that the voice was created outside the body. I was so aware of how it filled a space in the room. I now know that sound is created at the larynx and can reverberate throughout the body. (Adult recovering from SM)

Voice production

Relaxed throat muscles are essential for voice production

Referring to Figure 10.1, it can also help individuals to become familiar with the sensation in their throat when they produce voice, however quietly this may be. The resulting vibration can be felt against the fingertips when placed against the throat (close to the Adam's apple in males, and the smaller protuberance in females). After some practice, it can be felt as a vibration in the upper chest or throat alone. Young people can be encouraged to practise humming to experience this sensation. This can be done against background music in their bedrooms if they are concerned about being overheard.

★ Ensure that the shoulders and jaw are relaxed (pages 216–217) and posture allows unconstricted breathing.

★ Breathe out through the nose with lips together and, as gently and quietly as possible, hum 'mmmmmmm' on the outward breath, checking for vibration against your fingertips. The vibration tells you that your throat is relaxed and your vocal cords are moving. In a quiet room you will easily hear the sound you make because it is amplified as it reverberates inside your head (resonance). However, it is barely audible to other people. Even people who are close up would not hear the sound against other people talking or background music.

★ Practise producing a short hum at will – 'mm' – when you are out and about, walking the dog, waiting for the bus, doing the washing-up. Tune in to the sensation of your unconstricted, open and relaxed airway as you hum. Whenever you notice your throat muscles tensing and tightening up, breathe slowly in and out to release them, and try humming a short 'mm' again.

★ If you are preparing to read aloud or speak, you can first check that your throat is relaxed by focusing on your outward breath and humming a short 'mm' as you bring your vocal cords together. This is the equivalent of the throat clearing that many people do before speaking but only you will be aware of it.

If individuals like the idea of private voice-coaching, we recommend videos such as Jay Miller's 'Spinal Roll' on YouTube, which incorporates the three aspects of relaxation, breathing and resonance.

Daily voice use promotes and maintains familiarity

Sustained periods of silence do not weaken the vocal cords, even over many years, but for people with long-standing SM, the longer they don't speak, the less familiar the sound of their voice will become, which may impose an extra barrier to intervention. It has long been disputed that 'talking to yourself is the first sign of madness' – we highly recommend it on a daily basis! People should do whatever suits them, as often as possible, to become accustomed to the sound of their own voice. For example: talking to a pet; reading aloud from the newspaper; recording an online video journal; counting aloud while exercising; singing along to music or in the shower; or talking to the sat nav while driving.

Talking about feelings

Many young people who have SM do not express their feelings or explain what is making them anxious. Usually this is because they have not been enabled to communicate complex messages. They need the reassurance that their communication won't have undesirable consequences, such as disapproval, public attention or an extended conversation requiring a higher level of one-to-one interaction than they can currently manage. In addition, they may need a non-verbal means of expression, such as the questionnaires in Chapter 5 (page 85) and the strategies in Chapter 8 (page 126).

Identifying and managing anxiety triggers

Having established that a young person feels anxious, it is important to know the trigger, so that you can try to address it in one of the following ways:

★ provide help with advance rehearsal or preparation

★ change someone else's behaviour or a specific practice

★ help the young person to see that they are worrying excessively about an imagined, rather than likely, scenario (see 'Challenging unhelpful thoughts' on page 226).

Remember that asking anxious individuals to talk about a situation that is worrying them may trigger the same feelings of nausea and a racing heart as the situation itself. It is then not surprising that they would prefer *not* to talk about it. Indeed, a panic reaction will prevent analytical thinking, making it very difficult to contemplate a situation and possible solutions rationally. We find it is more successful to give students statements to consider about themselves. This is the basis of many assessments, as shown by Forms 7–10 and 15 (online).

For example, a student might justify avoiding a situation with a general reason, rather than confronting their SM, and resist going out because 'they hate crowds'. This could be unpicked to 'I hate crowds because …'

I get panicky and can't breathe.

I will be squashed.

I don't like talking near other people.

People get in the way and slow me down.

There's more chance someone will talk to me.

It feels like everyone's watching me.

The last statement above can also be unpicked if rated or selected as a key factor. Does the student feel that being watched poses a risk of being approached and spoken to, or do they feel that people are judging them?

It may be easier to deflect attention by considering an imaginary third party and asking which statements constitute the most likely reasons in their opinion. For example, 'Some students with SM don't like eating in the school canteen because …'

They feel too nauseous to eat.

They find social conversation difficult.

They can't choose who they sit with.

They don't like the food.

… and so on.

Similarly, if a student does not get on with a specific teacher, or is opting out of a particular activity, it may help to break down lessons or sessions into individual components or teacher behaviours and ask the student to rate each component for comfort level, as shown in Figure 10.2. Whenever possible, contrast a lesson or teacher they like with one that is causing anxiety. In this way, it may be possible to identify differences in management style and address the concern.

Difficulty acknowledging anxiety

Sometimes, students are clearly anxious – they may present with physical symptoms such as vomiting, sleep disruption or inability to eat – but maintain that nothing is wrong or disengage from attempts to identify the cause. It is possible that they genuinely do not know the exact cause of their anxiety; it is just always there in certain settings. When staff members are on board and everything has been done to provide an anxiety-free environment, it may be worth considering the following explanations, both of which result in the day-long conflict of wanting to fit in, while feeling that their SM sets them apart.

★ The student feels ashamed of their SM and sees it as a reason for people to have a low opinion of them. Therefore, they want it to be ignored as much as possible and both welcome and resent the efforts of teachers to make allowances for them. They are afraid that interventions from staff members will make their difficulties more obvious to their peers.

★ The student is trying to do just enough to blend in (they may even be able to speak a little), but not too much to draw attention to themselves. Being noticed runs the risk of being expected to speak more than they feel they can manage.

The student may agree to one or both of these explanations to a greater or lesser extent, each of which places them, without exaggeration, in an agonising position of constant vigilance as described in Declan Sharry's autobiographical account, *Persona Medusa: An Embodied Tale of Anxiety* (2015). There

This teacher …	Does this ✓	Does NOT do this ✗	I feel good about this	I feel OK about this	This bothers me a bit	This bothers me a lot
Calls the register at the beginning of the lesson						
Talks to me before or after the lesson						
Asks me questions in front of the others when I'm not expecting it						
Only asks me questions in front of the others if I put up my hand first						
Treats me differently from the other students						
Comes up to me and asks if I'm understanding the lesson						
Ignores me						
Asks me questions and waits for an answer						
Gets annoyed with the other students						
Asks students to read out loud during lesson						
Makes the lesson very clear and goes at the right pace						
Has had a chat with me to say it's OK if I don't say much						
Makes me feel like I should be saying more						
Looks at me quite a lot during lessons						

Figure 10.2: **Example of breaking down a situation to identify the source of anxiety**

are no easy answers here but, once staff members have reassured the student that no action will be taken without their agreement, essentially the student's options are as follows.

★ Do nothing and continue in a state of high anxiety.

★ Accept help to overcome their SM in the current setting, working on appropriate assignments at their own pace until their fear of talking dissipates.

★ Stretch themselves to face their fears in community settings, giving them confidence to transfer skills to their educational setting or hold their own in a different placement (see 'Talking to strangers' on page 162, and 'Making a fresh start' on page 247).

★ Do what it takes to ensure that no-one will find out they have SM (eg to participate in low-risk activities in the classroom) with the reassurance that

   (a) they do not stand out from other quiet students

   (b) their peers are used to some students being quieter than others and accept this without question. They are more interested in their own contributions than what the student with SM is doing

   (c) their SM will be sensitively handled by all staff members with no obligation to do more than the structured activities that have been agreed (see Table 10.4 on page 193 and 'Talking in the classroom' on page 209).

★ Challenge their belief that peers view them or their SM negatively by investigating their peers' views or giving them the opportunity to understand and provide support (see 'Involving the child's classmates' on page 207).

A point may be reached where an adult who has good rapport with the student sets out these options for the student to appraise. However, possible solution(s) may be introduced earlier, based on the adult's knowledge of the student. The last option is often a key factor because very often the students who make the slowest progress are those who are adamant that their difficulties are not shared with others.

We know about one keyworker who gave a girl aged 11 a series of questions to ask the few friends she spoke to. Having learned that they also had various fears, difficulties and coping strategies, she became much more outward-looking. She realised she was not so different and that people were far less aware of her own struggles than she had previously thought. Another keyworker asked a teenager to write down three words to describe a peer and a staff member they liked or admired. Once done, she presented the teenager with words that specially selected staff and peers had written about *her*. They were not asked to write only positive descriptions but invariably did so, boosting her self-image.

Meeting other people who have SM

Not all young people have difficulty opening up about the effects of SM on their lives, their hopes and dreams, their frustrations and achievements. For adolescents looking for a sense of self on the road to adulthood, it is particularly important to identify with other people in the same position. The benefits of group work are discussed in Chapter 9 (page 165). When face-to-face meetings and activities are not possible, the online forums listed in Appendix F ('Organisations' and 'Other websites') can provide acceptance, support and inspiration.

Taking a different perspective

We have used Activity 1 for many years and regret that we do not know the original source. It has been useful to reduce the pressure young people put *themselves* under to talk, by demonstrating that they will not be judged by how much they talk. It is the quality of their interactions, and more specifically their *responses*, that are important to other people. We tend to use it as a group activity with friends or family members.

Activity 1: Exploring communication styles

Using the four empty quadrants shown in Figure 10.3(a), participants (including the facilitating adult) supply words to describe people who (clockwise from top-right):

a) listen to what other people have to say and answer their questions or show they are interested, and make comments or ask questions of their own (**sociable**)

b) talk a lot, ignore what other people have to say and often interrupt to get their own point of view across (**own agenda**)

c) don't react when people talk to them and don't start conversations (**passive**)

d) say very little but respond when people talk to them by listening, smiling, nodding or looking interested (**shy**).

Words are added to the quadrants and then discussed. It soon emerges that personality types in the upper two quadrants are the most likeable; people who dominate conversations (bottom-right quadrant) are the least popular. Some words may be repeated, as shown

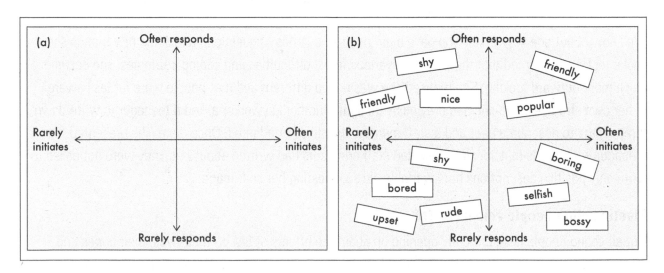

Figure 10.3: **Exploring communication styles**

in Figure 10.3(b), where the double use of 'friendly' emphasises that people prefer good listeners, whether they talk or not. Therefore, it is better to focus on *responding*, either non-verbally or verbally, and to allow spontaneous comments to develop later.

Sometimes it is necessary to challenge words that are generated, for example, when a participant places 'shy' in the 'passive' quadrant. Shy people may not initiate contact but they do respond when other people approach them. Individuals with SM often believe they look 'shy' because that is how they *feel*. It is possible to gently point out that other people can't see how they are feeling inside and can only go by their outward body language and facial expression. Unless they *know* that the young person is shy and would like to be friends, they could easily interpret their behaviour as a lack of interest. Similarly, the individual with SM cannot know what other people are feeling. They must not assume other people think badly of them. Judging by the words generated in this exercise, other people are far more likely to think they are quiet but calm, patient or nice.

The exercise could be concluded by agreeing what the student needs to do to ensure they are not regarded as 'passive' (which could be interpreted as rude, uninterested, sulky or depressed if people did not know better).

Having an escape route

Some adults are concerned that giving a young person with SM an escape route *enables* them to speak less. On the contrary, we find that it encourages them to take more risks and helps them to stay in a more relaxed frame of mind, which favours speaking. Paradoxically, in conjunction with target setting, we often remind young people that they don't *have* to speak and demonstrate various ways to escape if they need to. Depending on the situation, they could:

★ smile and shrug

★ hand over a written request

★ point to what they want (as non-English speakers often do) and let the other person talk while they nod or shake their head

★ present a brief explanation of SM (see the SM awareness cards in Appendix F)

★ produce their phone apologetically and pretend to take a call

★ shake their head and point to their throat (people will interpret this as a sore throat or laryngitis)

★ point to their watch and leave

★ smile or wave and keep walking

★ step aside and let the next person in the queue go forward.

Again, depending on the situation, we remind them that members of the public are used to people who don't speak the language, are hard of hearing, are too busy to stop or simply don't feel like speaking.

Being unable to speak feels unbearable to individuals with SM, so they put a lot of pressure on themselves to do well. This can raise their stress levels even further and result in complete avoidance of a situation. Escape routes enable them to *face* that situation and succeed.

Use role-play scenarios to practise non-verbal responses to the things that peers or strangers might say: pointing, shrugging, nodding, smiling and other facial expressions can all be used to good effect. The aim is to take the fear out of being approached because then speech may follow. More importantly, it could be the start of a good friendship!

Activity 2: Practising non-verbal responses

1 The adult sets the scene by asking the young person to imagine something like sitting in a café, waiting at the bus-stop for a friend, or attending a college open day. The adult then takes the role of a stranger and approaches the young person with a question.

For example:

Have you got the time please?	Where did you get the ketchup?
Do you know where the toilets are?	Could you watch my bag please?
What are the burgers like here?	Do you need any help?
Which tutor group are you in?	Is it OK to sit here?

2 Repeat with different voices or accents to represent different strangers!

3 Give the young person a list of questions and reverse roles. The adult responds non-verbally, using different types of body language.

4 Discuss which responses seem the friendliest and reverse roles again until the young person is responding quickly and confidently.

5 Finish by repeating the activity with *verbal* responses.

Challenging unhelpful thoughts

Perhaps the hardest thing to deal with when working with older sensitive individuals is the tendency to imagine the worst and project self-doubts onto other people. That is, to think and believe that other people view you in the same negative ways in which you view yourself. Young people with long-standing SM will frequently have felt embarrassed, stupid, ashamed or inadequate when unable to speak and, if no one tells you otherwise, it is easy to assume that other people also think you are weird, stupid or incompetent.

Reframing unhelpful thoughts as helpful, rational thoughts based on actual evidence, rather than imagination, is a fundamental strand of cognitive behavioural therapy (CBT). While aspects of this approach can be incorporated into sessions, as outlined below, it is essential to get help from professionals who are trained to practise CBT when progress is not made or you feel this is outside your remit or abilities. This is particularly true for individuals who have an additional diagnosis of social anxiety disorder (see Chapter 13, 'When it is more than SM', pages 271 and 278).

CBT is not always necessary. Some young people embrace the explanation that, as they got older, their attempt to make sense of their fear of talking led to distorted thinking patterns. They did not know they had a phobia of talking so they looked for other reasons and blamed themselves, or other people's reactions, or the specific consequences of talking.

The following activities have proved helpful.

Explain the science of how anxiety operates

This is covered in Chapter 5, Activity 5 (page 82) and the online booklet for teenagers and adults 'When the words won't come out'. More resources are suggested in Appendix F, 'Tackling anxiety'.

Identify unhelpful thoughts

Unhelpful thoughts (often called 'negative automatic thoughts') are the result of anxiety, low self-esteem and self-doubt. They make situations very difficult to deal with because they are not based on reason or reality. They may emerge when the young person completes Form 9, 'Worrying thoughts', or in response to questions about feared situations, for example:

★ What bothers you the most about this situation?

★ What do you think before/during/after this situation?

★ What are you afraid might happen in this situation?

★ What would happen if you managed to speak?

Most young people are much more forthcoming when able to express themselves through the written word (eg emails, flashcards, questionnaires) and may then be able to provide verbal clarification, as necessary.

Categorise unhelpful thoughts

Introduce young people to the types of unhelpful thinking most commonly seen with SM (see Table 10.7), and let them practise categorising 'your' negative thoughts before categorising their own. Don't be afraid to inject some humour to demonstrate irrationality, for example: 'The bus driver looked at me today – I'm sure he hates me'; 'There's a new chef starting tomorrow – I expect we'll all get food poisoning'. The message is *not* that thoughts like this are ridiculous; the mind is powerful enough to convince people that thoughts with no basis are true. Everyone needs to assume the role of detective to examine the evidence and sort fact from fiction.

Reframe unhelpful thoughts

Central to the process of cognitive reframing is the ability to answer the question, 'Is there another way of looking at this?' Sometimes young people need an adult they trust to tell them how it is. Some of these themes are touched on in Table 10.8, numbers 1–7. But once they have been introduced to the idea that SM can distort their thinking patterns, students can become very good at rewriting thoughts such as numbers 8–12 in a more neutral, factual and helpful manner themselves, often supported by activities to

Table 10.7: **Categorisation of unhelpful thinking patterns**

Category	Definition	Examples of unhelpful thought
Mind reading	Believing you know what other people are thinking	Everyone avoids me They think I'm weird
Fortune telling ('catastrophising')	Predicting only negative outcomes for the future	The whole class will laugh at me I'll never get into college
Labelling	Giving someone or something a label without taking the whole picture into account	That school is rubbish I'm no good at anything
Dismissing positive things	Telling yourself the good things that happen don't count	My teacher said it was good work but she just feels sorry for me
Unreasonable expectations ('should or must' thinking)	Having a fixed idea of how people should behave (typical of, but not exclusive to, ASD)	He should ask me to play with him She turned up late – she obviously doesn't care

challenge their perceptions, as described below. It can also help to ask, 'If someone you cared about was having these thoughts, what would you say to them?'

Having worked through and agreed more helpful ways of thinking, individuals need a visual reminder, such as a screensaver or a notice on their bedroom door, of two or three revised thoughts to repeat to themselves whenever they spot their automatic, unhelpful thoughts surfacing.

Test the theory

Young people can be helped to achieve a balanced view by writing down a thought with two columns below it for 'points for' and 'points against'. Before accepting the thought as true, it is important for them to 'put the thought on trial' and generate sufficient evidence to prove it, asking 'What evidence is there that this thought is (a) true and (b) not true?'. Feelings, while very real, do not constitute evidence. Initially, the facilitating adult may need to put forward their own observations, or prompt the young person to help them recall facts that they have discounted. It helps if the student takes 'ownership' by doing the writing.

Another useful exercise is to set the young person an observation challenge to see if what they predict actually happens. For example, how do peers react to other students when they make a mistake in class, and how is this influenced by the student's behaviour?

Sometimes, keyworkers can take up the challenge themselves. For example, one student was convinced that he would be ignored or laughed at if he could not place his order in McDonald's. The keyworker arranged to be filmed while she acted out her student's worst scenario – getting to the front of the queue and freezing on the spot. After staring at the person serving, the keyworker looked down and experienced at first hand her student's panic – her heart was racing, and she too became convinced that the person serving would walk away. However, after what seemed like an age, she pointed to the display menu and the person serving patiently looked, signed 'One?' and prepared her drink, completing the transaction with a friendly 'Thanks'. The video was the proof that her student needed that the people serving are trained to put the customer first!

Table 10.8: **Reframing unhelpful thoughts**

	Unhelpful thought	Another way to look at this
1	Everyone will stare at me when I go in	We have to check out the people in our environment – it reassures us that everything's OK
2	When they look at me, I know there must be something wrong with my appearance	It's natural to check out people. I look at other people too and often get ideas I'd like to try
3	There's no point asking, he won't hear me over this noise	He may not hear me the first time but I can repeat it and he can come closer
4	I'm no good at making friends	I find it hard to make the first approach, but I'm good at being friendly when people come up to me. I can smile and listen and sometimes answer
5	If I look down, people won't notice me and I won't need to talk	If I look down, people might ask if I'm OK. If I look up, I won't stand out
6	People will talk to me and I won't be able to answer	There's a chance that someone will talk to me but if I practise slow-breathing, there's also a chance I'll be able to answer. If I can't, I'll point to my throat and they'll think I've got laryngitis
7	I'm the only one who has difficulty talking	There are several of us who don't say much in lessons for lots of different reasons. The teacher's OK with that and we contribute in other ways
8	If I volunteer to answer and get it wrong, my teacher will show me up	My teacher doesn't make other people look stupid when they get it wrong. He likes it when they have a go and says it gives the class something to think about. It's safe to get it wrong
9	Everyone avoids me – they think I'm weird	They probably don't understand why I go off on my own and think I don't want to mix with them. I need to think about ways to make the situation better
10	The whole class will think my presentation is rubbish	I don't know that. They might think it's really good. I'll test it out on Mr Jones first.
11	I'll never get into college	I didn't go to the interview this year but there's no age limit and I can try again
12	She turned up late – she obviously doesn't care	We can't always be on time, but it doesn't make us bad people. It's good she sent me a message to let me know she was on her way – it shows she didn't want me to worry

Finally, we want to draw attention to the belief that peers will be horrified, repulsed, delighted to find a source of ridicule, or see it as a sign of weakness if the young person's 'secret' is discovered. In fact, peers are usually no more than curious when classmates can't get their words out and, generally, are extremely supportive when they recognise genuine difficulties. The YouTube extract from Channel 4's series *Educating Yorkshire*, 'Mushy Finds His Voice' (2013), demonstrates this beautifully and generates several talking points for young people who have SM – perhaps even gives a positive glimpse of their own future.

Sometimes, they can then be persuaded to test the water and share their difficulties with just one friend or new member of staff, to see what reaction they get, with a reminder that phobias are common and nothing to be ashamed of.

For example, one teacher skilfully engineered a classroom discussion around the topic of phobias, but not mentioning SM. The student with SM observed her peers' respect for the courage that individuals need to face and overcome their fears. This particular student did not reveal to her peers that she had SM. But she said she felt very much better after this discussion, knowing that she and the teacher had an explanation if it was ever needed. It was not long afterwards that she started volunteering answers in class.

Conversational skills

After years of being marginalised, some young people lack confidence in their conversational skills and feel unsure about *what* to say, rather than how to get their words out. Others may not be aware that their conversation is lacking; they have become so used to saying the bare minimum that, even when they are relaxed and able to speak, they say very little, not realising that they sound rude or uninterested. All of these young people may benefit from a few pointers or ongoing conversational practice, particularly if there are interviews or social events approaching.

The following guidelines may help and can initially be practised through instant messaging, texting or at a keyboard until the responses are more automatic.

1   Avoid answering with one word, unless you add another comment or question straight away.

2   Qualify 'Yes' or 'No' with a full sentence (eg 'Yes, I did', 'No, it wasn't'), or with more information: 'Yes, it was the best film I've seen for ages'; 'No, I wish I hadn't bothered'.

3   Keep the conversation going with one of the following options:

   • provide some information

   • ask a question

   • give a reaction, eg 'Oh no!', 'What a pain', 'I hope you find it'

   • agree or disagree with the last comment.

4   After you answer a question, it is even better if you follow it with either another question (*not* appropriate in an interview though) or more information.

5   End conversations with a short explanation or pleasantry before you say goodbye, eg 'This is my bus', 'I need to get on with my homework now', 'Good to see you'.

Each type of response can be explored individually; for example, young people could be given five different statements and asked to respond with five reactions or five questions. The next activity is useful for putting the guidelines into practice and building up speed.

Activity 3: Conversational practice

Aim: to converse in writing for a set time without returning a one-word answer. The activity takes place in either the same room (eg sitting at a keyboard) or different locations (eg instant messaging).

1   A scoring system is agreed: one point for giving more than a one-word answer; two points for keeping the conversation going with a new question or comment, and for taking a second turn after a long pause.

2   Conversational partners take turns at introducing a topic with a statement such as 'I've got my first driving lesson tomorrow'.

3   The turn now passes to the other person but, if there is a long pause, the first person may add a further comment or question such as 'Can you drive?'

4   If either person replies with a one-word answer, their partner has the option to either respond straightaway (this reduces the first person's score!) or to give them a little longer to expand on their reply.

5   Continue for an agreed time (eg 10 minutes) and then the person who started the conversation ends it. (This is excellent practice for escaping politely!)

6   When the time is up, print out the conversation if possible and get the young person to score it – this is more productive than telling them how they could improve their score. Now they have a baseline to beat next time.

7   If one-word answers persist, introduce a prompt system. If either person replies with a one word answer, they get an 'Uh oh!' emoticon or '+' in return. They should then expand their answer. (The supporting adult should 'forget' occasionally and type a one-word answer to see whether the student spots this and gives appropriate feedback.) Aim to complete the task with no prompts.

As students improve, extend their versatility by introducing topics they have no knowledge of – or interest in – such as your central heating! Progress from writing to talking, and from one-to-one to three-way conversations, which have to be carefully managed to prevent some young people feeling left out. The good news is that conversational flow really does improve with practice.

Letting go

Intervention can only be regarded as completely successful once a child or young person can communicate fully and spontaneously in all situations, including participating in groups and talking in public places. When the individual has reached this stage it will be clear that they need no further adaptations or additional support. Everyone who has been involved in the intervention can then let go and celebrate!

The following pointers may be useful to indicate that no further help is needed.

★ The child is not being held back educationally or socially.

★ The child can talk to strangers.

★ The parents and the school are no longer worried.

★ The child is happy to be discharged.

★ The parent and child or young person can carry on building confidence in social situations, aware of the underpinning rationale of treatment and the strategies that are effective.

However, sometimes the situation is not that straightforward.

★ If the individual has to make a transition soon – whether to another class, school, youth club, work placement or college – do not 'let go' until they have successfully settled into that setting. Before the transition, they will need to be introduced to the new setting and new people; and their progress should be monitored for a while once they have made the change. This can be complicated by the fact that some professionals will only concern themselves with the individual's functioning in one setting. And yet arrangements still need to be made to find a suitable other person to ensure that the individual can communicate fully in the new setting (see Chapter 11 'Making successful transitions').

★ Some professionals may need to 'let go' because they have reached the stage where they have done all that is reasonable within their remit. This may make sense but, if the individual's SM is not fully resolved, we suggest that they look carefully for someone else to provide suitable intervention or support.

★ If a young person has to move out of the remit of the professional after only brief contact, the priority is to equip them with a good understanding of their SM and what maintains it, and to prepare them with what might help them in the future (see 'Moving into adulthood' in Chapter 11).

★ Some individuals continue to tend towards mutism in a few situations. People closely involved with the child or young person in the future may need to be aware of this and adjust their style of interaction accordingly. For example, several adults who had SM as children have told us that it did not fully resolve until they left school and felt free of authority, more in control, and able to carve out a new image for themselves. Ironically, many of them are now in 'speaking' occupations, having pursued careers in teaching, law and event management.

Online resources for Chapter 10

The handouts, booklet, forms, Progress charts and appendices accompanying this chapter are available at www.routledge.com/cw/speechmark for you to access, print and copy.

Progress Chart 1 ONE-TO-ONE INTERACTION WITH A RANGE OF PEOPLE (Completed school example)

Name: __TS__   Keyworker: __Teaching Assistant (TA)__   Start date: __20 January 2016__

People and stage*	Year 2 TA	Year 2 Teacher	SENCo	Year 3 Teacher	Head Teacher	Peer 1 (name) Donna	Peer 2 Zara	Peer 3 Chelsea	Peer 4 Tyrone
1		✓ Sept. 15	✓ Sept. 15		✓ Dec. 15				
2	✓ Sept. 15	✓ Oct. 15	✓ 12/2/16			✓	✓	✓	✓
3	✓ Oct. 15	✓ 2/2/16	✓ 16/2/16			✓	✓ Dec. 15	✓ Dec. 15	✓ 7/3/16
4	✓ Dec. 15	✓ 3/4/16				✓	✓ 5/3/16	✓ 7/3/16	
5	✓ 1/2/16	✓ 3/4/16				✓	✓		
6	✓ 1/2/16 | ✓ 10/2/16	✓ 4/4/16				✓ 20/2/16 | ✓ 7/3/13	✓		
7	✓ 2/2/16 | ✓ 12/2/16					✓ 20/2/16 | ✓	✓		
8						✓ Jan. 16			

* See reverse for the key to stages of one-to-one interaction. Tick and date each box as each stage is achieved.

Note: where cells are split, ☐ = with supporting adult, ✓ = without supporting adult.

CHAPTER 11

MAKING SUCCESSFUL TRANSITIONS

Introduction

A transition is a big step for all children and young people, whether it is a change of school, class or teacher; starting for the first time at preschool, school or college; or joining a new social club or activity class. For understandable reasons it can be particularly significant for someone with selective mutism (SM) and their family. They may dread a change even more than other people, particularly if a child is doing well and the parents are afraid of losing momentum. However, a new beginning can be the fresh start that is needed; a chance to leave old memories and associations behind and gain confidence and independence in the new setting. Perhaps the most difficult transition, if support has not been available, is the transition into adulthood.

This chapter focuses on how to make transitions as smooth and helpful as possible for the child or young person who has SM by looking at:

★ general guidelines for all transition planning

★ starting preschool, school, a social club or an activity class changing school, class or teacher

★ transition to middle, secondary or high school

★ transition to college and work-related settings

★ making a fresh start

★ moving into adulthood.

Where appropriate, you will be referred to other parts of this manual where there are more details.

General guidelines for all transition planning

The following recommendations summarise the areas that need to be covered in a well-managed plan for *all* transitions.

Prepare the child

Prepare the child several weeks in advance of the transition by making positive comments about the move and familiarising them with the building, staff and rooms, as appropriate. For example:

★ Take the child on social visits with their parents for events such as the summer fair, concerts or play schemes.

★ Have a look round when the building is either empty (eg during holidays or after school) or quiet, so that the child experiences talking to their parents on the premises.

★ Encourage young children to take photos and make a booklet about 'My New Class or School' to show their friends and relatives.

Meet key members of staff in as informal a situation as possible. Include the child's younger siblings, if they are available and it is appropriate. Warn staff members not to be surprised if the child or young person speaks. It is important to recognise that this is down to everyone's careful handling of the situation which needs to continue, rather than a sudden 'cure' or an exaggeration of the child's difficulties.

Educate staff members

All staff members in the new setting must be educated about the nature and implications of SM *before* the child arrives, so that there will be no pressure to speak until the child is ready. Both parents and key staff should reassure the child about this, with an equally confident assurance that this time *will* come. If other staff members have understood the principles of SM and how best to manage it, their approach to the child will demonstrate and reinforce this understanding; they will not need to raise the issue of SM with the child themselves. In addition to discussion, and a chance for questions and answers without the child present, we recommend that a written summary of the child's profile is made available with an explanation of SM and how the child's needs are best managed. Ask the person in charge for their agreement that this document will be updated as necessary and passed on to new or temporary staff, as appropriate.

The example in Figure 11.1 overleaf was written by a parent, who tailored the advice in this manual to her unique knowledge of her child. It was folded in half and laminated as a helpful A5 diary-sized reminder for the class teacher and visiting music teacher, and a copy was kept in the school office for supply teachers.

Registration

Day one sets the tone for the rest of the term, so it is important for staff members to think about how they will handle registration if the child either has no experience of this or has not responded to roll-call in their previous class. Rather than exclude the child, agree an age-appropriate strategy such as self-registration, collecting a name badge (followed by answering in unison to 'Is [N] here?' on day two), or giving *all* of the children the option to put up their hand or say 'Here!' (they will answer if they can, with no loss of face if they can't).

Identify a supportive adult

Staff members must understand that the majority of individuals with SM find *all* initiation difficult, not just starting a conversation. Asking questions, reporting difficulties, seeking help or clarification, approaching other people, standing up for themselves, correcting or contradicting others – these can all be problematic, even if the child is invited to email or text a staff member rather than speak.

Hello!

I am
[child's name]

Child's photo
(optional)

I am a happy, energetic, inquisitive and bright [age]-year-old girl.

I happen to have an anxiety disorder called **selective mutism**.

This means that I get so nervous and anxious at the thought of speaking in some social settings that I literally cannot talk. I often have difficulty even smiling or looking you in the eye. Responding to directions may take a long time when I'm scared that I might do the wrong thing, but sometimes I can answer 'yes or no' questions with a head nod and can point to the right answer.

Please understand that I am not being stubborn, controlling, wilful or purposely ignoring you. Sometimes I stand motionless or expressionless, sometimes I have a 'fixed' smile to cover my embarrassment. I will often whisper to my Mum if I want her to ask you a question. Sometimes I will be able to talk easily when we go out, other times not at all. The good news is that I speak well at home. I can be just as animated, silly and dramatic as any girl my age. This is when I am comfortable, secure and relaxed.

Please read on to see how you can help ...

The best thing you can do to help me is ...

- Talk to me often, even if I don't always respond, so that I feel included.
- When first trying to engage me, focus on the activity and materials we are using, rather than on me. Focusing attention directly on me can make me uneasy.
- Welcome my efforts at non-verbal communication, such as head nodding, pointing or gesturing.
- Avoid direct and open-ended questions. **'Yes or no' questions are the best.**
- If children ask why I'm not speaking, explain to them that I talk plenty at home, but sometimes find it difficult to speak when other people are around. I will be fine if they let me join in quietly and wait patiently until I'm ready to talk.
- Carry on as normal when I manage to talk and don't make a fuss – I just want to be treated the same as the others.
- Increase my self-esteem by commenting on all the things I can do – I worry a lot about getting things wrong.
- Remove expectations for talking by not pressurising me to speak, bribing me, or making me the centre of attention.
- Understand that changes to routine, new situations, meeting new people, making mistakes and transitioning from one activity to another make me more anxious. Please use simple language and explain things gently.
- Loud noises, sudden changes and unexpected physical contact are very difficult for me to tolerate – please remember this.
- Be patient and understand that I really do want to speak. I am going to try to be brave and maybe join in when everyone's saying the words together or singing. I love telling my parents what I've learned when I get home!

Find out more at [**add favourite websites**].

Figure 11.1: **Introducing a child who has selective mutism**

Therefore, it is important to identify a supportive adult in the new setting who will:

★ approach, meet or email the child or young person regularly to check how they are managing

★ ensure they are as happy as possible and not being teased or bullied

★ oversee their inclusion and participation

★ liaise with home

★ arrange any extra strategies, as needed, to build independence.

> *Time invested in agreeing and implementing a transition plan will ensure that the child adapts quickly to a new environment, builds on any progress made and develops in confidence and independence.*

It will help if the designated adult in the new setting can meet the child early on – *on a one-to-one basis* – to carry out as many of the following actions as the parents (or young person) and staff members agree are appropriate. Much will depend on the child's age and the stage they have reached in their previous class or a similar activity. This will also be an opportunity to build rapport and provide the opportunity for the child to speak, using the commentary-style technique on page 122.

★ Reassure the child that they will check they are OK, have a friend to sit with, understand the work, have been to the toilet, and so on.

★ Give the younger child confidence to respond by playing games that initially only require non-verbal responses such as pointing, nodding or shaking their head.

★ Enlist the child's help with routine tasks and then praise them for a job well done.

★ Explain that the adults may need to use a loud voice sometimes, just to make sure that children are listening, but this is nothing to be frightened of.

★ Reassure the child that they will *not* be picked for demonstrations or to answer questions in front of other people unless the child volunteers.

★ Reassure older children that they can contribute or ask questions in writing until they feel relaxed enough to talk.

★ Establish how and when they will meet or contact the child.

★ Offer a bolthole or a procedure for when the child needs some 'time out'.

Make links with other children

Foster friendships with other children as actively as possible, particularly outside school by inviting peers home to play or have tea. Try to find out in advance whether there are children nearby who attend the setting and contact their parents. Teachers can help by suggesting which children would make good friends and introducing parents if the parents have difficulty making the first move.

Monitor progress

Continue to monitor the situation after any transition. With a warm welcome and sensitive handling, many children overcome their SM in a new environment. However, if this is going to happen, small signs of progress will be evident right from the start. If there is no change within a few weeks, school and family will need to take a proactive role in devising a programme to help the child or young person move forwards. Therefore, the situation should be reviewed about six weeks after transition, or sooner if there is apparent regression or distress.

Relax!

Try to relax and *don't convey your own anxiety to your child*! If everyone is positive about this big step, it may be exactly the fresh start that your child needs. Remember that many children do not speak for the first month in a new setting, so this is a time to alleviate anxiety and ensure a positive experience, rather than focus on talking.

Starting preschool, school, a social club or an activity class

Separating from parents

Parents should stay with their children in preschool settings until the child is beginning to engage with staff members, other children or activities and is comfortable for them to leave. However, don't delay the initial separation too long because it is only by successfully coping on their own that children learn not to be afraid. Do not *expect* the child to be anxious because this will be conveyed to the child. Parents can help to inspire confidence by smiling and making positive statements. This is better than asking questions which are often accompanied by raised eyebrows and, therefore, convey worry and uncertainty; for example, try saying 'You can build me a tower, just like at home', rather than 'Would you like to play with the building bricks?'

Separations can be planned *within* the session (eg the parent leaves to go to the toilet or make a drink). Praise the child for being brave and staying on their own for longer each day and let them hear you describing their adventurous behaviour to other people.

Home visits

It often helps if staff members arrange a home visit to meet the child informally, so they present a familiar face in the new setting (see 'Meeting the child for the first time', page 70 and Box 10.1 on page 181).

Before starting school, Neil's teaching assistant visited us a couple of times over the summer and established a very good bond with him. We used the informal 'sliding-in technique' with me then 'sliding out', which worked great.

The teaching assistant also prepared a little book with some pictures of herself, the teacher and the school which we then read every day.

Neil speaks freely to her now and there have been no worries as the September term approaches.

Parent involvement

If children are finding it hard to join in, it may help if parents arrive early to collect them and join in the last few activities with the child so that they leave with a positive experience. Alternatively, a parent could stay for the first half an hour, joining in the activities and helping the child to integrate, make friends or build rapport with a designated adult. It will encourage independence in the child if their parent is seen to be a *general* helper; through interacting with other children and adults, the parent models and mediates sociable behaviour.

Changing school, class or teacher

Arrange a handover meeting

The importance of a good handover from one setting to the next cannot be overemphasised. Parents and professionals such as SLTs can be instrumental in ensuring that schools fulfil their obligation to pass on and share information about a child who has additional needs when there is a change of school, teacher or class. Rather than risk this not happening because of an oversight or overwork, there is no harm in checking whether a handover meeting has been arranged, or photocopying useful materials to circulate to the relevant new staff. An introductory or updated report or letter is always useful to accompany the child's file. This should summarise the key background information that the new setting needs to know, and the main points about how to approach and work with the child or young person.

Ensure continuity

Whenever possible, arrange for children to meet staff members from their next year group *before* they move up. For example:

★ Even if the current class routinely visits the next class towards the end of the school year, add an extra visit or two with a familiar adult or friend.

★ Invite the new teacher or teaching assistant (TA) to visit the child either in their current class or at home.

★ Slide in the new teacher or TA in the last few weeks of term (see Chapter 10).

If it is not possible to meet new staff members in advance, try to ensure as much continuity as possible by doing one or more of the following:

★ keep the child with a best friend

★ arrange for the previous teacher or TA to spend some time with the child in the first week of term

★ 'borrow' the previous keyworker for a few sessions in the first fortnight of term to hand over to the new keyworker

★ keep the current keyworker (but beware of the child becoming too dependent on one adult over a long period of time: aim to change keyworker every 12–18 months, and always have a back-up keyworker for when the main keyworker is absent').

Thinking about a fresh start

Changing class is always an opportunity for a fresh start when the child understands that their SM is a fear which has built up and persisted out of habit, but can be overcome in small steps when supported by staff who won't rush them. So it helps to find out how the new teacher carries out registration, so that the child is aware of what is required and has a chance to practise their response before the move. By speaking on their first day, they will have started the process of turning things around.

Transition to middle, secondary or high school

Make an informed choice

Most education systems require children to change schools around 11 to 14 years old. Parents will want to be reassured that the new, and usually much larger, school has a good record for pastoral care and that key staff members sound knowledgeable and experienced about supporting anxious and vulnerable pupils. While parents are responsible for the final decision, it is important for them to listen to and take into account their child's wishes. The child may:

★ want to go to the same school as their friends

★ be looking for a fresh start where no one will react if they talk

★ pick up on a particularly welcoming atmosphere at the prospective school's open day

★ be drawn to a particular aspect such as the music or the sports facility.

Once students have found their own incentive, they often surprise their parents by taking challenges such as the size of the school in their stride.

Having found a school that seems to meet all, or most, of the family's requirements, there is then the possibility that the child is offered a place at a different school. By taking a calm, factual approach with the aim of demonstrating that their child's needs cannot be appropriately met elsewhere, parents can appeal this decision, ideally with the support of their child's current school.

Box 11.1 overleaf is a sample letter written by a professional which formed part of the evidence compiled by a primary school SENCo for such an appeal.

Box 11.1: Sample letter from professional to primary school SENCo about secondary school transfer

Background summary

B was referred to the speech and language therapy department in 2011 because of her phobia of talking in certain situations (selective mutism). Over the last four years we have watched her develop from an excessively anxious and self-conscious child, who found any form of interaction outside her family difficult, to a child who is happy to be involved in non-verbal activities and is beginning to speak to trusted friends and adults. Most of the gains in her spoken communication have taken place in the last year since assigning her a one-to-one keyworker at school. So, clearly, this is a critical time for B, in terms of both maintaining the progress she has made and building on her current success. As her confidence grows, we are beginning to see the outgoing, talkative child that her family and friends see. It is essential that the gap between her relaxed and 'frozen' personas continues to close, so that she can achieve her academic and social potential without long-term effects on her mental health.

Recommendations

As with any anxious child, it is essential to ensure continued confidence building and self-esteem through:

- a sense of being valued

- a sense of achievement rather than failure

- structured support to gradually face their fears rather than finding comfort in the status quo (avoidance strengthens fear).

This means that all changes need to be planned and carefully managed so that B does not become overloaded and overwhelmed. A good method is to take small steps forward, changing only one thing at a time, so that anxiety is controlled at a manageable level.

Success at secondary school will depend on four factors.

1   As few changes as possible for B at any one time. Her secondary school therefore needs to be as close as possible to her primary school in terms of size, structure and ethos.

2   The support of a mentor from student support or special needs department – ideally, someone who has training and/or experience of working with selective mutism (SM) and appreciates that the difficulty in speaking is very different from problems caused by shyness, traumatisation, emotional difficulties or absent parenting.

3   The full understanding of all staff about the nature of SM and how to handle it on a daily basis, so that B's access to the curriculum is not compromised. This will require ongoing efficient communication and networking; as any person who does not appreciate that SM is a genuine phobia and anxiety disorder can unwittingly undo everyone else's good work, and make a child who has SM afraid to go to school. In time, B's performance anxiety and SM may need to be taken into account in connection with public examinations and oral tests.

4   A sympathetic peer group with minimal to zero levels of teasing, bullying, disruptive behaviour and rudeness – all of which put anxious children in a heightened state of tension throughout the day.

I do hope this information is helpful; please do not hesitate to contact me again if needed.

Build confidence

While some children look forward to changing schools, others are less confident. Many anxious or vulnerable children benefit from transition groups during their last term to prepare them for secondary school. These are generally organised by the sending primary school, with or without input from the secondary school. Typical topics include learning new vocabulary for secondary school life; practising reading timetables; looking at photos and maps of the new schools before extra orientation visits; and even learning how to do up a school tie!

The summer holidays are a good time for shared activities and trips with friends who will also be attending the new school. Practise making the train or bus journey to school with a friend or sibling and meeting new people who know nothing about the child's difficulties. Remind the child that if they can talk to strangers, they will be able to talk to the people they meet for the first time at their new school (see 'Making a fresh start' on page 247).

Ensure a united approach

Some children are very confident that this is the move they need, having proved to themselves that, when they are with strangers, they have no difficulty in talking. They have a deep conviction that they will be fine in a new school; they are adamant that they don't want staff to know about their difficulties; and they don't want to look back. Others need more of a helping hand and the reassurance that staff will be looking out for them, while being careful not to draw attention to them. This is best achieved by agreeing simple strategies *before* the move.

Box 11.2 (overleaf) is a sample plan that was written by a secondary school SENCo after a handover meeting during the student's last term at primary school. It was distributed to all staff in the secondary school after a short information session and DVD about SM at a staff meeting.

Transition to college and work-related settings

Make a moving-on plan

A moving-on plan, written jointly with the student and sent in their name, can be very powerful and effective, not only for the staff members in the new setting but also for helping the students themselves to understand their SM better. Box 11.3 (page 245) is a helpful template which can be adapted in any similar circumstances – work experience, meeting a career adviser, visiting the job centre, and for new employers. Also see 'Making a fresh start' (page 247).

Prepare for interviews

When a college interview is looming, contact the student support department and request a copy of the questions so that the young person can practise with a parent or mentor. Staff members may be unable to guarantee the order of the questions. However, they should be able to accommodate the young person's social anxiety and history of SM in this way, if evidence of their difficulties is provided by the young person's school or an outside professional.

Box 11.2: Sample education plan for transition to secondary school

Name: C R

Information

C has been diagnosed with selective mutism (SM) and severe social anxiety. This sometimes causes her to 'freeze' when compelled to speak or if she is watched too closely by other people. The same condition often causes her to speak at barely audible volumes to some people, notably authority figures. C may become very distressed if overwhelmed by a situation. C is terrified of getting anything wrong.

Objectives

- For C to feel positive about her return to mainstream education.
- For C to participate fully in the curriculum, using non-verbal means, as required.

Strategies

Don't pressurise C to speak. The focus should be on welcoming C into the class, making her feel happy, safe, involved and that she can make a valuable contribution to the lesson.

Don't ask direct questions of C such as 'How did you do that?!' but make them rhetorical, eg 'I wonder how you did that'. This takes away any pressure from C feeling that she has to answer your question.

Wherever possible, ensure that C sits with a friend (we will know more about her friends after the first two days of term). C does not tend to have difficulty communicating with other children.

When instructions have been given, quietly ask C if she understands the task or homework and accept a nod or shake of the head as an answer. C cannot initiate conversation and will need to be given the opportunity to return to you with her questions written down.

When starting any written task, C will take longer than the others because of her fear of getting it wrong. Advice on how to start, or a first sentence, will make this less traumatic for C, but the main point is she needs not to feel rushed and assurance that we all make mistakes.

It is important that C has regular contact with a member of staff. Alongside her fortnightly tutor meetings with CB, she will meet with AF at least once a week initially.

Having said all this, don't feel that you have to tip-toe around C. She will respond well to patience, understanding and humour just like any other student.

Here are some tips given by children who have SM on how you can help them.

* They do want to talk, and will talk as their anxiety levels drop, as long as there is no pressure to speak.

* Don't single out children in public to praise them for talking or rebuke them for not talking.

* Be encouraging, patient and positive.

* Be prepared for a long haul to the 'cure'.

* Close collaboration is needed between home and school.

For further information about SM, please see the training notes, copies of which are held by [person] and in [place].

Box 11.3: Sample moving on plan written by a teenager with adult support and made available to college before transition

Educational background and current situation

I always found it very difficult to talk at school and would usually freeze when teachers asked me a question. I left [XXX] School during Year 11 when I started having panic attacks and became too anxious to attend. I couldn't take my GCSEs but, up until then, I was coping well with my course work and was on track for at least Cs in my basic subjects. I particularly enjoyed English and ICT and would like another chance to take these, along with Maths.

Some work experience was planned for me with deaf children and animals, which I was really looking forward to but, for some reason, it was left too late to organise. I would love another opportunity for work experience as I enjoy being busy and doing something practical. Other things I enjoy include looking after my young nephews and nieces, taking care of all our animals, walking friends' dogs, going to the gym, spending time with my friends (I talk easily to them!) and computing.

Since leaving school I have started rebuilding my confidence and now go out much more, use the telephone, shop independently and communicate with people who I've never managed to talk to before. I feel ready to resume my education and am looking forward to a fresh start at college, even though I am nervous about this too. If I can just get through the first day, I know I will be OK!

Where I see myself going

I would love to follow a career with animals, so I have applied for the Animal Care course at [YYY] College. [ZZZ] College is full of people I used to know at school – it will be much easier for me to start again with people who won't question me about why I missed so much school and what I have been doing since I left school.

I would also like to pick up my GCSE course work and think the part-time GCSE option would work well for me if the timings fit in with the rest of my timetable. I also hope that going to college will help me make new friends and build on the progress I have made this year, so that I have the confidence to travel on my own and become more independent.

The support I need and what I am doing to achieve my goals

I used to attend [specify service] but left just over a year ago as it was not helping me. Since then [youth worker/counsellor/SLT/voluntary agency] has helped me with my communication and anxiety and I have made good progress.

I have reached the point where my main fear about college is the first day. It was very helpful to talk to [Head of Learning Support] earlier this week and look around the college site. If I get a place I will visit a few more times to familiarise myself with the buildings and get used to being around other students again. I don't want to be seen as 'different' from the other students and would like to integrate with as little attention drawn to me as possible.

Specific things to help me

- Knowing that I can contact [Head of Learning Support/Learning Mentor] if I need to talk (she has given me her email address).

- Attending Enrolment on the same day as my friend if she gets a place too (I am going to let [Head of Learning Support] know her name so she can organise this).

- Being introduced to other students on Day One and at the team-building events, so that I am not on my own and relying on other people to make the first move.

- Very clear instructions about timetable arrangements and changes because I hate to get anything wrong and get panicky if I am uncertain about anything.

- Friendly staff who chat to me normally but don't mind if I don't say much back at first.

- Staff who let students email them if they have any concerns or questions. I find it a lot easier to answer emails than to initiate them, though.

- Staff who don't press me for more information if I can't think of anything to say.

- Time to settle in at my own pace.

- Rooms with enough seats so I don't have to go to another room to collect a chair.

- Being told which seats are free so I'm not worrying about taking someone's place.

- Being paired with other quiet students who are looking to make friends.

- Sitting with friends.

- Talking in small groups of peers rather than in front of the whole class.

- Writing things down to help me gather my thoughts.

- Knowing I don't have to do presentations. I need to talk to tutors privately about when I feel ready for this.

- To get used to talking to tutors in small groups, or at my seat, before I talk to them in front of the whole class.

- Having somewhere to go if things get too much and I just need to sit quietly and get my anxiety under control. I don't think I will need this, but it would help to know that there is somewhere to go and that my tutors would understand and know where to find me.

- Travelling to and from college with my friend or one of my parents.

- Staff who understand that, when I'm anxious, I find it very difficult to initiate communication. So, if you don't hear from me, please email or text me and don't think I am deliberately missing a lesson.

What will *not* help me because I want to be the same as everyone else:

- Individual meetings with learning support or tutors (other than the routine meetings that *all* students have).

- Being singled out or treated differently in front of other students, eg someone saying 'Claire, you can write it down if you find it easier.'

Support independence

Never dismiss the idea of work experience for students who don't speak in classroom settings. They often flourish in a more practical working environment with a sympathetic supervisor.

Student support departments may be able to implement or share a travel training programme to support a young person who is not travelling independently.

Making a fresh start

Timing

If children have less than a school term left in one class or setting when starting an SM programme, we recommend focusing on their *next* setting to expand their talking circle. General anxiety reduction will be needed in the current setting, in terms of talking to the child and modifying the environment (see Chapter 8). However, it may not be worth setting up a programme to help the child talk there if this time can be channelled into preparing for the next setting.

Similarly, a young person who has not spoken at secondary school for several years will probably make this breakthrough at college or university more easily.

Rowena (Ro) had never spoken at nursery. The following intervention started soon after Easter to coincide with school entry.

- The TA (Janet) from Ro's new school visited Ro at home a few times during her final term at nursery.

- Ro began talking to her Mum in front of Janet, and then to Janet directly.

- Ro visited her new school one evening, and chatted to Janet in the classroom and the empty playground.

- Ro visited the reception class with Janet towards the end of term and joined in a craft session. She spoke to the teacher at her table, and to another TA in the playground (staff were advised to avoid direct questions).

- Ro's Mum invited future classmates round to tea during the summer holidays.

- Ro made a smooth transition to her new school in September.

Whenever appropriate, remind the child or young person that the setting is new for *everyone*. Everyone else will be nervous and looking for friends, not just them, and it is to be expected.

Leave the phobia behind

Young people preparing for transition to secondary school or college need a good understanding of SM as a phobia which can be overcome, rather than seeing it as part of their personality (see Chapter 5, page 81). In this way, they can regard their fresh start as a chance to leave their phobia behind in the old setting.

While it is important to know that they will be made welcome, without any uncomfortable pressure to speak, young people need to understand that even managing a single word such as 'Hi' or 'Yes', or answering the register, is the way to reinvent themselves in their new setting and leave their phobia behind.

> The BBC documentary *My Child Won't Speak* (which is available on YouTube) shows how a 14 year old transferred to a new secondary school and was able to speak from day one.
>
> She knew that if she could just get one word out, she would not be labelled as 'the kid who doesn't speak'. Although her heart was racing, she got out that one word 'Hello' in response to her head of year's greeting. And, for the first time, she felt 'free'.

Talk to strangers

The best preparation for a fresh start at secondary school or college is to focus on developing independence and shared interests outside school and the confidence to talk to *strangers* (see Chapter 9, pages 161–165). Strangers don't expect a sustained conversation, and the young person has much more control over initiating and ending the exchange; for example, 'Do you have the time please? Thank you'.

Encourage young people to challenge themselves in as many ways as possible, on the understanding that the initial panic will pass with perseverance. For example:

★ make phone calls

★ order pizza

★ buy sweets, a magazine or cinema tickets

★ go on errands

★ walk the dog

★ earn money from car washing and babysitting

★ go swimming, or join a gym or a cycling club

★ develop interests at evening classes

★ join a volunteer programme.

Every trip outside the front door and every few words spoken are a step towards overcoming SM. Remind the young person that no one likes a talkative person who dominates every conversation; equally, no one objects to a quiet person who does not initiate conversation. Simple responses such as gestures and a smile are all they need to get started!

Classroom management

Having chosen to make a fresh start, young people will not want their peers to know about their history of SM. They simply want to be treated fairly and included in the same way as everyone else (except that they may not talk), without a big fuss being made of them. They want their teachers to make it acceptable for some members of the class to be quieter than others, and to find ways of involving them in activities that don't show them up.

A positive attitude to quiet students in general will greatly enhance their experience. For example, 'Some students like to talk, some like to think – I don't mind which as long as you all contribute in some way'; 'I want each group to decide which slides to include in your presentation, who will advance the slides, who will read out the bullet points and who will take questions at the end'.

Think hard about switching school

Finally, although a fresh start often works to the child's advantage in our experience, especially when managed in the ways described here, a change of school at an unnatural time needs to be considered very carefully. It cannot be assumed that this is what every child needs or naturally means an end to their SM. If a child is struggling at a particular school, it is important to know exactly what the issues are, in order to ensure that things will be different in a new setting.

Moving into adulthood

Clearly, and logically, some people move into adulthood with unresolved SM. We are paediatric therapists but, through our teaching and advising, we have met a significant number of adults who have only recently recovered or still have SM. Some of their stories are included in Chapter 15. Here, we briefly discuss some of the issues around SM in adulthood with suggestions for possible ways forward.

General issues of SM in adulthood

★ *It is not known how common SM in adults is* because the little that has been written about it focuses on individual case studies and recollections, rather than prevalence. A survey by Carl Sutton is cited in Sutton & Forrester (2015) and summarised in *Finding Our Voices*, issue 4 (2015) (see Appendix F, 'Resources'). It had 83 participants over the age of 18 who reported that they had SM. They came from 11 different countries and there were four times as many females as males. Based on current estimates for children and documented rates of recovery, Sutton suggests that SM prevalence is at least one in 2,400 young adults and this figure is probably higher, due to low profile SM (see 'Prevalence' on page 36).

★ *There is no clear model for how SM in adults should be managed or by whom.* Because of its nature and invisibility, adult SM is below the radar. Relatively few medical professionals, therapists or staff in tertiary education will meet an adult who has SM; and the condition probably won't have been mentioned in their training in relation to adults.

★ *It is vital to raise awareness within adult services*, for when a professional does meet an adult with SM (probably with coexisting conditions) the identification of SM will influence both the treatment process and the possibility of a better outcome.

Specific issues for adults with SM

★ Lack of public awareness means that adults may not even be aware that they have SM. In the absence of a rational explanation, many feel ashamed and try to camouflage their difficulty talking, rather than consider seeking help. For those who do suspect SM, difficulty coming forward and communicating their needs is part of the condition, so it is not always easy to seek help or support.

★ There may not have been a diagnosis (only 25 per cent of the adults in Sutton's study received a diagnosis of SM in childhood). So it is important to clarify whether the mutism fits the criteria for SM (see Chapter 3) or is it better described in another way. The online booklet for teenagers and adults with SM, 'When the Words Won't Come Out', was written in conjunction with adults who have SM. It may help individuals and practitioners decide whether SM seems 'a good fit'.

★ There may be other coexisting (sometimes called *comorbid*) conditions to consider. These may have been present from childhood and overlooked, ignored or misdiagnosed; or ones that started later. Indeed, there is a greater chance of coexisting conditions in people who experience SM into mid-teens and adulthood, as discussed in Chapter 13.

★ Long-term SM can have a debilitating effect on self-confidence and self-esteem. As one woman who recovered from SM in her forties put it, 'It has a huge impact on the development of one's true self/ identity that is imprisoned behind the silence.'

★ In addition to the SM, there may be unresolved emotional or psychological issues associated with either early contributing or maintaining factors, the effects of years of misunderstanding and mismanagement of the SM, or the longstanding deprivation of freedom of expression.

Recommendations and resources

SM affects adults with varying degrees of severity and impact on their lives, and a holistic and person-centred approach to assessment and treatment is essential. It is not possible or appropriate to recommend a single treatment path: for many individuals, the issues are complex and a coordinated package of care addressing a range of issues with SM at its core is needed. We urge practitioners and policy-makers in adult therapy services and multidisciplinary mental health teams to broaden the scope of their care planning and provision to include SM. They should seek the views of adults who have SM, and liaise with colleagues in children's services who have SM expertise. Similarly, we urge paediatric practitioners to educate their colleagues in adult services and work together to improve transitional care for 16–25 year olds.

We hope that adults with SM will find the following suggestions useful.

★ Consider asking for a diagnosis to confirm, rule out or highlight relevant issues and, where appropriate, to facilitate access to services and entitlements to assist independent living. An SLT or a psychology department may be able to help.

★ Long-term support may be provided by volunteers from befriending services or mental health charities such as Mind, Together or Rethink Mental Illness in the UK.

★ To avoid the isolation of feeling that you are the only one who has SM, we recommend the website Finding Our Voices and their magazine and chat forum for young people and adults, together with the iSpeak website and SM Space Café Facebook group (see Appendix F, 'Websites'). Work is currently being done to develop adult SM peer support groups in the UK, locally and then nationally. These groups aim to provide face-to-face support for adults with SM as a step towards acceptance and recovery. See Appendix F 'Resources and useful contacts' for further information.

★ You may be able to plan recovery for yourself, as indicated by some of our contributors in Chapter 15 and in the BBC Radio 4 programme *Finding Your Voice* (2015). Invariably, this involves understanding the role that anxiety plays in SM and a deep conviction that the condition can be overcome by pushing yourself beyond your comfort zone. The online booklet for teenagers and adults with SM 'When the Words Won't Come Out' may be useful here, combined with the programmes in Appendix B and Handouts 16–18 if you find phobia management techniques appealing. Chapter 10, 'Additional considerations for adolescents and young adults' (page 214), provides complementary information about breathing and voice production.

★ It can help to have someone who can act as a support or mentor while you seek help or set yourself graded targets to overcome on your road to recovery. This should be someone who believes in you and your SM, listens to you and encourages you.

★ Long-standing SM may leave you feeling out of practice with general conversation and you may feel more confident with someone who needs help to improve their language skills. Organisations such as Couchsurfing bring together people from all over the world, or look out for opportunities to provide conversation practice for migrants on a voluntary basis.

★ You may be looking for a particular type of therapy. Since SM is a recognised anxiety condition linked to social anxiety, the recommended traditional treatment is cognitive behavioural therapy (CBT) (see Chapter 13). To overcome SM using CBT, you need to understand and face the fear of talking; to challenge unhelpful thinking patterns that impede progress and the build-up of self-esteem; and to work out a hierarchy of situations which can be tackled in a graded way. An experienced therapist, who is able to draw from a range of therapy techniques, should be able to work with you despite the usual expectation to talk in therapy.

★ CBT is usually offered as a short course, more likely to provide the tools to continue to work on SM than to overcome it. However, CBT focuses on current thinking patterns and behaviours, rather than the role of past experiences in shaping your beliefs, attitudes and behaviour. Other forms of counselling or psychotherapy may initially be more helpful in addressing deep-rooted feelings and conflicts which are preventing progress.

★ Equally, you may want to try a so-called 'alternative' therapy. Adults with SM find a variety of styles helpful. A common theme in successful alternative therapies is the combination of feeling accepted by the therapist, externalisation of the SM as something that can be overcome, and a form of physical release. However, we strongly advise against any therapy which encourages the adult to take responsibility for their SM as a result of their own life choices.

★ As with many parents of children who have SM, you will need to be ready to educate the professionals or practitioners you approach, perhaps using the online booklet for teenagers and adults with SM. It is particularly important to explain how you will find it easiest to communicate with them initially. Whichever method you choose, the most important elements in your recovery will be:

– the therapist's understanding of SM and appreciation that in any treatment, social comfort precedes speech

– a shared understanding of your SM in relation to other emotional or psychological issues which may need to be addressed alongside the SM

– your relationship with the therapist as someone you can trust, who understands you and only wants you to be able to communicate more fully and freely.

Online resources for Chapter 11

The handouts, booklet and appendices accompanying this chapter are available at www.routledge.com/cw /speechmark for you to access, print and copy.

PART 4

REFLECTIVE PRACTICE: LEARNING FROM EXPERIENCE

CONTENTS

CHAPTER 12

TROUBLESHOOTING: WHY ISN'T IT WORKING?

Introduction

You may have come to this chapter feeling stuck, frustrated or disheartened because the small-steps programme is not working. So, first, here is a positive message: we must stress that, although many factors can impede progress, *they can all be resolved*! It is never too late to repair the situation after a setback, with open discussion between everyone involved, to identify and modify the relevant factors.

This chapter may be useful to people who supervise less experienced colleagues as well as those who directly experience or manage selective mutism (SM). It can also be used in workshops or on training days to promote understanding of the principles of SM management or for people who need a refresher session.

Specifically, this chapter looks at:

★ common practices which prevent or hinder the progress of an intervention programme, along with some possible solutions

★ situations where children appear to have regressed

★ identifying and addressing the reasons for the setbacks.

The various accompanying materials for this chapter are in the online resource library.

Practices affecting progress in small-steps programmes

We see lack of progress with intervention programmes in one of two ways:

★ children fail to meet the targets set, resulting in either the school or the child opting out of the programme

★ children repeat the same or similar targets at every session, resulting in the programme coming to a halt.

In every case, we have identified one or more of the following practices which contradict the advice provided in this manual.

1 Inadequate assessment before the programme

Inadequate assessment before starting the programme may lead to an inappropriate diagnosis and/or intervention plan.

a) Factors at home or at school which may be reinforcing the child's mutism or raising their anxiety may not have been fully explored and addressed.

b) The child may have additional problems such as autism spectrum disorder or language difficulties which need to be addressed alongside the mutism.

c) The child's reluctance to speak may result from cultural or personal inhibitions which need to be addressed in the first instance.

It may help to revisit (or use for the first time) the extended parent interview form, the school report form, the record of speaking habits, the checklist of possible maintaining factors or the reactions of family/ friends/staff form as tools to either obtain more information or discover other concerns (in the online resource library). In addition, Form 16 (a staff questionnaire) may reveal inconsistencies in teaching styles or attitudes which could account for slow progress or a child's reluctance to attend school.

2 Lack of teamwork and information sharing

An ongoing team approach involving both home and school is paramount. Sufficient time must be invested in information sharing, joint planning and monitoring to avoid the loss of momentum or the programme being abandoned. Any unaddressed anxiety or inconsistent handling will undermine the effectiveness of direct work with the child. For example, if one person is offering money, computer games or a meal out as a reward for speaking, it should not be surprising that someone else's stars appear less exciting and even negotiable. Furthermore, using rewards as a *bribe* conflicts with acknowledging and celebrating achievement. This results in mixed messages and increased anxiety for the child. (See Chapter 10, page 191 for more about rewards and incentives.) Even when parents cannot contribute to the programme directly, every effort should be made to forge a home–school link to ensure as united an approach as possible.

Similarly, there should be a procedure in place to routinely bring new staff on board; ideally, before they come into contact with the child. An information sheet of agreed management strategies should always be available (see Chapter 11, Figure 11.1 and Box 11.2 for examples). Checks and reminders may be needed to ensure consistency.

3 The family is inadvertently supporting a pattern of avoidance

Home interventions need to run alongside school-based programmes, to help children overcome their fear of talking with new people both at home and in the community. If the family is maintaining old patterns – for example, answering for their child, or allowing them to whisper or use gesture with them – this could be holding up progress at school by increasing the child's dependence on their parents and strengthening patterns of avoidance. Parents and close family members may not have had sufficient information and support to gradually extend their child's talking beyond their comfort zone.

See Chapter 9 and the online resources for suitable strategies and handouts, especially Handout 12 'Do I answer for my child?', Handout 13 'Easing in friends and relatives' and Handout 14 'Talking in public places'.

4 Insufficient keyworker support and reviews

Working with children who have SM is emotionally draining and keyworkers need ongoing support and regular opportunities for reviewing progress and sounding out ideas with the school SENCo, class teacher or visiting specialist. Time must be factored in for this, not just for face-to-face contacts with the child. Outside agencies should note that leaving a programme in school without building in this support is rarely successful. Inexperienced keyworkers will need help, encouragement and reassurance to plan targets and to maintain momentum. Never put the onus on a keyworker to make contact only if they have a problem, which needs courage to admit and can imply failure. Review meetings must be frequent enough for the keyworker to feel well supported and any difficulties with the programme should be fully discussed and resolved. (See Chapter 7, page 104, for more about frequency of review meetings.)

5 Inadequate discussion about the intervention and the optimum length of sessions

Some schools may have been unaware of the time commitment required to successfully address SM. If they are concerned about this, they may not appreciate that a relatively small time investment now will eliminate the need for prolonged intervention and anxiety in later years. Other schools may be committed to the long haul but have allocated a keyworker to the child for only one or two overly lengthy sessions per week.

Frequent individual sessions lasting 10–15 minutes are required to establish speech initially (a minimum of three times a week) and then a gradual reduction in frequency in the generalisation phase (when sessions can be increased to 20–30 minutes). It should take no longer than a term for schools to slide in the initial keyworker and slide out the parent. Subsequent generalisation to other people and situations, and the transitions into new classes and schools, must be managed as part of the intervention plan.

6 Intervention started too early before the child was prepared

There is no point in starting an intervention programme without discussing with the child the nature of their difficulties, as set out in the Pep Talk (page 73). The child needs reassurance that progress will be made by moving one small step at a time, at their pace. They also need to know where each activity is heading, in order to avoid heightened wariness and anxiety, a sense of being 'tricked' into talking and a dread of further consequences. Many children fear that if they talk to one person, they will immediately be expected to speak to everyone else as well – their secret will be out! They need to hear from everyone involved – parent, keyworker and teacher are the usual minimum – that there is no rush, and that they can get used to talking to just one new person at a time.

Children can also feel more in control and confident if they are consulted and allowed to make choices, even in small ways: for instance, which child will join the talking circle next, or whether to use reading or counting for a warm-up activity.

7 The child is not comfortable with the designated keyworker

Young children need very regular contact with a keyworker, in a familiar place, to gradually feel comfortable and confident in their company. Therefore, sessions need to be either at home or in school in the early years with an appropriate adult who is part of the child's everyday routine. It usually helps if the keyworker is someone attached to the child's class, rather than an adult who they see only for their one-to-one sessions.

There may have been insufficient time to develop rapport before attempting the sliding-in technique or the keyworker may have little understanding of the condition and conveys impatience or insensitivity. Sometimes the keyworker has not been particularly sympathetic to the child in the past and the child has a clear memory of this. A genuine apology and fresh start can work wonders!

8 Insufficient or broken trust between keyworker and child

Children will only relax sufficiently to take new risks when they trust that what the keyworker says will happen actually does happen. For example, if the child has been assured that everyone at school understands their difficulty, and that they need only talk to their keyworker for the time being, valuable trust can be lost if other staff members try to elicit speech. Is more staff education needed? Equally, if the child is told they will be working alone, they need to see a 'Do Not Disturb' sign on the door, rather than worrying that someone will come in at any moment. It only needs someone to barge into the room a couple of times for the child to stop talking during sessions.

9 Plans are not shared with the child

Frequency of sessions

The child may have no clear indication about how often the sessions will happen. There may be no warning that sessions are about to take place or no explanation if sessions are missed. Children who have SM need to know exactly what is happening, otherwise they worry, which is counterproductive to 'having a go' and taking risks. Many have a heightened sense of 'abandonment', so it is vital they believe that their keyworker won't let them down without sufficient notice or, at the very least, a good explanation and an apology when a session is cancelled.

Timing of sessions

The child may have no clear indication about how long the sessions will last. Open-ended sessions increase their uncertainty and anxiety. The child will be less inclined to take risks if they don't know how long they will be required to keep pushing themselves. Fixed times for the sessions ensure that the end is always in sight and motivate the child to make the most of their time with the keyworker. We usually recommend 10 to 15 minutes for the target component of each session (page 188).

Content of sessions

The child may be unclear about the content of sessions. Minimise their uncertainty by providing an outline of the session at the beginning (eg 10 minutes on targets, complete a questionnaire about bullying, check to see how course work is going) and give students the option of choosing the order (they may prefer you to choose). Younger children may simply be working on targets.

10 Inappropriate strategies

Sometimes the keyworker tries to make the sessions more interesting, personal or general, based on their experience with children who do *not* have SM. Strategies that are effective with shy children, or children with ASD or language difficulties, for example, are often stressful for children who have SM. It will *not* help to do any of the following.

★ Attempt to build rapport by starting or finishing with a general chat and asking about the child's weekend, for example. Everyday conversation and sharing personal information are extremely difficult for children who have SM.

★ Focus on social skills training (eg making eye contact, greetings and initiating conversation) rather than anxiety management and specific interventions for SM.

★ Introduce 'motivating' activities with little regard for their position in the 'social functioning' quadrant of the confident talking model (see Chapter 10, page 210). Children who have SM need activities that cause the minimum of anxiety. Sometimes these may seem boring to keyworkers or parents, but they are designed with phobia management in mind, rather than language development or stimulation.

11 The parent or keyworker did not slide out

If the child becomes dependent on the parent's presence, they may get into the habit of only talking when the parent is there. Therefore, it is very important that the parent is used only as a transitional person in the programme. As soon as the child is talking in sentences to a school keyworker, for example, the parent should start to slide out. This enables the child to become used to talking to the keyworker, whether their parent is present or not.

Similarly, the child can become dependent on their keyworker's presence and only talk during planned sessions; this delays the further generalisation and spontaneous use of language. After introducing each new person, it is important for the keyworker to leave the room, or move out of sight, while the child and the new person do one or more activities which can be extended as appropriate. This is equally true when a parent takes on the keyworker role in order to slide in a succession of new people.

See Chapter 10 (page 200) and Handout 16, step 17 (online) for more details about sliding out.

12 The keyworker enjoys having a unique relationship with the child

It can feel very special to be the only person a child talks to in the school setting. Subconsciously, a keyworker may delay the generalisation phase to hold on to this privileged position. The keyworker genuinely believes that the child is benefiting from the sessions, and from having a go-between, but is confusing SM management with general nurturing and advocacy. The child will only overcome their difficulties by facing their fears with more stretching targets. A keyworker knows they have been successful when the child they support no longer needs them!

13 The keyworker follows the child's lead, not vice versa

It is not appropriate to hand control of the programme to the child by asking or allowing them to set their own targets; this conveys uncertainty and raises anxiety. When put in this position, most children choose to repeat 'easy' activities, rather than take risks, or they don't respond at all. They need the adult to take a strong lead and say 'Now you are ready to ...'.

As discussed on page 129, it is important for children to be given *options*, but only within an overall progression which has been set by the keyworker. The keyworker may need to remind the child that they are there to help the anxiety (the 'nasty feeling') go away, so that the child can have friends and fun, get help with their work, and so on. It is useful to have the phrase 'I can't do that because then I wouldn't be helping you' ready! Use the child's favourite activities as *rewards* rather than time-fillers, and *end sessions early* if the child is not ready to try something new (see page 192).

14 The keyworker lacks confidence

The keyworker may repeat the same or similar activities at every session because they lack the confidence to move the child on. Usually the keyworker is afraid to set the child more challenging tasks in case of failure. Perhaps this happened in the past and the keyworker was unsure how to deal with it. In effect, the keyworker's own fear of failure is holding back the child.

It is essential to repeat the last two or three activities from the previous session, provided they are very short. Then it is important to move forwards each time with a clear aim for the next few sessions; for example, to slide out the parent, increase the group size, or transfer sessions to the classroom. See Chapter 10, page 192 for information about what to do if the child does not meet a target.

15 The target is too difficult

More than one variable was changed when setting a new target

The keyworker may not appreciate how subtle some of the variables are, so they may have inadvertently changed more than one variable at a time, making the target too difficult. Chapter 10 (page 190) lists the possible variables with examples of how to move forward. See also the scenarios at the end of this chapter.

One variable was changed but it was too much for the child

When a child fails a target, it often helps to share ideas with a colleague about how the step could be broken down into even smaller steps. For example, if the child does not manage to sustain voice when their teacher enters the room, consider:

★ Has good rapport previously been established so that the child can comfortably communicate with their teacher without talking?

★ Could they work on leaving the door open wider before the teacher enters the room?

★ Could the teacher join in the talking before they enter the room?

★ Could the teacher enter the room backwards so there is no eye contact?

★ Could the child make a voice recording for the teacher?

★ Would it be better to slide in another child or more familiar adult before the teacher?

16 Sessions lack a warm-up or are too far apart to capitalise on progress

When a child has overcome their fear of speaking, and can talk spontaneously to their keyworker without hesitation, they will be able to resume each session where they left off, even after a long gap of weeks or even months. Until then, it is necessary to ease into each session with a warm-up activity which the child has previously managed easily, such as reading aloud or reciting the letters of the alphabet together.

When working on targets, it is always necessary to warm up by repeating the last couple of targets from the previous session before moving on. When sessions are more than a few days apart, it may be necessary to go back even further, to gradually build up to the point the child previously reached.

17 Tasks are too vague or too long

Keep tasks short and specific. Otherwise, there will only be time for one or two more after the warm-up, and the child will be overwhelmed by their open-ended nature. Choose tasks such as 'read five words', 'read aloud for one minute', 'count to 20, taking it in turns', and 'give and solve two clues each'; and *avoid* tasks such as 'read to me', 'talk to each other for five minutes' or 'tell me about your holiday.'

18 The child was rewarded after failing to meet a target

When children fail to meet a target, it is counterproductive to (a) let them think they have succeeded by giving them a token or a sticker, or (b) put the targets away and spend the rest of the session doing something easier. These actions reinforce avoidance. They also lead the child to see the keyworker as someone nice to spend time with, rather than someone who is there to help them move forward by tolerating a little anxiety and taking on a new challenge. There is no incentive for the child to rise to this challenge if both achieved and failed targets are handled in the same way. See Chapter 10 page 192 for information about what to do if the child does not meet a target.

19 The child has used a whispered voice throughout the programme

This relates to the above point but is worthy of specific mention because whispering can become an extremely difficult habit to break. It is very important *not* to give a sticker or to aim for whispered or 'mouthed' words as part of the programme. Children can become very comfortable with whispering, just as some become comfortable talking with their hand in front of their mouth or with their lips closed. In all cases, the phobia of talking still exists. The adopted safety behaviour is an anxiety-free alternative to releasing their voice into the public arena.

Whispering indicates audience-awareness and extreme tension around the vocal cords. It will be necessary to backtrack with the sliding-in technique to the point where an audible, albeit quiet, voice is produced; and then to move slowly forwards again, acknowledging only an audible voice (see Chapter 10, page 192).

Note that it is perfectly acceptable for children to whisper at other times *outside* the special time allocated to working on targets. *Any* communication in natural settings is acceptable until the programme helps them to feel better about using a stronger voice.

20 The programme ended too early without actively managing transitions

It cannot be assumed that, once a child is talking to one or two people, they will now improve spontaneously and transfer easily to a new class or year group. Change can sometimes be an advantage, as discussed in Chapter 11 'Making successful transitions' but generalisation usually needs to be closely monitored and facilitated, especially when transitioning from one year group to the next within the same school.

21 The child is worried about the next session rather than pleased about the previous one

It is important to finish each session on a high note, even if the child has failed a target (see Chapter 10, page 192), and to let them know when you will see them again. The child will know you expect to continue working in the same vein towards an agreed long-term goal, but they should not feel under any time pressure, or be told the details of the small steps targets you have planned. Remember that when new targets are tackled in a session, each one builds on the last, so the child is never looking further ahead than one step at a time. If they are told several steps in advance, without the benefit of a gradual warm-up, the task will feel unmanageable.

Similarly, it is tempting, but extremely daunting, to give the child a list of targets for 'homework'. It is better to set either *one* target to be achieved between sessions or one target with the instruction to report back when it has been achieved. Of course, other targets may be set for parents and staff.

22 The child is worried about their peers' reaction
Children may do well in their individual sessions with a keyworker but resist speaking to other children or talking in the classroom. It is important to ascertain their fear of a negative reaction from other children and to address this, as explained in Chapter 10 (page 206).

When children appear to have regressed

The following scenarios are examples of how individuals may report their concerns that a child has regressed. If not dissected and addressed in a different way, the programme could grind to a halt or be abandoned. Whenever you encounter this sort of situation, you need to ask for more details – for what exactly happened. This fuller information usually shows up inconsistencies and reasons for the setback. The resolutions are given at the end of the section because you may like to use the scenarios for problem solving *before* looking at how each one was handled.

Scenario 1 (as reported by a mother)

'Cristina (aged 4 years 9 months) finally read to me in front of her teacher and was thrilled. She wanted to do it again the next day. However, she did not speak at all the next day and has since regressed. She never speaks to me at school now. How do we deal with this?'

What actually happened

Day one
Cristina was reading to Mum in the home corner of the classroom at the end of the day. The teacher came in unexpectedly and, to Mum's surprise and Cristina's delight, Cristina carried on reading with her teacher in the room.

Day two
The teacher sat in the classroom while Cristina and Mum went into the home corner. However, Cristina was unable to read and she went home in tears.

Scenario 2 (as reported by a mother)

'Maddy (aged 7) is doing really well at school but regressing at home. She's always spoken to her maths tutor who comes every Saturday but didn't speak to her this week. She spoke a few words to me in front of her but that's all. I just don't understand it.'

What actually happened

Most Saturdays
Mum welcomes the home tutor and has a cup of coffee and chat with her before Maddy starts her lesson. Mum then leaves them to it.

This Saturday
Mum needed to go out, so Dad let the home tutor in. Maddy was silent during the lesson. When Mum got back, Maddy spoke to her in front of the tutor.

Scenario 3 (as reported by a keyworker)

'Kelly just blanked me. I couldn't get a word out of her. Do you think she's annoyed with me because I had to cancel her session?'

What actually happened

Most Fridays
Kelly had a one-to-one session with her keyworker in the interview room to discuss any school or homework issues.

This Friday
The keyworker sent a note to Kelly in the morning to explain that she had to cancel their session in the afternoon. At lunch-time, she happened to see Kelly and stopped her in the corridor to apologise and ask if there was anything she had been hoping to discuss.

Resolutions

Scenario 1

Several variables had changed on day two. The activity had changed from an 'unplanned' to a 'planned' event; the starting position of the teacher had changed; and Cristina had no opportunity to warm up by reading to her Mum first. Therefore, Mum explained to Cristina that there was a good reason she had not managed to read in front of her teacher. Mum and the teacher should have repeated events in exactly the same way but they had done it wrong, so it was not surprising that Cristina hadn't managed to talk. Cristina was then prepared to try again.

The next day, Cristina got used to reading to Mum in the classroom again. The following day, Cristina read to Mum alone and, after a few minutes, her teacher came into the classroom and sat at his desk while Cristina finished the story.

Scenario 2

Again, several variables had changed on the second occasion. Maddy was expected to go straight into the session with the tutor because her father did not offer the tutor a cup of coffee. She had no warm-up time to (a) talk to her father in front of her tutor and (b) talk to her tutor in her father's presence.

Over the next few weeks:

★ Dad joined his wife and the tutor for a cup of coffee before Maddy's session

★ Maddy's mother went out after the session had started

★ Dad joined Maddy at the end of the session to go through what she had done with the tutor

★ Dad welcomed the tutor on days when Mum could not be there.

Scenario 3

Kelly had only spoken to her keyworker previously during arranged sessions, when she was alone in a room with the door shut. Expecting her to talk to the keyworker in the corridor without warning, with other people walking by or overhearing was a huge step.

At their next session, Kelly's keyworker apologised to Kelly for talking to her in the corridor. She told Kelly that she understood how difficult it must have been for her. As a result, they agreed to work towards holding their sessions in more public places, starting with leaving the door to the interview room slightly ajar.

Online resources for Chapter 12

The forms and handouts referred to in this chapter are available online at www.routledge.com/cw /speechmark for you to access, print and copy.

CHAPTER 13

WHEN IT IS MORE THAN SELECTIVE MUTISM

Introduction

Chapter 6 looked at extended assessment. This included the extended parent interview; ways to tackle speech, language, cognitive and literacy assessments which are most likely to be picked up in the classroom and dealt with in school or at a local clinic; and, briefly, how to make effective onward referrals to specialists, if needed. This chapter focuses on coexisting conditions more fully. Specifically, it looks at the following topics:

★ what it means to have more than selective mutism

★ why we need to know

★ how to find out more and get help

★ what other difficulties are most likely to occur alongside selective mutism

★ tackling the subject of mental health issues and referral to child and adolescent mental health services (CAMHS)

★ identifying and managing coexisting anxiety conditions

★ the question of medication

★ tips for managing additional anxiety alongside SM

★ identifying and managing autism spectrum disorder (ASD)

★ identifying and managing speech, language and communication difficulties

★ bilingualism and English as an additional language (EAL).

What it means to have more than selective mutism

As a parent or teacher of a child who has selective mutism (SM), you may be concerned in other ways about their development or how they present. You may feel that the term 'selective mutism' does not cover the whole picture. You may also wonder whether they might have an additional emotional, behavioural, developmental or learning difficulty. The technical term for having more than one diagnosis is *comorbidity* but don't be put off by this rather grim name which is used by medical or psychology professionals; it simply means *coexistence*. It is very common for a child to have more than one difficulty (or disorder).

Why we need to know

Certain professionals, usually a doctor, psychologist or other specialist, have the specific role of assessing and diagnosing other difficulties that children may have alongside SM. However, the people who are closest to the child are in the best position to recognise signs of additional complications and they should discuss their concerns with clinicians. The label as such may not matter but it is important that everyone who comes into contact with a child who has SM has as complete a picture of that child or young person as possible.

Some basic knowledge and awareness of other difficulties may help to explain slower progress with overcoming the SM and will ensure a coordinated approach to management. It may be necessary to adapt the strategies being used, or to incorporate other aspects into the child's SM intervention. It will also help when considering whether and when more support may be needed for parents.

> *The presence of an additional difficulty must not distract people from addressing the SM.*

However, don't forget that early identification and intervention are universally acknowledged to be crucial for the good management of SM (see Appendix E). It follows that the presence of an additional difficulty or diagnosis must not distract the family or professionals from addressing the SM. There may be a need for modifications or extra strategies to accommodate or manage the additional difficulty, but these *must not* replace the SM interventions.

How to find out more and get help

Here are a few practical suggestions for anyone who suspects that a child might have something more than SM.

★ Write down what you notice about the child that concerns you.

★ Look for more information on certain conditions from websites such as NHS Choices.

★ Find out whether trusted family members and friends share your concerns.

★ Talk to professionals the child already knows (eg the teacher).

Then if you think you should pursue this, you could consider a referral to a professional who can carry out further assessment. The most likely people who could help are as follows.

★ A school psychologist assesses and advises on additional learning, emotional and behavioural difficulties. This can be arranged through the school's special needs department.

★ A speech and language therapist assesses difficulties with speech pronunciation, the understanding and use of language, voice and fluency. Again, this can be arranged through the school's special needs department, or through the family doctor, but many speech and language therapy services have an open referral policy and can be contacted directly.

★ A paediatrician will look more widely at the different aspects of a child's development and will also assess and diagnose more serious general learning difficulties and autism spectrum disorder (ASD). In the UK, a doctor's referral may be needed.

★ A clinical psychologist, a child psychiatrist or, in the UK, a Child and Adolescent Mental Health Services (CAMHS) team should be consulted if the child has more serious emotional or behavioural difficulties, especially if they interfere significantly with the child's ability to socialise and learn, or if the child is older.

★ A physiotherapist or an occupational therapist will assess and advise on difficulties with movement and coordination. In the UK, the referral generally needs to be made by a doctor.

★ Many localities also have multidisciplinary teams comprising a child psychiatrist or paediatrician, a psychologist and a speech and language therapist, for example. They will carry out a joint assessment for social–communication difficulties and ASD.

Other difficulties that occur alongside SM

Research indicates that a child or young person with SM often has another anxiety disorder, a communication disorder, ASD, oppositional behaviour, or developmental delay affecting their motor coordination (see Appendix E).

In our experience, ASD and the following mental health conditions most often coexist with SM:

★ separation anxiety

★ other phobias such as eating in public or using toilets outside the home

★ generalised anxiety

★ in older children, social anxiety disorder (SAD).

We have also encountered young people who have become depressed or started to self-harm after living with undiagnosed SM for many years.

Tackling the subject of mental health issues and referral for specialist support

Mild-to-moderate emotional and behavioural difficulties are recognised and managed every day by teachers and therapists working at 'grass-roots' level. The child's needs are described, some strategies are put in place to manage them, and an education plan is drawn up. To help the teachers do this, they may have some additional training, experience and skills, or the support of a specialist teacher or the school psychologist. The more that all of the professional people can contribute at this level, to prevent anxiety and behavioural issues escalating to crisis point, clearly the better it is for the children and families. To help with this some pointers are included in the next section.

More serious emotional and behavioural difficulties, which have a significant effect on the child's well-being, education, social or family life, may be called mental health disorders. These need to be assessed and diagnosed by the local CAMHS or its equivalent. This also applies to any child or young person who is either significantly depressed or self-harming. When such a referral has been agreed, it may be necessary to explain about CAMHS and dispel any myths about it that might be off-putting.

Unfortunately, the phrase 'mental health' is often misunderstood, with too much emphasis on the word 'mental'. For example, a child might say 'I'm not mental' after hearing the word used either in connection with adult mental illness or as a form of taunt. It may help to:

★ emphasise the word 'health'

★ talk about the importance of looking after both our physical and our mental health

★ equate mental health difficulties with more commonly used words such as stress, worries, feeling low or not enjoying life as fully as possible

★ describe what many people do to counteract stress, eg meditation, yoga, mindfulness or counselling.

Pursuing a referral to CAMHS

This works best if you are aware of how your local mental health service works. It helps to have established contacts. Otherwise a telephone call could clarify:

★ whether a potential referral would be accepted

★ what referral information is required

★ what steps might be taken when it is received

★ broadly what might be offered to the child and family.

Identification of coexisting anxiety conditions

In this section a few important points are made about anxiety disorders, followed by a description of the most common anxiety disorders which occur alongside a diagnosis of SM.

General points about the presentation of anxiety disorders

★ A diagnosis will only be made if the symptoms are sufficiently severe to be causing significant distress or impairment in the child's routine, functioning at home and school, and social relationships; and if the symptoms are sufficiently persistent to be regarded as more than just a passing phase.

★ The signs of a possible anxiety disorder are both physical (eg headache, stomach ache, vomiting) and psychological (fear and worry).

★ Children express their anxiety through their mood – in general, crying, irritability, clinginess and anger (tantrums) – and avoidance behaviour which may be misunderstood as disobedience or defiance (also known as *oppositional behaviours*).

★ Anxiety may be associated with a generally low mood or depression but usually it precedes depression.

Separation anxiety

This causes the child to show excessive distress either before or during times of separation from their parents or carers. It is the most common anxiety disorder in young children, lasting six months or more. They may have difficulty being alone, falling asleep alone or going away from home. They may refuse to go to school or to another activity where they might need to separate from their parent. They may worry about losing an important person, or that some harm will come to them; or that an event such as getting lost would cause separation; and they may have nightmares about separation.

Specific phobia

This is identified by excessive fear in the presence of, or in anticipation of, a specific object or situation. Common phobia triggers in children are dogs, being alone in the dark, thunderstorms, vomiting and heights. When faced with these events, the child becomes intensely distressed, which is expressed by crying, tantrums or clinging behaviour; but the most common way of coping is avoidance. Children who have SM often have a phobia of eating in public or using the toilet outside home, and if their SM is poorly managed, they may also develop school phobia.

Social anxiety disorder (SAD)

Previously known as 'social phobia', SAD is characterised by anxiety about social situations through a fear of appearing foolish or being criticised or ridiculed by other people. The anxiety is out of proportion with the situation and significantly interferes with the individual's ability to lead a normal life. The onset is usually during adolescence, and it must occur in the presence of peers as well as adults to be diagnosed as SAD.

Typically, the young person will avoid social gatherings and volunteering answers in class, and hates being watched while working or simply going about their daily business. As with SM, SAD often involves avoiding situations where speaking is expected, but the fear is that their *contribution* will be poorly received, thus causing shame or embarrassment. Feared situations are not related to the act of speaking as such, but to the type of interaction involved and the risk of being negatively judged.

Generalised anxiety disorder (GAD)

GAD causes anxiety about a wide range of situations and issues, rather than one specific event. While it is normal for children to have frequent fears and worries, GAD may be diagnosed when they are present for at least six months and are difficult to control. Young people affected by GAD feel anxious on most days and often struggle to remember the last time they felt relaxed.

Effective management of anxiety disorders

This section describes some of the approaches used in anxiety management that we have encountered and found helpful, either in our own practice or as reported by other people. As SM is an anxiety disorder, it will not surprise you that the management strategies we recommend for SM in this manual originate from some of these methods. You may find the summaries useful to expand your understanding of the terminology. Alternatively, some young people or adults with SM may like to explore them further for their own use.

Cognitive behavioural therapy (CBT)

CBT is a talking therapy that can help you manage your problems by changing how you think and behave. It is based on the concept that thoughts, feelings, physical sensations and actions are interconnected, and that negative thoughts and feelings can trap you in a vicious circle of safety behaviours (avoidance) and increased anxiety. CBT aims to help crack this circle by breaking down overwhelming problems into smaller parts, challenging negative thoughts, and showing that these negative patterns can be changed to improve how you feel mentally. CBT also involves *graded exposure* to help build up the individual's tolerance of the anxiety-provoking stimulus in small steps; this method underpins all of the intervention programmes in this manual.

Unlike some other talking therapies, CBT deals with *current* problems, rather than focusing on issues from the past. A CBT course typically involves around six to 15 hourly sessions, in which you set goals with your therapist and carry out tasks between the sessions. CBT is the recommended treatment for phobias, SAD, generalised anxiety, panic attacks and post-traumatic stress disorder (PTSD).

Solution-focused therapy

Various techniques such as *the desired situation question*, *scaling* and *the miracle question* are used to focus on constructing solutions with the clients, rather than gathering information about the problem.

Externalisation

Children are helped to see the anxiety condition as separate from themselves — they are not the problem and the problem is not inside them. This enables them to take control of the difficulty and overcome it more easily, rather than blame themselves for the difficulty (see 'The pep talk' and the speech bubbles in Chapter 5, pages 73–75).

Neurolinguistic programming (NLP)

NLP uses techniques such as visualisation and Timeline Therapy® to help clients replace unhelpful habits and limiting beliefs with more effective behaviour and supportive beliefs.

Parenting work

This umbrella term covers both specific and general ways to empower parents to manage children who are difficult to parent. With many anxious children, some work will be needed to teach the parents various strategies to help their children cope with anxiety and gain confidence; also to help the parents recognise their role in inadvertently strengthening the child's fear. This is described in detail in Chapter 8 and on Handouts 6–8.

The question of medication

In the UK, the use of medication to manage anxiety disorders, including SM, in children is rare. The National Institute for Health and Care Excellence (NICE) guidelines state clearly that 'pharmacological interventions should not be offered routinely to treat anxiety disorders in children and young people' (NICE Guidelines for social anxiety, 2013). However, medication is used much more frequently in the USA.

The most likely drugs to be prescribed are SSRIs (selective serotonin reuptake inhibitors), especially fluoxetine – also known as Prozac®. SSRIs are a type of antidepressant medication which is also used to treat various anxiety conditions, including panic attacks and phobias. SSRIs work by increasing the levels of a chemical in the brain called serotonin which reduces inhibition in children. It is thought that a rise in serotonin levels can improve symptoms and make users more responsive to other types of treatment, such as CBT.

> *Medication should not be offered routinely to treat anxiety disorders in children.*

SSRIs are usually taken as tablets, starting on the lowest possible dose and increasing as needed. They must be taken for two to four weeks before any benefit is felt (it can take longer in adults). They are not generally recommended for young people under 18 because there is an increased risk of serious side effects, although exceptions can be made if the benefits of treatment are thought to outweigh the risks. The prescription of medication is recommended and managed by a child and adolescent psychiatrist.

Another medication called diazepam is occasionally prescribed. This powerful sedative is used short-term for faster relief of severe anxiety.

It is difficult to find sufficient evidence for using medication to manage SM. In spite of a steep increase in more carefully controlled research, no large scale controlled clinical trials of any form of drug treatment have been done specifically for SM. The results of small or single case research studies and anecdotal feedback on the success of medication in the treatment of SM vary considerably, from reports of no noticeable effects to significant effects. Where medication *appears* to have been effective, it is difficult to gauge whether it is indeed the medication that made the difference or other factors that played a part alongside it.

The following guidelines may help to decide whether to go down the medication route. It should only be considered:

★ for older children and adolescents

★ *and* where recognised intervention measures for SM are not working because of severe anxiety

★ *and* when additional anxiety-reducing techniques such as relaxation and cognitive-behavioural therapy are also unsuccessful.

Tips for managing additional anxieties alongside SM

Parents may need support to:

★ understand that anxiety is normal and should be managed, rather than eliminated

★ work out how anxiety operates in their child

★ learn what they can do that is and is not helpful.

Listening to anxieties for just a limited time is recommended while acknowledging the distress. Measuring how big it is can help the child achieve a greater sense of control (see 'externalisation' on page 272), perhaps using a worry thermometer or a rating scale (see Chapter 8, page 126). It may also enable the child to put the worry into perspective.

As Leila's example below shows, talking to children about both their role and the parent's role in anxiety management is crucial because it is not helpful for children's confidence, or their independence, to rely on their parents to fix everything. From about five years old, simple metaphors can be used to convey anxiety as something that makes us hold on and be afraid to let go. But when we are brave enough to try on our own, we practise and improve and the anxiety goes away.

Choose something that the child can relate to, for example:

★ holding on to the side when you can't swim or ice-skate

★ getting stuck on a ladder or platform and being too afraid to move or jump

★ gripping the sides at the top of a slide or water chute and being afraid to let go.

Then link it to the child's first-hand experience or observation of how good it feels to conquer anxiety.

Using a step-by-step approach

We have often seen children with SM who have fixations and a tendency towards rigid behaviour patterns, particularly around:

★ eating

★ using the toilet (especially outside their own home)

★ bedtime.

These may be thought of, or diagnosed as, phobias. They can be managed by a small-steps programme (graded exposure) in the same way in which the SM is managed; and they can run alongside the SM interventions. The following examples may help to show how to manage a problem with eating in public, using the school toilet or sleeping alone.

Example 1: Jonny

Jonny was 'refusing' to eat at lunch-time in school.

The targets included:

★ to eat in a separate room from his peers

★ to introduce an adult to eat lunch in the separate room

★ to go to the dining hall with the adult before the other children, eat lunch and leave before the hall got too busy

★ to go to the dining hall with the adult before the other children, and leave with other children

★ to introduce a peer

★ to go to the dining room with a peer.

Example 2: Richard

Richard would only use the school toilet if his mother took him.

The targets included:

★ Richard to develop total independence at home (eg shutting the bathroom door and wiping himself).

★ Mum to take Richard and a peer to the school toilet and wait outside the cubicle

★ Mum to wait in the corridor while Richard uses the school toilet accompanied by a peer.

★ Richard to use the school toilet accompanied by a peer without his mother being present.

Example 3: Leila

Leila would only fall asleep if her mother was also in her bed.

The targets included:

★ Leila to choose a bedside lamp to be left switched on throughout the night.

★ Parents to adopt a consistent bedtime routine, to include a story with the bedside lamp on.

★ Parents to establish that there will be no more chat or stories after 8.30 p.m. because this was 'grown-up time' for work or relaxation. Leila to be praised for being old enough to understand this.

★ Leila's anxiety around falling asleep alone to be acknowledged. It was natural for her to feel worried at first because this was something new that she had never done before. Parents to explain that, by being brave and having a go, Leila would soon stop being worried, just like she learned to swim by practising without her armbands. Leila to be reassured that her parents would help her, just like her swimming instructor had done.

★ Mum or Dad to go into the next room after story-time and then look in every 10 minutes until Leila fell asleep. (It was also agreed that, if necessary, Mum or Dad would read a book or do the ironing on the landing outside Leila's room, rather than in the next room, but this wasn't necessary.) There should be no talking during these checks other than 'You're doing really well. It's time to sleep, I'll be next door' if Leila tried to talk.

★ Mum or Dad to go downstairs and look in every 10 minutes.

★ Mum or Dad to look in less frequently.

★ Bedside lamp to be switched off when Leila was asleep but landing light left on.

★ Door to be gradually shut.

Other anxieties may require the same step-by-step approach Simple graded programmes may be devised by school staff, perhaps with the help of the school psychologist. Alternatively, a specialist health visitor could advise on anxiety management in the early years.

Identifying and managing a specific anxiety trigger

Sometimes just one aspect of a task or situation causes the child distress. Once the specific anxiety trigger is identified and understood, steps can be taken to modify the environment, or conquer the fear, as shown in the following examples. The specific trigger could be identified by comparing the feared situation with a similar situation that the child finds manageable, as in Example 4 below. At other times, the child may provide the clue; in Example 5, Jack often held his chest when he felt distressed. But often children cannot calmly unpick a situation and pinpoint the problem. It may then help to break down the task into very small steps, using pictures or short sentences on sticky notes, for example. Each step can be mimed, discussed or walked through with an adult, the child rating each one for how easy or difficult it is, or sorting into 'Like' and 'Don't like' piles. In this way, you might discover that a specific requirement like locking the toilet door, or finding somewhere to sit in the canteen, is triggering the avoidance behaviour.

Example 4: Vikram

Vikram would not use the toilets at school but he had no difficulty in other people's homes. The sudden and unexpected noise of the hand-dryer alarmed him. For a while he was allowed to use a separate staff toilet while he went into the main toilets with his teaching assistant just to get used to switching on the hand-dryer himself. He also practised drying his hands at home while instructing his mother to switch her hair-dryer on and off.

Example 5: Jack

Jack was returning distressed after any activity which involved running around and he did not want to join in any physical games at school. At first, his parents thought he was scared of being chased or getting hurt. Then they worked out that it was the pounding of his heart. Jack had previously only experienced an increased heart rate in association with anxiety.

So Jack and his Dad had lots of fun playing 'tag' with water pistols and took turns feeling each other's heartbeat. Jack learned that this is what happened when he ran fast, so that his muscles would get more energy and he could run for longer.

Example 6: Bethan

Bethan cried every time the class got changed for PE. This was not about her SM or the changing itself; it was the fear of being asked to perform in front of the class. She showed no anxiety after her teacher promised he would only ask her to demonstrate an activity if she put up her hand.

Example 7: Pria

In addition to her SM, Pria had developmental coordination disorder and hated taking longer to change than everyone else. While the other children lined up and waited for her before walking round to the school hall, she felt that everyone was staring at her. By getting a 10-minute head start on the others, she was ready for PE at the same time as the rest of the class. (She was also allowed to use wet-wipes rather than toilet paper at school because of her coordination difficulties.)

Positive problem solving – or not giving up at the first hurdle

Older children can take a more proactive role in problem solving by being routinely encouraged to break down overwhelming big problems into smaller manageable chunks – none of which will seem as scary on their own. They can then focus on just one thing at a time – for example, getting a prospectus – before dismissing the whole idea of going to college completely. Teaching positive problem solving is a way to move on and instil valuable coping skills for when something occurs in future.

Visualisation

Just getting circular repetitive thoughts and anxieties out of your head and onto paper, where you can *see* them, is the first step towards putting the problem in a place where you can deal with it – or putting it to one side to deal with later. If children or young people can't sleep for worrying thoughts, try this first.

Visuals are always helpful for understanding abstract concepts and anxiety is no different. Simple pictures like those below speak volumes.

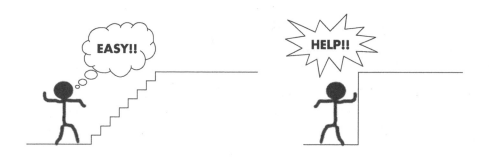

Many of the parents we work with have reported that their children have found books, worksheets and visual exercises helpful as a way of picturing and managing their anxiety. See Appendix F 'Books, Tackling anxiety' for examples. Similarly, teachers recommend the Worry Wheels in Appendix F, 'Therapy resources'.

Visuals also provide a powerful memory trigger when children are too anxious or overwhelmed to process or retain spoken information. It often helps to write things down as a reminder or a checklist for children to refer to and to keep this in a prominent place. It can also save endless nagging! Many children get into the habit of asking questions for reassurance but gain reassurance from the routine of asking, rather than the answer. When this happens, try to break the cycle by giving a written answer, drawing or picture in response, or make sure that they can look up the answer, such as on a timetable or an invitation. Then, when the child repeats the question, direct them to their visual reminder, so that they can find the answer for themselves.

Managing SM plus social anxiety disorder (SAD)

All children who have SM are socially anxious but this does not necessarily mean that they have SAD. In practice, particularly when SM is addressed within a few years of onset, usually their social anxiety will subside as their SM is treated. However, in older children social anxiety may go beyond the fear of being unable to speak and may need specifically addressing alongside the SM. Chapter 9 discusses this issue in connection with Form 15, 'Talking to strangers' (page 162) and, in Chapter 10, 'Additional considerations for adolescents and young adults' (page 214) suggests suitable approaches and techniques.

If the social anxiety does not ease, it may help to query a diagnosis of SAD which might need to be treated independently. Where there are indications from their profile that a young person may have SAD, a preliminary screening could be carried out using Form 9 'Worrying thoughts' in Chapter 5.

Managing SM plus general anxiety and GAD

Many children who have SM seem to be 'born worriers'. Handouts 6–8 which accompany Chapter 8 are designed to support anxiety in general. Some schools run excellent evidence-based programmes based on CBT approaches which are designed to prevent and actively break the cycles of stress and worry in children. Children are helped to externalise and take charge of their anxiety, using a set of tools or coping strategies. The group aspect of such interventions is beneficial as children learn that they are not alone and gain strength from each other. However, care must be taken that children who have SM feel under no pressure to contribute verbally before they are ready.

Where available, some of our older students have benefited from a short course of CBT to address general anxiety, before working on SM assignments. This has enabled them to recognise and understand their anxiety as something that is uncomfortable but will pass, rather than being a cue to escape. They learn that the steps they have taken to avoid perceived, but non-existent, danger have, in fact, increased their anxiety, and they are better prepared to face their fears. Other students have gone on to treatment for GAD after their SM has been resolved.

Autism spectrum disorder (ASD)

There has been much confusion about the similarities between SM and ASD, and whether a child can be diagnosed with both conditions. Both DSM-5 (APA, 2013) and the previous edition, published in 1994, exclude a dual diagnosis, yet before the publication of DSM-5, a significant number of children and adults were given the dual-diagnosis of SM and Asperger's syndrome.

Asperger's syndrome is now included in, and named as, 'autism spectrum disorder'. Significantly, children who would previously have received a diagnosis of Asperger's syndrome have superior verbal skills and this must be specified when making the diagnosis (DSM-5, page 32).

We believe we have encountered several verbal children with a valid dual diagnosis of SM and ASD. In all cases they meet the DSM-5 criteria for ASD. And yet there are situations where they 'have an established capacity to speak', but only with certain people in certain situations, thus also meeting the criteria for SM (DSM-5, page 197). In this section we discuss some of the issues involved and share our experiences on identification, assessment and management.

Identifying ASD

ASD is a developmental condition that affects social interaction, communication, interests and behaviour. It covers the whole range from high-functioning autism to people who have severe learning difficulties and no speech. ASD can cause a wide range of symptoms from an early age. These are divided into two main groups.

★ Problems with social interaction and communication, including: problems with understanding, developing and maintaining relationships; deficits in non-verbal communication; and an inability to initiate or respond to social interactions or take part in easy to-and-fro conversation.

★ Restricted and repetitive patterns of thought, interests, activities and behaviours, including: making repetitive physical movements, intense and restricted interests; and becoming upset if set routines are disrupted.

Young people and adults with ASD often have difficulty speaking which should not be confused with SM. They may be unsure what to do and what to say in social situations and find it difficult to deal with intense emotion, leaving them too angry, upset or overwhelmed to speak.

Assessing a child who may have *both* SM and ASD is complex for various reasons. In some settings some of the symptoms of the two conditions can appear to overlap, such as a reluctance to communicate and deficits in social communication. The most commonly used methods for assessing children for ASD are not fully accessible to a child with SM who cannot interact comfortably with unfamiliar people; for example, the Autism Diagnostic Observation Schedule (ADOS, Lord *et al*, 2000). And, unfortunately, professionals who assess children for ASD may have little or no experience of SM. These complexities are discussed in more detail in 'Exploring the relationship of SM to ASD' in Smith & Sluckin (2015, pp97–111).

> *The assessment of a child who may have both SM and ASD is complex.*

If you are wondering whether a child who has SM might also have ASD, we suggest looking out for the following indicators in the situations in which the child feels comfortable:

★ rigid behaviour patterns or rituals

★ no interest in social chat, even with familiar people

★ lack of empathy and appreciation of other people's needs (eg conversational topics)

★ poor 'mind-reading' skills (eg assuming that other children at activity club already know each other, because they know each other's names, but everyone wears a name badge)

★ additional fears around sensory or body issues (eg terror of loud noises or having hair or nails cut).

If, after discussion with other people who know the child well, you decide to pursue an assessment for ASD, the following guidelines may be useful to ensure that it is as effective as possible:

★ involving more than one professional, from a team of a paediatrician or child psychiatrist, a clinical psychologist and a speech and language therapist

★ ensuring that the professionals have some understanding or experience of SM (see Chapter 3, page 58 for questions to ask)

★ asking questions about the content of the ASD assessment and what modifications will be made to accommodate a child with possible or identified SM

★ the possibility of using a one-way viewing mirror, seeing a recording of the child at home, or the additional use of questionnaires completed by people the child speaks to freely.

General management of ASD

There is currently no 'cure' for ASD but a wide range of educational and behavioural interventions can improve the skills of people who have the condition. The most common programmes focus on social awareness and interaction, improving communication skills, and educating and training parents. There is much information about these interventions on the web or from organisations supporting people with autism, such as The National Autistic Society in the UK.

Managing SM plus ASD

The crucial factor when planning and carrying out an effective programme for a child who has both SM and ASD is that everyone understands the nature of the *two* conditions and the strategies that will help. In general, we recommend handling the child's SM in exactly the same way as for any other child but, when direct work on the child's SM is indicated, some features of the child's ASD may dictate some modifications. For example, the difficulties that the child may have with understanding abstract language or the language of emotions could be partly overcome by using additional visual material (stick people, line drawings, cartoons, expression faces) or social stories for younger children.

A child with ASD, because of their rigidity and love of routine, will have a particular need for a consistent programme and explicit new talking rules. However, this also means that a specific graded programme will appeal to the child and give them a feeling of success and confidence. Again, these points are discussed more by Wintgens in 'Exploring the relationship of SM to ASD' in Smith & Sluckin (2015, pp97–111).

Because of the problems with social interaction and communication that all children with ASD have, social skills training is a core part of their management. Once the SM has been resolved, children who had this dual diagnosis will need ongoing social skills training. Indeed, now that they can talk freely, this area of work can be addressed in a way which was not possible earlier.

Identifying and managing speech, language and communication difficulties

The terms 'speech', 'language' and 'communication' are widely used every day in a variety of contexts. To avoid misunderstanding we will briefly define how they are used technically to describe the developmental impairments that some children experience, plus other terminology that is used in this field.

★ *Speech impairment* means difficulty in pronouncing speech sounds (*articulation*) or using them effectively in words or sentences (*phonology*).

★ *Language impairment* can be divided into *receptive* or *expressive* difficulties (difficulties *understanding* or *formulating* concepts, words and grammatical sentences).

★ *Communication impairment* is a broader concept, meaning difficulty with using speech, language and non-verbal communication to interact appropriately and effectively.

★ *Stammering*, or *stuttering*, is a fluency disorder in which words, or parts of words, are repeated and certain speech sounds are prolonged. There is associated tension and the speaker may also have difficulty starting some words, resulting in intermittent silences while speaking.

Sometimes we also refer to *speech, language and communication needs* (SLCN), which is an umbrella term for all of those above. Children can have various combinations of speech, language and communication difficulties.

The assessment of speech and language difficulties is covered in Chapter 6 'The extended assessment' (page 94).

Managing SM plus speech and language difficulties

As discussed in 'How to reach a diagnosis of selective mutism' in Chapter 3 (page 53), it is important to establish how aware the child is of any difficulty they have with pronunciation, expressive language or fluency. A reluctance to talk that can be fully accounted for by self-consciousness about speech or fear of correction excludes a diagnosis of SM. However, reluctant speakers with spoken language difficulties will also benefit from the strategies outlined below.

If a child has SM plus some speech and/or language difficulty, here are some general tips for management.

★ Again, it is important that everyone who comes into contact with the child is aware and has sufficient knowledge about *both* conditions.

★ There must be general strategies at home and in school to tackle both the SM and the speech or language difficulties.

★ In some situations, perhaps where the child has mild-to-moderate speech or expressive language difficulties, the emphasis on intervention should be on the child's SM. Once the child is starting to speak comfortably, specific sessions can be introduced for the speech or language work.

★ If the speech or language difficulties are more severe, direct work to address these will be needed earlier. More competence with their speech and language skills may lead to more confidence in talking, as with Stephen in the example on the next page.

★ General strategies should include reassurance that everyone has difficulty explaining themselves at times and it is nothing to be ashamed of if people don't understand you at first. Children and adults alike can learn to give and ask for clarification through gesture, drawings, finger spelling, definitions, and so on, and by playing games that suit children with word-finding difficulties, disordered speech, limited vocabulary and SM. (See 'Active listening for active learning' in Appendix F, 'Therapy resources'.)

★ While bearing in mind the general strategies for managing both conditions, a clear distinction should be made between *specific* work on the speech and language difficulties and a *specific* SM programme to elicit speech. Don't mix the two specific interventions in the same session.

★ Children who have SM respond better on a one-to-one basis than in group sessions where there is an emphasis on taking turns to speak. Therefore, group work for their delayed language development should be considered only if the group leaders are knowledgeable about SM and the child is reassured that speaking is *optional*. Activities should focus on receptive language work or judgement tasks (see 'Children who have SM and additional speech difficulties' below), where children can respond without talking, and could include opportunities to perform actions, sing or chant *in unison*.

The main (and obvious) difference when working on speech and language difficulties with a child who has SM is the child's lack of participation in expressive tasks during the session. The speech and language therapist (SLT) or the teaching assistant (TA) carrying out the programme will need to make adaptations. If there are expressive language or speech difficulties, the sessions need to be viewed as training sessions, passing on to the parent, carer or TA the skills of the SLT, with the emphasis on motivating homework in the form of worksheets, games and activities. The accompanying adult needs to have fully understood what they are aiming at, be sure that they have the capacity to fit the work into their normal routine, and be keen to try it with the child at home or somewhere the child feels comfortable.

It may help to run through the recommended games and activities during the session, with the accompanying adult taking the *lead* role, as they would at home. In the next session, ask the adult to show or tell you exactly how they got on with the homework, so that the next stage can be planned effectively. Some therapists routinely film new activities for the child and parent to watch at home and vice versa. This enables the therapist to see whether activities were done at home as intended. We have found that children do not usually object to being filmed when they are very clear about how the film will be used and who will see it. Adults and children should be told that, if they encounter any difficulties, they should stop, especially if either party is not enjoying it, or they get stuck.

Children who have SM and additional speech difficulties

Initially, these children benefit from listening tasks in sessions focused on auditory discrimination and phonological awareness, rather than speech production. Listening tasks include sorting, sequencing and matching activities, and judgement tasks in which the adult, or a suitable toy or puppet, says a word or sound and the child decides whether it was right or wrong. When discussing homework, include a casual 'and when you're at home, you can see if you remember the words/sounds too'. Start with items that the child can say easily, to build confidence and familiarity with the activity formats, which may encourage the child to speak in the sessions without any prompting. Later, when working on speech sounds or sequences that the child has difficulty articulating, therapists should demonstrate them either on themselves and/or the adult or using a toy such as the Big Mouth Crocodile Puppet (see Appendix F, 'Therapy resources'). Again, the child can then be asked to try it at home. Usually, as the child succeeds with listening tasks in the session, and the accompanying adult reports on how well they are doing at home, the child begins to speak in the session over a few weeks.

> At 5½ years old, it was difficult for other people to understand. Stephen's speech. Alongside the general management of his SM, he attended several sessions of speech work with his aunt.
>
> After he proudly showed off his speech book to his teacher, and gave her whispered examples of his improved speech sounds, he started to talk to her and his peers in a quiet voice. He went on to talk fully and freely to everyone at school within a few weeks.

Children who have SM and additional language difficulties

These children need language enrichment and/or work on specific comprehension deficits and should be given this help immediately. With no demands placed on the child to speak, this may take the pressure off the selective mutism. As described above, the initial focus should be on activities in which the child can respond by participating and communicating non-verbally. Comprehension tasks are good for this approach, while expressive language may be supported with sorting, sequencing and judgement tasks in the session, and spoken language practice with the accompanying adult between sessions.

As spoken language emerges – either spontaneously or through the techniques described in Chapters 9 and 10 – everyone involved with the child needs to be aware of how the child's comprehension difficulties will affect the likelihood of a response. Typically, the child will respond when the language level is simple enough and they feel able to respond correctly. As soon as they are confused, or perceive that the task has become more difficult, they will become silent again. Similarly, they may happily offer spontaneous comments when they can be in control of a familiar topic of conversation, but clam up as soon as they are asked direct questions which require a higher level of language-processing. Table 10.4 'Classification of activities by level of risk' (page 193) will help teachers match their expectations to the child's comprehension and confidence levels.

SM and stammering

Practitioners report that SM and stammering can and do occur together but there is a lack of research or case examples. What is helpful for people involved in the SM field is that there are similarities between the two conditions in terms of contributing factors, presentation and management. Both conditions:

★ can reduce the child to silence

★ are associated with anxiety and self-consciousness

★ are influenced by the reactions of other people

★ are managed or maintained by avoiding potentially distressing speaking situations.

Also, many of the interventions for anxiety conditions are used to manage stammering and SM. Stammering, with its overt symptoms and longer history, is better recognised than SM, consequently it is researched and managed more thoroughly and rigorously in most countries and services. The level of recognition of the importance of intervention for stammering can be used as an argument for more recognised management of SM. Indeed, in the UK, some therapists specialising in stammering also specialise in SM because they have the appropriate skills.

As with other speech difficulties, individuals who have SM and also stammer will need a coordinated approach to intervention which includes aspects of the two different treatment regimes. For more information, see 'Selective mutism and stammering' by Jenny Packer in Smith & Sluckin (2015, pp112–15).

Bilingualism and English as an additional language

First, a word about terminology: in this section, for simplicity, 'bilingualism' refers to people who acquire skills in more than one language. 'English as an additional language' (EAL) is used when English is taught or exposed to people who have moved to an English-speaking country and whose first language is not English. Although we refer to English, of course the same principles apply for any additional language which a child is introduced to in similar circumstances.

In all cases, it is important to have a clear history of language exposure, competence and needs, that is:

★ which language(s) the child has been (and will be) exposed to

★ at what ages

★ in what contexts

★ how well they can understand and use the languages.

The 'silent period'

Additional language learners sometimes go through a 'silent period' as they acclimatise to an unfamiliar language and setting. All being well, after a period of watching, listening, engaging and learning, they will then start to use the new language; initially, to copy words and gradually to communicate with other people. The silent period may last anything from a few days to a year, but it is usually less than six months and is most common in children aged 3 to 8 (see Appendix E for references).

Just as there is no single reason for SM, a variety of factors may contribute to the silent period. Certainly, children need time to process and understand a new language and some are more confident than others about throwing caution to the wind and having a go. However, children may also be confused, anxious and overwhelmed by the setting itself and by other changes in their lives. For example, they may have picked up on their parents' stress and uncertainty in a different culture or be feeling different and self-conscious. They may even associate the new language with an incident of teasing. In short, the silent period should not be regarded as inevitable, and it cannot be assumed that, with improved language competence, children will speak. On the contrary, the silent period marks a vulnerable time for young language learners, as is borne out by the much higher incidence of SM in bilingual and immigrant populations (see Appendix E). Any pressure to talk when the child is already feeling uncomfortable risks a negative association with the expectation to speak.

Managing SM plus bilingualism and EAL

When a bilingual child is silent on entering a new setting, and the parents confirm that the child understands and speaks the language of the setting at home, or with certain relatives for example, this could be natural shyness. If so, the child will be talking within a few weeks. However, if parents have already noted selectivity in speaking in *either* language, and if the child has spoken in some situations but not others for more than a month, we advise proceeding as for SM.

Similarly, we recommend that children who do not speak English *and* appear anxious or frozen should be treated as though they may have SM. Rather than accepting their silence as a natural pre-verbal stage, strategies that are helpful to create an anxiety-free environment for children who have SM will help them to relax and enjoy school with the opportunity – but *no pressure* – to talk (see Handouts 9, 10a and 10b).

Using the child's first language in informal situations at school could be an important part of the settling-in process, so involving family or staff members who speak the same language should be encouraged. However, care must be taken to ensure that children do not use *only* their preferred language at school or in other social situations. We have known many bilingual children who were not necessarily mute in certain situations; they used the language that would not be understood by other people in that setting, in the same way as other children with SM might avoid anxiety by whispering or using an altered voice. These and other safety behaviours can be expected to decrease as children respond to SM intervention to overcome their fear of using their natural voice or a certain language in specific communicative contexts.

Support strategies

In addition to the strategies described in this manual, we have found the following tips particularly helpful for children who are exposed to more than one language and show reluctance to speak in certain settings or situations.

Imperfect English is better than silence

Parents who lack confidence in English themselves may not attempt to speak English to teachers or other parents, which their child is likely to witness. Rather than modelling avoidance in this way, they should be reassured that it is more helpful to give their child a clear message that it is best to speak, and that it *does not* matter if you don't always say things completely correctly. To help things along, parents could show an interest in learning or improving their English and ask their child to teach them a song or some new words every day, perhaps by sharing their school work, a fun educational app or their reading book. If parents can make it fun and laugh as they make mistakes, they will teach their child valuable lessons in learning and participation; this is even better if they can team up with other parents and children in the same position.

One social situation, one language

Some bilingual families with parents whose first language is different adopt the 'one person, one language' rule where each parent speaks in their first language. This suits most children very well. They are exposed to more than one language simultaneously and have the capacity, adaptability and social awareness to acquire and use them appropriately. In contrast, children who have difficulty using more than one language, because of underlying anxiety, rigidity or specific language learning difficulties, can be greatly helped by the 'one social situation, one language' rule (which is also useful for parents wanting to maintain sufficient exposure to a minority language). Here, the whole family tries to use the same language in a given situation. The child therefore hears only one language at a time and witnesses both parents smoothly transitioning from one language to another, depending on the social context. For children who have SM, the particular advantage of this is that the parents consistently use the language the child is resisting, across a range of contexts.

For example, when the family is at home, the language used at mealtimes might depend on who cooked it, who leads a conversational topic or which set of grandparents are present. But when a school friend is invited round, the school language is chosen. The school language is also used as far as possible when assisting the child with homework. Parents talk to their child in their home language as they take the child to school, but swap to the school language when joined by other children in the car or playground, or when addressing their child in front of the child's teacher.

Children who have SM can find it quite alarming when a parent suddenly addresses them in the 'wrong' language and they may not want other people to discover that they speak this language too. They may answer in a different language or not at all which is fine. Just ask a simpler question where they can nod or shake their head (see Handout 14 'Talking in public places'). However, if the parent shows no anxiety and persists with this rule, calmly explaining if necessary that it is polite or sensible to use a different language at times, the child will gradually find it easier to make the same transition.

Watch out for bullying or teasing

Finally, it may be important to look out for the possibility of bullying or teasing. The child may have commented on this to their parents, or tried to stop a parent accompanying them to school if they have become aware of negative comments from other children who thought they sounded 'funny'. By investigating how aware the child is that their speech is different, because of a strong accent or difficulty using certain sounds outside the repertoire of their home language, it may become apparent that issues need to be addressed both with the child individually and with the class as a whole. It is important for the child to feel proud of their culture and a valued member of the class.

Online resources for Chapter 13

The forms, handouts and appendices for this chapter are available online at www.routledge.com/cw /speechmark for you to access, print and copy.

CHAPTER 14

EXAMPLES OF INTERVENTIONS

Introduction

This chapter looks at examples of children and young people who have received treatment for selective mutism (SM). We have included a wide range of ages, some with SM alone and some with additional difficulties. Their management illustrates the ideas from this manual, under the headings:

★ Background

★ Assessment

★ Intervention

★ Outcome.

As with a review of most interventions, inevitably there are lessons to be learned and things that, in an ideal world, could have been done faster or better. Indeed, some of the examples date from early on in our practice. At the end of each one we suggest what, with hindsight, might have been done differently. Occasionally, the therapist's, teacher's and/or parents' comments are also included.

Below are listed the eight children and young people (whose names have been changed), their age at the start of effective intervention, their difficulties and the style of intervention. It is unusual for there to be more boys than girl, the reverse of the usual ratio.

1   Adam (3 years): pure SM; building rapport.

2   Aidan (4 years): pure SM; intervention initiated by mother; informal sliding-in.

3   Leonardo (6 years): SM + English as an additional language (EAL); shaping followed by sliding-in.

4   Daniel (6 years): SM + specific language impairment (SLI); shaping followed by speech and language therapy to address expressive language and speech disorder.

5   Robbie (6 years): SM + autism spectrum disorder (ASD); sliding-in.

6   Natia (7 years): SM + oppositional behaviour + urine infections; advice and support for emotional and behaviour problems.

7   Lisa (15 years): entrenched SM + SLI; speech and language therapy for poor speech rhythm and pronunciation, followed by assignments in community settings.

8   Sander (16 years): entrenched SM; intervention initiated by mother; sliding-in.

1 Adam (3 years 11 months)

Background

★ Adam was referred to a speech and language therapist (SLT) by a health visitor who heard about his playgroup leader's concerns. He did not talk at playgroup and the inducements to get him to talk had all been unsuccessful.

★ Mum was more embarrassed than concerned, but she agreed to the referral, especially as Adam was due to start school soon after his fourth birthday.

Assessment

★ Adam spoke to his immediate family, grandparents and a neighbour in his own home. He spoke freely to family members outside the home, but stopped if anyone joined in or overheard him.

★ He did not use any toilet outside his home.

★ During the initial appointment with the SLT, Adam talked quietly to his sister while the therapist talked to Mum. He was unhappy about participating in formal assessment on first meeting; he made no eye contact but used Mum's finger to point at pictures during a comprehension test.

★ Mum made an audio recording of Adam speaking at home; there was no evidence of speech and language difficulties.

Intervention

★ The SLT gave general advice to Mum and playgroup staff about removing the pressure to communicate, and providing a structured programme for a one-to-one helper (keyworker) at the playgroup (building rapport, stages 2–3 from this manual, pages 123 and 124).

★ The keyworker explained to Adam that she understood how hard it was for him to speak, and that she would not expect him to talk to her until he felt ready. She reassured him that this was perfectly OK, and that he would be fine if they took things very slowly. Clearly, this was a great relief to him and he hugged her, much to her surprise.

★ The keyworker saw Adam for 10 to 15 minutes of 'special time' at every playgroup session. There were no rewards other than Adam's enjoyment of the sessions, his relationship with the keyworker, and his ability to communicate with her non-verbally, before progressing to speech.

Outcome

★ Adam spoke to the keyworker after four weeks. When he was using sentences confidently, the other playgroup leaders and helpers were invited to join in the special time. This generalised spontaneously to the main playgroup setting, and he spoke freely, apart from when direct questions were asked and when answering the register.

★ As speaking increased, Adam gained in confidence generally and began to use toilets outside the home.

★ When Adam began to attend his local infants school, he continued to attend a playgroup session once a week on the same site as the school. His playgroup keyworker also worked as a support assistant at his school, so could see Adam in class twice a week as part of the main group.

★ In the first week, Adam's class teacher put pressure on him to answer the register, much to the keyworker's dismay. Adam hung his head and looked extremely distressed. After a chat, the teacher and the keyworker agreed that Adam should sit at the side of the class, out of the teacher's direct line of vision, and could answer when he felt ready. Having had the opportunity to talk to his teacher more informally, Adam was able to speak when his turn came, first in unison with his keyworker, then alone.

★ Three months later, Adam was discharged from speech and language therapy when he was: volunteering information in group situations; talking freely to adults and children; answering the register; attending parties and forming friendships.

Therapist's comments

The playgroup had no experience of selective mutism, and benefited from having a structured programme to follow, with clear goals. The keyworker couldn't believe what a difference it made to take the pressure off and play games that required non-verbal communication. Adam started to progress once family and playgroup had a shared understanding of the nature of his difficulties.

Authors' comments

★ Adam was very lucky to get prompt, appropriate help at such a young age, thanks to the initiative and close working relationship between his playgroup, health visitor and therapist. This no doubt also accounted for the successful outcome.

★ Formal assessment was not necessary: the informal gathering of information would have been sufficient, as was discovered by the audio recording.

★ As the mutism was not long established, a progression of rapport-building activities was enough to elicit speech. We would also recommend the informal involvement of a parent whenever possible.

★ The turning point was when Adam's difficulties were highlighted by his playgroup keyworker. Again, he was extremely lucky that she could provide continuity when he started school, especially as the new class teacher had not fully understood the nature of his difficulties.

2 Aidan (4 years)

Background

★ When Aidan was nearly 3 years old, he spoke only to his parents, brother, paternal grandparents, and two close friends with whom he always used a 'strange' voice.

★ There was an earlier period when Aidan would speak to other people. His SM was possibly triggered when he was 2 years 4 months old by an adult he didn't know shouting at him at a party when he 'did something wrong'. It was so inappropriate and disproportionate that everyone in the room, not only Aidan, was shocked and went silent.

★ Some time after he was three and had started nursery, Aidan's parents saw a television programme about SM and realised that this was what Aidan was experiencing. They recorded it and passed it to his sympathetic nursery teacher, who spotted a seminar on SM, which his mother attended with a friend.

★ At 3 years 9 months old, Aidan was referred by his doctor to a psychologist, who assessed him, and concluded that 'he was not at all traumatised or suffering from any emotional problems'. However, a two-year course of psychotherapy was suggested but declined by Mum who felt that something more cognitive was required. Aidan was then put on the waiting list to see a behavioural psychologist.

★ In parallel, Aidan was referred to the speech and language therapy service. They organised a case conference at the school with the SENCo and the psychologist when Aidan was in reception aged about 4 years 3 months.

Intervention

★ The SENCo bought *The Selective Mutism Resource Manual* (SMRM) and Aidan's reception class teacher read it and volunteered to be his keyworker. She and Mum worked out an informal sliding-in programme and started to implement it.

★ One day a week, Mum took Aidan to school early and played simple games with him in his classroom. Each session, Aidan's teacher got progressively more involved until, after about four weeks, he finally spoke to her, with a look of delighted relief on his face.

★ Aidan's teacher arranged an informal sliding-in session with each of the other adults in the school who he had contact with (lunch staff, other reception teachers, classroom assistants, etc).

Outcome

★ From the start of the intervention programme, progress was very quick and Aidan was talking to his teacher within just a few sessions. By the time he finished in reception class, before his fifth birthday, he was talking to everyone.

★ Aidan then started telephoning various family members and, by the end of the summer before entering Year 1, there was no one within his wider circle of acquaintances who he could not speak to.

★ In the following year, there were times when Aidan looked anxious and worried when a stranger, or someone he didn't know well, spoke to him; but gradually that anxiety faded and, within two years, you would not know that he ever had SM.

Parents' comments

We are so pleased that we discovered the SMRM and were able to get such a fantastic result from the tools you developed. The methodology worked so well for Aidan and we are all just so grateful that we were able to help him through that worrying period of mutism. Aidan's reception teacher should certainly receive a lot of the credit for the good results we achieved, as should the school for the resources they committed to helping him.

He is now 12 and a very confident, thoughtful and articulate boy. He has never had any kind of relapse. He was very young and his memories of that time are hazy but he says he can remember feeling like he was being 'squashed' when people expected him to speak. Strangely, the experience of being mute has shaped his character in some positive ways – he is a good listener, perceptive, quite considered in his speech, and also is very resilient. We are aware it could have been very different if we hadn't intervened and the mutism had persisted and become more entrenched.

Authors' comments

★ This is a lovely example of parents taking the initiative and getting on with it, with excellent results. To refuse psychotherapy, and to press on with educating Aidan's school about SM and intervention, were wise decisions.

★ It is very fortunate that the school staff members were willing to work closely with Mum and put in place the help that she requested. Also, because it was common to have children with EAL, who spoke little when they started nursery, the school's initial relaxed approach meant that they did not put pressure on Aidan to speak, which was helpful.

3 Leonardo (6 years)

Background

★ EAL: only Italian was spoken at home; English was first introduced at 3 years old when Leonardo went to school.

★ At 4–5 years old, Leonardo was referred to an SLT, a specialist teacher for language impairment, and an educational psychologist. While they acknowledged that Leonardo had SM, their assessments were inconclusive and no effective programme was put forward to reduce his SM.

★ Aged 6, Leonardo had still not spoken to anyone at the school and was referred by them to an SLT experienced in SM. Leonardo's teacher questioned his knowledge of English since he did not appear to understand some mathematical concepts.

Assessment (by SLT experienced in SM)

★ Mum was seen alone. In-depth (rather than screening) information was gathered using the extended parent interview form (Chapter 6) in view of the lack of progress.

★ Initial meeting with Leonardo: informal rapport building (during which he gradually spoke freely) and assessment of receptive language skills using the British Picture Vocabulary Scales and the Test for Reception of Grammar (showing some mild language comprehension deficits).

★ School meeting to gather information, using the school report form (Chapter 4) and environmental checklist (Chapter 8), and to provide information about SM.

★ Teacher was advised how to help with Leonardo's understanding without putting pressure on him to talk (Chapter 13).

Intervention

★ Shaping programme introduced (in view of the lack of concern from parents, Mum's working hours and Dad's limited English). Carried out by keyworker three times a week in the library, starting with Stage 3 activities (non-verbal communication).

★ Two school visits each term to review progress and discuss programme.

★ At 6 years 9 months old, Leonardo was significantly ill and missed several weeks of school.

★ In-school review meeting at 7 years old, involving both parents, head teacher and class teacher: school was concerned that Leonardo had not progressed beyond Stage 5 (using his voice to make animal and vehicle sounds); SLT was concerned about inconsistency of shaping programme (sessions were cancelled because the keyworker had to fill in elsewhere; sessions were interrupted by other people working in the library).

★ Formal sliding-in programme was introduced, supervised by the head teacher, involving Dad, Leonardo and sibling coming into the empty classroom daily before the start of school for 10 minutes.

★ Telephone support given by SLT in the first week.

★ Four in-school reviews each half-term.

Outcome

★ Rapid progress once the sliding-in programme was introduced, with other children joining one by one; keyworker sliding in; Dad sliding out by the end of the second week.

★ Transfer to classroom and other locations and people was followed steadily.

★ At the last school meeting, the SLT was told by the keyworker that Leonardo had been shouting across the football pitch that morning.

★ Discharged at 8 years 3 months, after a successful transfer into the new school year.

Authors' comments

★ This example illustrates: the greater effectiveness of sliding-in over shaping; the difficulties of ensuring regular consistent management of a programme; the importance of regular planned reviews; and the importance of the interest and commitment of the head teacher.

★ With hindsight, more could have been tried to get Dad involved in a sliding-in programme earlier. This would have needed more time spent on helping the parents to understand the concerns better.

★ It was unfortunate that the three professionals Leonardo was initially referred to did not have sufficient knowledge or experience of SM to offer effective help earlier.

★ Although covering two years, this works represents only 10 sessions of SLT time, split between the clinic and school, along with the important telephone support – with the SLT acting in an advisory capacity.

4 Daniel (referral at 6 years)

(Source: adapted with permission from Carole Davies and Pauline Winters, *RCSLT Bulletin*, June 1996)

Background

★ Daniel had a history of severe speech and expressive language impairment, diagnosed at 2 years old by an SLT. Therapy had focused on stimulating language development and improving articulatory control. Daniel had been participating but either whispered or used a very quiet voice.

★ From 2 years old he had spoken freely at home (despite his poor speech and language) but was mostly silent with strangers and at nursery school. However, no diagnosis of SM had been made.

★ Aged 4, Daniel went to a designated school for children with specific speech and language disorders but, at 6 years old, the school voiced concern that all of his speech in school was whispered and asked whether this could be addressed.

Assessment

★ Assessment of Daniel's speaking habits showed that he talked a lot at home, using his voice appropriately, but in school he had no spontaneous speech; answered direct questions in a whisper; only whispered to adults, not children; and was generally reticent to join in with activities.

★ His expressive language was disordered, he used three- or four-word utterances consisting of key words only, with no grammatical development.

★ He had a disordered sound system, vowel distortions and consonant substitutions and omissions.

Intervention

★ The SLT instigated a daily shaping programme as Mum, although happy for the school to do what was necessary, could not travel to the school regularly (see Appendix B 'Shaping programmes').

★ There were daily 10-minute sessions with a specialist teacher (keyworker) during Daniel's playtime; and twice weekly visits from an SLT to discuss targets. Sessions began with non-verbal activities and were extended to 15 minutes after a few weeks.

★ Daniel was involved in setting his own targets and agreeing rewards which ranged from pencil sharpeners to tubs of bubble mixture.

Outcome

★ After one week, there was: a change in body language; a broad smile when it was time for sessions; larger, relaxed movements; and growth in self-esteem.

★ After six weeks, Daniel was much more confident generally and eager to whisper answers in group sessions.

★ After 12 weeks, Daniel used his voice for the first time in single sounds with the keyworker; and, one week later, the first real words in relaxed conversation in the one-to-one withdrawal room.

★ Generalisation followed: other adults and children were brought into the withdrawal room; sessions gradually moved into the classroom; and new locations were introduced, including the street outside the school and the local shops.

★ Three months later, Daniel began talking spontaneously to other adults and children, including the person who would be his class teacher in the following year.

★ In his new class, Daniel read to his new teacher at her desk, using his voice. The same afternoon, after three refusals to accept a whispered voice, Daniel read a story he had written, this time with the rest of his class around him.

★ Then Daniel's individual programme was discontinued, with no repercussions, and the programme to work on expressive language and disordered speech was reintroduced. Daniel was extremely cooperative and spoke freely in school.

★ Progress continued: Daniel spoke in class assembly in front of the whole school, At 8 years old, he returned to mainstream school where he received continued support to develop literacy.

Teacher's and therapist's comments

This was our first experience of SM and we felt very tentative about starting the programme. The emotional involvement of the specialist teacher was higher than expected and frustrations were sometimes difficult to rationalise. Having two members of staff involved to share the load and discuss every stage was, therefore, extremely valuable. It was important to hold on to the idea that Daniel was stressed about using language, and therefore had a huge hurdle to overcome.

We learned that we could not rush the generalisation phase and frequently had to backtrack and take smaller steps. Daily sessions were very effective, as long as the keyworker remained in control. It worked well to return to class when Daniel could not manage a target, and to resist when he tried to extend a session.

Authors' comments

★ This example illustrates how an interest in SM can lead to effective therapy even without previous experience.

★ It was impossible to give Daniel therapy for his expressive language and speech disorder until the mutism was addressed. However, Daniel's whispering had been accepted for so long that it had become quite entrenched, so progress took time.

★ As parental involvement was not an option, voice was elicited through shaping; full use was made of an audio recorder so that he would not have to speak directly to adults to begin with.

★ Close liaison between everyone involved meant that Daniel's whispered voice was not accepted in his new class. This decision was reached because he had used voice with the teacher, and spoken in front of the class on other occasions. It was very wise not to let this habit return.

★ Daniel was lucky; few children have the quality and quantity of support he received.

5 Robbie (6 years 3 months)

Background

★ Robbie had a history of normal speaking in nursery class at a small preparatory school but, aged four, he found the transition to main school frightening and confusing. Robbie did not speak again at school and soon stopped speaking to his grandparents. Within three months, he would only talk to his parents in his own home.

★ There was a history of severe anxiety and resistance to change, for example: terrified of loud noises; unable to cope with other children; very rigid eating patterns; would only use the toilet when accompanied by Mum in his own home.

★ Aged 5, Robbie was referred to a family mental health centre where 'voluntary mutism' was diagnosed, followed by referral to an SLT who suspected autism.

★ Aged 6, a multi-agency assessment resulted in a diagnosis of Asperger's syndrome and SM. The team called in a second SLT who had experience of SM.

Multi-agency assessment

★ Living alone with parents, Robbie spoke comfortably to them at home and in the car. He no longer spoke to them in public but, occasionally, whispered to them outside the home.

★ Robbie cooperated fully with assessments, where he could respond by nodding, shaking his head or pointing. When spoken answers were required, he whispered answers in Mum's ear. These responses were quite audible at times but directed only at Mum.

★ Understanding and use of language was within the average range, but limited to concrete experience. Very poor understanding of implied speech, inference and abstract language. Little empathy or ability to take another person's perspective. Excellent rote memory.

★ Presented as serious and rigid, rather than shy; stared at examiners with little expression, but was much more relaxed and interactive with his parents.

Intervention

★ Initial long session at multi-agency centre with SLT, clinical psychologist (CP) and both parents. It involved the Pep Talk (see Chapter 5); Robbie helping the SLT make a talking map (Chapter 5); and explanation of the Sliding-in Technique (Chapter 10). Using this technique, with a star given as Robbie achieved each target, succeeded in eliciting sentences at normal volume in simple talking games, with his parents, the SLT and the CP (see targets in Appendix C).

★ Session at home: the Sliding-in Technique was repeated and the parents were faded out; Robbie answered simple questions on his own with the SLT.

★ Session at school with Mum: activities were repeated in the homework room. Robbie spoke to the SLT spontaneously for the first time. The SLT met Robbie's teacher afterwards to discuss the implications of both Asperger's syndrome and SM.

★ Session with Mum and teacher in the homework room at the end of the school day: the Sliding-in Technique was used to elicit speech with Robbie's teacher and activities were repeated in his classroom. Mum and the SLT were then faded out. The teacher was given simple verbal games to play with Robbie in the lunch-hour over the next 10 days. They met four times for a five-minute session before he went out to play.

★ Lunch-time session with teacher and SLT: another child successfully slid in. Robbie was beginning to answer the SLT's and teacher's questions outside the formal structure of a games session, but he was still very wary of other people overhearing, unless it was part of a game. Over the next 10 days, the teacher acted as the keyworker and slid in four more children, until Robbie was playing games and working on phonic activities in a small group at lunch-time.

★ Walkabout (see Chapter 10) at school: Robbie spoke easily to the SLT within earshot of other children, parents and staff members in various parts of the school. Robbie agreed to invite his class teacher for the following year to the next session. Soon afterwards, his teacher held a small group-games session during class-time; Robbie spoke in the classroom with all 15 class members present.

★ Setback: after the classroom session, children surrounded Robbie in the playground, excited that he could now speak. Terrified by the sudden noise and close proximity of the children, Robbie told his parents that evening that he could not talk to his new teacher, and did not want to talk to the other children any more. He maintained this position throughout the summer holidays, dreading going back to school. His parents had great difficulty reassuring Robbie, as he had little concept of past and future, and could relate only to his present anxiety state.

★ The SLT visited Robbie at home a few days before he returned to school. They had a relaxed session in the garden, playing football and chasing his rabbit. Robbie spoke freely and was happy to discuss his return to school. An action plan was agreed: there was no need to talk to his new teacher until he felt ready; the other children would be instructed to keep calm when they were near him; plus visits to his old classroom to see his previous teacher.

★ Session at school in his *new* classroom with his *old* teacher: Robbie talked freely and happily, having settled into his new classroom well. SLT used a timeline to illustrate what he had achieved over time, and to separate past, present and future. Positive thoughts were planted in his mind.

★ At the next session, Robbie spoke freely in the classroom, with other children present, with the SLT and his new teacher. During the last week, she had attended a session with his previous teacher, and then taken over as keyworker, sliding in a new child each lunch-time. This was unprompted by the SLT and showed a real understanding of both general treatment principles and Robbie's readiness to move forwards.

Outcome

★ Three weeks into the new school term, Robbie participated in all classroom activities and talked to other children as well as his teacher.

★ He also started drinking water at school and using the school toilet for the first time. Dinner-time remained problematic – not eating pudding at school (afraid of the other children's reaction if he did something different) and eating only a narrow range of food – but Robbie himself said that he would 'do it in tiny steps'.

★ School staff reported that Robbie was doing new things every day and were happy for the SLT to review the situation in four months' time.

★ Robbie began talking to his grandparents again about halfway through the programme and, by the end, he talked freely to his parents outside the home.

Parents' comments

Robbie is a different child – for the first time in almost three years, he is enjoying going to school and talking about the other children. He is keen for them to visit and play with him at home. The diagnosis of Asperger's syndrome made a lot of sense and helps us explain his embarrassing behaviour at times. It's wonderful that he's talking now, but he can be so rude without realising it! We can see that the difficulty talking was just one part of his very rule-bound behaviour.

Authors' comments

★ It is unfortunate that Robbie was passed from agency to agency before the right help was secured. However, the thorough assessment and case history which preceded speech and language therapy involvement were invaluable in planning intervention, understanding Robbie's response and counselling his parents. The SLT's knowledge of both autism spectrum disorders and SM was also an advantage.

★ Robbie overcame his SM but his diagnosis of Asperger's syndrome means that he will continue to experience difficulties with socialisation and reciprocal conversation.

★ This represents 10 sessions of SLT time plus telephone calls between school visits to update his parents on progress and get feedback from home. A very visual approach was used throughout to compensate for Robbie's difficulties with abstract language.

★ This account perfectly illustrates what can be achieved in a short space of time if the school is open-minded to a new approach and can provide support on a regular basis. Extra help at lunch-times for four weeks, planned continuity between Year 1 and Year 2, and close liaison between home, school and therapist, led to a successful outcome.

6 Natia (7 years 5 months)

Background

★ When Natia was 6 months old, the family came to the UK as refugees, suddenly leaving everything in their homeland. They had a long and frightening escape from their country and five different hostels or homes before being given a council flat on a rough housing estate.

★ Natia's maternal grandmother joined the family in the UK when Natia was 2 years old.

★ Natia was referred by her SENCo to a specialist SLT on a Child and Adolescent Mental Health Service team because of her SM. She spoke to adults in reception class but only to a few peers since; in response to adults, she whispered to a friend or nodded or shook her head. There was no previous referral or intervention.

★ The referral stated there were no behaviour problems at school but Natia 'could be difficult at home'. She was doing very well academically.

Assessment

★ The extended parent interview (Chapter 6) was carried out with Mum who spoke English well. She was not worried about Natia's lack of talking – 'It's her personality'.

★ Mum was concerned that Natia was stubborn, challenging and defiant, taking out her anger on her parents and grandmother; behaving like a teenager; not respecting any boundaries they tried to set; occasionally physically aggressive when she did not get her own way.

★ Natia was also described as creative and imaginative; she had four friends but could be controlling with them; she did not attend groups or after-school activities.

★ Natia could hold in urine for up to 36 hours two years ago and, at the time of referral, only went to the toilet a maximum of twice a day, causing urine infections every two weeks. She never used the school toilets and could not go to the toilet independently at home.

★ Natia had a history of poor sleeping: up to the age of 7 someone had to lie with her until she fell asleep; she often woke at night, sometimes screaming for 30 minutes or more.

★ She had a history of separation difficulties: soon after her grandmother arrived, Natia could be left with her but had never been left with anyone else. They tried three nurseries from 2 years 6 months but Natia could not stay without her grandmother; she was very slow to settle in nursery class at school and in reception.

★ There were no concerns about her speech and language development or her learning of English; Natia was bilingual and spoke her first language to her grandmother.

★ Mum described herself as shy when young and very anxious during their move to the UK; she described Dad as a very strong personality and socially shy.

Intervention

★ Educate family and school about SM.

★ Liaison with doctor and specialist health visitor in enuresis clinic to help with urine infections.

★ Parental sessions to discuss behaviour management strategies and consistency in limit setting.

★ Shaping was used to elicit speech with keyworker – Natia's excellent, newly qualified class teacher who was fascinated by SM and taught Natia for two years. Then the Sliding-in Technique was used to generalise Natia's speech with adults and other children in school.

★ Some individual sessions to work on Natia's anxieties.

★ Occasional family therapy sessions, including Natia's maternal grandmother.

★ Assessment meeting with child psychiatrist and a trial period of the SSRI fluoxetine to relieve anxiety around going to secondary school at 11 years old.

Outcome

★ Natia made good progress with talking to her keyworker and an extended number of peers. But, when she reached Years 5 and 6, she stopped progressing further and resisted going to school in the mornings.

★ However, Natia started talking to people outside school who did not know her, and she benefited greatly from a fresh start in secondary school.

★ Her SM had totally resolved six months into secondary school, except for continued anxiety with three people she associated with her SM phase – the SLT, Mum's best friend and her best friend's mother. However, Mum asked for Natia to be discharged.

★ Slightly improved management of emotional and behavioural problems.

Authors' comments

★ Using the extended parent interview elicited much very helpful assessment information which was crucial to understanding the complexities of Natia's history. To summarise, Natia had SM, behaviour problems at home, toileting and urinary problems, and emotional problems in the context of migration, loss and stresses, family anxiety, issues of control and inconsistent parenting, and the family's struggle to rebuild their lives.

★ With hindsight, intervention could have included more emphasis on Natia's anxieties, helping the parents understand the relationship of her difficulties with talking, separation, sleeping and toileting.

★ Sadly, in spite of the keyworker's attempts at handover, the school staff in Years 5 and 6 were not prepared to offer Natia the help she needed.

★ The five-year intervention for Natia could have been more effective and carried out over a shorter time had it not been for her parents' heavy work programme, driven by their efforts to rebuild their lives.

★ Mum was not clear about what part the medication played and decided that Natia should stop using it after three months.

7 Lisa (15 years 10 months)

Background

★ Lisa was initially referred to speech and language therapy at 2 years 10 months old because of a general delay and reluctance to speak. Lisa was discharged at 6 years 3 months old, still delayed with 'immature speech' which was considered in line with her slower learning rate (the conclusion of an educational psychology assessment).

★ Lisa attended a mainstream secondary school with a special needs statement for moderate learning difficulties (MLD) and dyslexia. She was extremely distressed by school attendance, so attended part-time with tutor support in school and had 6 hours of home-tutoring. She was excused from all physical activity.

★ Self-referral to her doctor at 15 years old, who referred her on to a clinical psychologist (CP) in the private sector because of 'severe inferiority complex, lack of confidence, nervous tic (head and neck) and extremely limited nasal speech'.

★ Four sessions of cognitive behavioural therapy (CBT) with CP for social anxiety, low self-worth and negative (distorted) body-image. CP thought Lisa's confidence and social presentation would benefit from SLT to improve pronunciation.

★ Referred to and assessed by an SLT from the Adult Team who identified SM, in addition to a speech disorder. Transferred to a paediatric SLT with experience of SM.

Assessment (at hospital's adult speech and language therapy clinic)

★ Mum provided most of the background information. Lisa had two friends she saw in and outside school (normal interaction) and a cousin she got on well with, but generally had great difficulty making friends. Loud and demanding at home but often hard to understand as she spoke rapidly and indistinctly. Spoke minimally (one- or two-word responses) to some teachers and to her parents' friends. By this time, the tic was gone but Lisa would immediately hunch her shoulders, hang her head and clench her fists in the company of anyone other than close family and friends.

★ Lisa presented as chronically anxious. She answered the SLT in single words with inconsistent nasality, always preceded by a forced 'um' with head down, very limited eye contact and fixed smile. Completely froze when asked to imitate movements (for breathing awareness) and appeared to be dyspraxic. No initiation or spontaneous comments made.

Assessment (at home by paediatric SLT with experience of SM)

★ Lisa was assessed over two sessions with Mum in attendance. Lisa was invited to point or gesture her responses and to speak as much as she felt comfortable doing. Information gathering revealed a significant incident with a teacher at 8 years old. Lisa was kept in school for one hour until she clapped her hands (she never did). This resulted in cowering body posture (which never went away) and no more speaking at primary school. The teacher had to admit to Lisa's parents what she had done.

★ Lisa preferred her home-tutoring sessions to being at school but both she and Mum thought her tutor was quite formidable. Lisa was embarrassed that her tutor sat with her all the time at school but knew she couldn't manage without her. Other children had teased her in the past but this was no longer a problem; and yet Lisa still felt permanently self-conscious.

★ Mum thought her husband had unrealistic expectations that Lisa would go to university. She and her two daughters were much more relaxed when Dad was away on business.

★ Rating scales and ranking were used to establish Lisa's perception of her situation and priorities (Chapter 5). Lisa was more relaxed and answered in sentences, with no nasality. Poor intelligibility because of loud 'Um', poor rhythm and intonation, some vowel distortions and weak articulatory contacts at speed. Flat intonation and very poor timing when reading aloud. Unable to control pitch of voice but some control of volume. General body coordination was poor. All consistent with a diagnosis of articulatory dyspraxia and, probably, developmental coordination disorder (DCD).

★ Between assessment sessions, Lisa wrote down five wishes which she prioritised as follows.

1 To speak clearer.

2 To be less shy.

3 To stop worrying about my speech.

4 To be happy with my appearance.

5 To be better at school work.

★ Using a solution-focused approach (see Chapter 5, page 87), the SLT helped Lisa to convert priorities 2 and 3 into measurable targets, for example:

SLT: 'How will you know that you are less shy?' **Lisa:** 'I'll look natural'.

SLT: 'So you'd like to have good eye contact and posture?' **Lisa:** 'Yes.'

SLT: 'What are you thinking when you worry about your speech?' **Lisa:** 'People won't understand me. I'll have to repeat myself.'

SLT: 'How will you know you are less worried?' **Lisa:** 'I'll just speak.'

SLT: 'So you'd like to join in more and not worry about repeating yourself if necessary?' **Lisa:** 'Yes.'

Intervention

★ Explanation of avoidance cycle and phobia (Chapter 5); impact of anxiety on school work; reframing unhelpful thoughts (CBT influence); anxiety reduction by facing fear one step at a time.

★ Ten sessions, each lasting at least an hour, over 8 months focusing on priorities 1 and 2 at home, through reading (pausing, hard contacts), conversation and honest feedback about her posture and use of the telephone (volume, clarity, posture). Relaxation work was very difficult because of DCD – it just seemed to make things worse.

★ Then tackled priority 3 with targets to speak in shops, cafés and fast-food outlets (Chapter 9). Lisa now had a positive mind-set and believed that, if she had to repeat herself, people would always understand her the second time. Practical sessions continued every two to six weeks, fitting in with school holidays.

★ During the community phase Lisa got to know a local boy. She progressed from instant messaging to live webcam conversations and finally talking face-to-face at her home. At 16 years 8 months old, she announced that she had a boyfriend, which seemed to take care of priority 4! He was instrumental in supporting Lisa's community programme and took over the SLT's 'hands-on' sessions once Lisa left school and went to college on a full-time basis, aged 16 years 11 months.

★ Priority 5 was tackled by helping Lisa break ties with her home tutor, who was not helping the situation, and managing a careful handover to college.

★ Once Lisa was at college, the SLT stayed involved, but at a distance, meeting once a term for a chat.

Outcome

★ Almost immediately at college, Lisa was making new friends, shopping and ordering food, and taking the initiative in making phone calls (eg making hair appointments, looking for a part-time job).

★ As Lisa became more confident and chatty, her speech became more rushed and she appeared to develop a stammer. Her SLT sought a second opinion and was advised this was more cluttering than stuttering. Lisa and the SLT discussed the effect of general poor coordination on her speech and the need to consciously slow down.

★ After a year, Lisa passed her driving test and temporarily left home to attend college in a different part of the country. She said 'I think I'll be all right now' even though she clearly still became nervous with new people and had difficulty controlling her breathing and speech delivery at these times. Significantly, she now saw this as something she could deal with, rather than a reason for avoidance.

★ The SLT discharged Lisa when she was 18 but would still chat online occasionally.

★ Aged 20, Lisa requested to be referred again to the adult speech and language therapy department for her stammer. She had four sessions which she found helpful. It seems she could cope better with relaxation techniques than when she was younger.

Authors' comments

★ This example illustrates several useful techniques for approaching, assessing and engaging with young people (see Chapter 5).

★ Speech awareness played a major role in Lisa's SM as confirmed by her priority list. Therefore, the SLT decided to focus on speech production initially, but it was essential to manage this within the context of chronic anxiety and fear of speaking.

★ All sessions (apart from college liaison and community targets) were held at home. This may not be possible for some professionals but undoubtedly contributed to Lisa's ability to relax and engage with therapy.

★ After her second year at college, Lisa gained a place at university, indicating that earlier assessment results had been negatively influenced by anxiety. Clearly, she did not have moderate learning difficulties and her father's expectations were not unrealistic after all!

8 Sander (16 years)

This example describes intervention in Norway, carried out largely by a parent who gave email feedback to one of the authors.

Background

★ Sander didn't speak out fully from the age of two. His parents' worries started when he was about four and didn't speak to several adults and unfamiliar children in kindergarten. When he was six, the only adults he spoke to were his parents; but he spoke, played and moved freely during break-time.

★ Referral to a specialist concluded that he had general anxiety but *not SM* because children with SM 'don't speak to anyone'.

★ Sander had no other problems except with the mechanics of writing and drawing. In Mum's words: 'There was no separation anxiety or sign of any other anxiety besides talking out loud; he was very social after school, and during break-time; always had friends visiting us, preferring our house because he couldn't talk to his friends' parents.'

★ At about 10 years old, when Mum was looking for help, she was told 'No worries, he will grow out of it, he is just shy.'

★ A year later, a specialist gave him the diagnosis of SM. But, in spite of guidance, the teachers still described him as 'lazy' and 'demotivated'. At this point, Sander gave up mathematics, which he had struggled with earlier, saying 'I'm just stupid'.

★ Aged 15, Sander would speak to six or seven peers and his English teacher (his favourite subject was English, taught in a class with different students). He isolated himself increasingly at home, but was active on social media and online games. He started to speak in English online with a Danish and a British internet friend.

★ Also aged 15, Sander was referred to a therapist – a psychologist. He met her initially once a week, later every other week.

★ Aged 16, Mum was very worried because Sander had all but given up; he could not speak to his grandparents; he was making no progress with his therapist; and was not getting help at school.

★ Mum contacted one of the authors by email for advice, having seen her on a television programme five years previously and bought a copy of *The Selective Mutism Resource Manual* (SMRM).

Intervention

★ Mum and Sander were recommended to watch the Saki Galaxidis video (a 22 year old talking about his recovery from SM) on YouTube (see Appendix F, 'Audio-visual resources').

★ Mum also got the *Silent Children* DVD from SMIRA and watched it with Sander. Mum commented, 'It is so important to learn about other people suffering from the same condition. And, of course, to learn that it's possible to overcome it.'

★ Mum was also advised about an SM training day for older children, run by the authors, which she attended a month later.

★ A week after the course, Mum emailed: 'I told my son about the Sliding-in Technique, and he is totally in! "Yes, mom, I know I can do this." And this is the boy who had given up, because he "didn't want any help"! And for the first time my son started talking after his session with his therapist. As soon as we closed the door, he started talking. This has never happened before! He always waits until we are back in the car before he starts talking again. I do really see a change in him. He is so positive and optimistic, so now is the very best time to start our journey working our way out of silence.'

★ A further week on, Mum wrote: 'The London trip already paid off! We've started the Sliding-in Technique with my mom, and we had so much fun! We used the rote speech, counting and days. Today his grandfather was here when I got home from work, and my son answered him in sentences! And I've noticed he is speaking generally more at home (like Saki recommended). Why didn't I do this years ago? I bought the SMRM back in 2009, and read it too, but using so much effort trying to get the school to buy in to your Sliding-in Technique (neither the school nor the therapist would), I couldn't see clearly. No intervention was done, only struggling.'

★ Three weeks later, Mum wrote that Sander had been offered a new therapist, starting in about 10 weeks when he began at a new school (in August).

★ Meanwhile, they continued working on sliding in with good progress reported – eg chatting while helping grandparents move house. Mum said: 'The Sliding-in-Technique is fantastic! My son has reached so many goals!'

★ Mum used ranking to help Sander prioritise two goals – going to the shop and having good health (see Chapter 5, page 89); and a quiz game for more in-depth conversation with his grandparents.

★ On the first day at the new school, Mum gave the staff information on SM and a few tips about her son, and what he might benefit from. She told us: 'All his new teachers were there – because they want to do everything to make his start as good as possible. Totally new experience to me, the teachers want to learn and listen! I lent them my SMIRA DVD – they were eager to watch it as soon as possible. That never happened before either!'

★ Mum described Sander's first two weeks in the new school: 'His anxiety level was above anything he ever experienced. But still he continued. The third week I saw a difference in him: he was smiling more, he told me about school and new subjects, and in general he looked much happier. He told me in his first weeks he was totally panicking, and then it was much better. He even got a six (the same as an 'A') in a test.'

★ The family also got a dog. Sander had been asking for one for a while and he convinced Mum by promising to walk the dog – so he would have to go out every day, and maybe talk to strangers – which he did.

★ The new therapist – a social worker – had knowledge of *and* experience in working with children and young people with SM. She told Mum that Sander had already taken some huge steps in the treatment. She also had a dog, so they met outside, in different places, and Sander spoke to Mum in her presence.

★ Early in the new school year, Sander had to do some tests, requested by his previous therapist. Apart from language, which was assessed non-verbally and in which his score was above his age, the results were devastating. The psychologist said he would never be able to live on his own, have an education or a job. Mum did not believe the results could be right. She got Dad to check how Sander was doing in school, and they heard 'Well, he is doing great! He even speaks to some of the students, and the teachers when nobody else can hear; he is working on what he is told to do; nothing different about him from the other students. The only thing was, the teacher wanted him to put his hand up in the class when he knows the answer'.

Mum summarised by saying: 'So, he is handling school all right; he is taking the bus; he even goes to the shop now with other students; he is walking the dog; he is motivated for treatment; he has got himself a few new friends on Facebook; he is talking more at home – I see a happy teen'. She was comforted by the new therapist suggesting that the test situation, and the fact that the psychologist had never tested anybody with SM before, could have affected the results.

★ A month later, Sander had spoken to their neighbours and his aunt: 'He talked more to her that day than he had done for 16 years!! He also had a group presentation at school – in front of the whole class!!!'

Outcome (10 weeks after the start of the new school)

★ Mum reported on the review with Sander's teachers: 'He is doing great! His grades are fine – most of them average, some above average! And, best of all, he is really a part of his class socially; they couldn't tell him apart from the others; he smiles and laughs and talks! He even did something out of the ordinary earlier this week. The class had another group presentation, and my son took leadership of that one, spontaneous, suddenly he simply began talking in front of the whole class, so he was the one that talked in his group. Of course, the three other students talked too, but not as much as my son!'

★ Mum reported just one problem (as well as needing some continued help with his anxiety). Sander was not participating in gymnastics with a group of 10 students who all had some difficulties, whether physical or mental. If he didn't join this group, they could not give him a grade in this subject. (Sander watched and familiarised himself with what was required in the gym class but didn't want to join in part-way through the year. He participated fully the following year.)

Authors' comments

★ Sadly, this example illustrates, on several occasions, the effect of ignorance about SM, causing a delay in referral and the appropriate identification and action, resulting in a worsening of Sander's condition.

★ It shows how much a parent can do when they are given the right advice. It is a great example of someone attending an appropriate training course and really understanding and putting into practice the course contents.

★ The real turning point for Sander was understanding that SM was a phobia which could be overcome in a logical, methodical way.

★ The attitude of the new school was most helpful – what a setback it could have been otherwise.

★ Sander was fortunate to find a therapist who had experience of SM. Although his recovery was already being well managed by his mother, she found the involvement of a like-minded professional an enormous support – and relief.

CHAPTER 15

LEARNING FROM PEOPLE WHO HAVE EXPERIENCED SELECTIVE MUTISM

Introduction

This chapter looks at the life stories of adults who had selective mutism (SM) as a child and, in some cases, into adulthood. They answered a series of questions about:

★ their age when the SM started

★ their earliest memories of being unable to speak fully and freely with everyone

★ when and how they realised that they had SM

★ what they think caused their SM

★ whether they had any other difficulties as a child

★ their experiences of not being able to speak comfortably

★ who and what helped and how

★ which strategies and attitudes did not help

★ whether they are completely over their SM or have any lasting effects.

We are very grateful to our contributors for the time and thought which they all put into this chapter, especially bearing in mind that, for some, it brought back rather painful memories. Although we have had to shorten some accounts, we have left each person to tell their own story, in their own words. Obviously, their experiences and interpretations differ. But we feel sure that you will find interest, encouragement and some very helpful advice from the experiences of people who know most about what it is like to have SM.

At the end of the chapter, we have added our comments: some are general; some relate to the points in the stories marked with an asterisk (*). You might prefer to look at the authors' comments section first.

The contributors to this chapter are Maria (19), Katie (26), Rachel (33), Carl (45), Sarah-Jane (50) and Vivienne (55). They chose whether to use their real name or not.

Maria (aged 19)

Age when the SM started

From what I can remember, I was around four or five, just starting reception at school. This was when I was first aware of it as an issue. But it must have started earlier as I couldn't speak to one of my nans or my grandad at that time.(*)

Earliest memories of being unable to speak fully and freely with everyone

My earliest memory of being unable to speak is when I was in my early years at primary school. My teacher (Miss A) bribed me into saying 'glove', in order to throw a big party. As much as I wanted to, the word just would not come out. Being under so much pressure, this just freaked me out, almost put me in shock.

I remember being at my nan and grandad's and the only person I would talk to was my nan. I would have to shut the door so my grandad would not hear me.

When and how I realised that I had SM

I had always been shy as a child, but I think I was always too young to understand that I had SM. It wasn't until I was older that my speech therapist made me more aware of SM; and when I was over it, I learnt more about the causes of SM and the possibility of why people get it.

What caused my SM

I'm still not sure to this day what started my SM. The only possibilities I can think of is that we had a lot of trouble with my brother in the family, and maybe his anger and actions put me in shock.

Any other difficulties as a child

No.

Experiences of not being able to speak comfortably

In my younger years at primary school, some of my teachers used to make me say 'Yes' to my name in the register. This made me feel very uncomfortable, as I knew myself there was other ways of communicating with the teacher, such as putting my hand up.

Another time I remember is when I used to get questioned constantly from children in my class, why I was the way I am and why I couldn't speak. This made me feel very under pressure and upset.

Who and what helped and how

My speech therapist helped me so much. She used to visit me in school, and helped me talk to a classroom assistant, who got a small group each week out of the class, and we used to do different games and tasks. This helped a lot because doing the things I liked gained my confidence, and also gave more of an understanding to the people in my class of why I was the way I was. The teacher drew a birthday cake and, every time I spoke to a new child, they wrote their name on a paper candle and stuck it on the cake.

From what I can remember, my speech therapist used to do a strategy to help me talk to my grandparents where she would organise a few members of my family together, and make them take a step closer every time I spoke.

Being praised by my speech therapist and at school (everyone clapped when my birthday cake was full of candles; and I was given a certificate when I first sang in assembly) helped me a lot. It made me feel like I was gaining back my confidence and I could do something right.

Strategies and attitudes that did not help

I had two other speech therapists when I was younger and both of them quit.[*] This made me feel like the progress I made was a waste of time because I never fully gained back my confidence.

Being pressured to speak all the time by my friends did not help. It made me not want to speak all the more.

Whether I am completely over my SM

I was fine by the end of Year 6, around 10 or 11 years old and didn't have any problems at secondary school. I would say I am totally over my SM. I would happily speak to a stranger if they asked me in the street what the time was. I'm studying art at university and have a part-time job and social life, so having SM has not held me back.

Katie (aged 26)

Age when the SM started

I think it was something that I was born with and became worse and more pronounced as I got older. My mum recalls how I was more reserved than other babies and she noticed how I would freeze and go quiet when I started school.

Earliest memories of being unable to speak fully and freely with everyone

I think I remember not being able to speak the same way as anyone else would remember being able to speak, as it started when I was so young. In my earliest school memories, I remember being too scared to put up my hand in class, or to speak to the people next to me or even leave my seat! In primary school, I had a couple of friends who I could speak to at school, if only quietly but, once I moved and started a new school, I couldn't speak to anyone.

When and how I realised that I had SM

I knew that I was different and that something was 'wrong' with me but I thought I was the only one who was going through what I was suffering from, which was very lonely. A teacher suggested I had SM when I was about 10 but it wasn't until I was in Year 8, at about 12 years old that I saw a speech therapist and was 'diagnosed'. It was then that I came across SMIRA (the Selective Mutism Information and Research Association).

What caused my SM

Some people think that SM is caused by some kind of trauma, but I don't think this is true in my case. I think it was partly inherited as I have family members that are also very shy. I think it is partly down to my nature but could have been triggered by a traumatic birth.

Any other difficulties as a child

No.

Experiences of not being able to speak comfortably

School was really difficult for me and I dreaded going in every day. There isn't really one bad experience that stands out, just lots and lots of daily experiences that I became used to. I was always by myself, last to be picked in group tasks, and people would always make a fuss if they had to work with me. They would talk about me as if I wasn't there and treat me as if I was a liability; for example, complaining if they were paired up with me or saying things like 'We only have three people in our group' if there were three people plus me. Teachers even joined in on occasion and told me that I was letting everyone down and that I was difficult to work with. Sometimes the other kids at school would take things that belonged to me or be rude to me, knowing that I would not tell anyone.(*) It was also frustrating in class, knowing the answer to questions and not be able to put my hand up and tell the teacher the answer, or to ask for a new exercise book or to ask to go to the toilet.

Who and what helped and how

Positive attitudes from other people make all the difference. Even if it didn't make me start talking, having people be nice to me and include me made me feel a lot happier and more comfortable around them. I'm not sure if there were any particular strategies that worked; I think it might have been different if I had been 'diagnosed' when I was younger but, by the point I knew what was wrong, it felt a bit too late.

It was very isolating and confusing not knowing what was wrong with me and not knowing how to fix it. I had never met anyone who was suffering from the same thing and there was nobody that I could relate to until I came across SMIRA. For the first time, I felt like I fitted in and was part of some kind of club. People wanted to know me, include me and hear about my experiences, and I felt useful and accepted for once. SMIRA introduced me to different techniques I could use to make speaking easier and also to people that were going through the same thing. I wasn't ashamed any more and didn't feel like a failure. Even though I wasn't 'cured' of my SM by finding SMIRA, it made me feel like it was going to be OK which, in turn, probably helped me get over it. It also helped my family and the school understand more about my situation too.

Strategies and attitudes that did not help

Bribery or putting any kind of pressure on me did not help. If I felt like people were trying to force me to speak, I just felt even more isolated, upset and misunderstood. In a way it made me not want to speak at all. A lot of people seemed to underestimate how hard it was for me to speak and kept saying things like 'just speak' which was very frustrating.

Whether I am completely over my SM

As soon as I started college at 18, I was able to speak freely, but was still very shy. I think I was ready to start talking before then but, as I had spent so long not speaking at school, it was so hard to break out of it.(*) I was fine at uni but, a few months later, when I had started my first proper job, I began to feel panicky and dreaded going to work. I felt extremely anxious, shy and self-conscious all the time and it reminded me of how I felt when I was at school. I went to the doctor's who gave me some beta-blockers and I also saw a cognitive hypnotherapist.

I think the effects of having SM for so much of my childhood, and the way people have treated me, may have affected my confidence. However, I am a lot more confident and less anxious now and feel like I am getting more confident as I get older. I am naturally quite introverted and think that being shy and quiet is perhaps part of my personality, rather than a side effect of having SM. I don't feel like I have been too affected by it.

Rachel (aged 33)

Age when the SM started

When I started playgroup, just before my third birthday, I would talk to the other children when no adults were present but refused (*) to speak if I was aware of any adults being nearby. When I started school, I refused (*) to talk at all, to the point that I would be talking to my Mum on the walk to school, but would freeze up when we got near to the site.

Earliest memories of being unable to speak fully and freely with everyone

My earliest memories are probably from Year 1 at primary school where I wouldn't (*) read to the teacher in class, so we would record me reading and then I would sit with my teacher and follow the words on the page as my recorded voice played.

When and how I realised that I had SM

At her wits' end, my Mum wrote to a parenting magazine when I was about six years old and they published her letter. Alice Sluckin (the founder of SMIRA) read the article and responded to the letter which led to my diagnosis.(*)

What caused my SM

I honestly have no idea. I think I was shy, but not exceptionally so. I now realise that my father suffers from anxiety but I don't know whether this would have had any bearing on it. There wasn't any particular life event or anything that could have caused me to suddenly stop talking.

Any other difficulties as a child

None that I am aware of!

Experiences of not being able to speak comfortably

The most concerning experience was probably when I cut my head open in the playground at school. I must have been around seven years old. No matter how hurt I was, I wouldn't cry so I would have held it all in. My head was bleeding but I wouldn't talk to give my grandparents details so that they could come and collect me from school (Mum was not contactable on that day for some reason). In the end, they sat me down with a friend for company and I found my grandparents' name in the phone book and pointed to it.

Other examples of difficult situations:

★ I was short-sighted but couldn't tell anyone that I couldn't read the blackboard ... mind you, I'm not sure how they would have performed the eye test without me reading out the letters!

★ I hated going to the dentist. I would refuse [*] to open my mouth and definitely wouldn't say 'Ahh'.

★ I wet myself in school assembly because I couldn't ask to go to the toilet.

Who and what helped and how

My teacher gave me cards with useful phrases on them, eg 'Please can I go to the toilet'. I'm not sure if this was particularly helpful long term because it made it possible for me to manage without talking but it certainly made life easier in the short term. One positive was that it enabled me to be more like the other children and I wasn't totally set apart by my silence.

I had a fantastic teacher when I was seven or eight years old who included me in the play by giving me a non-speaking part. She enabled my Mum to have reading sessions in the library with me and a small group of friends and I began to read with them in a non-threatening environment. This led on to me reading to Mum in the classroom while my teacher pretended not to listen. Over time, my voice wasn't such a whisper and I eventually read to the teacher. Ultimately, I read out some of my work in the full school assembly, much to the disbelief of the other teachers.

'How scary is it on a scale of 1 to 10?' This was a strategy that Mum used (I think on the advice of a psychologist that we saw). If there was a situation coming up that I was anxious about, we would discuss how scary it was on the scale of 1 to 10 and then try to rationalise the anxiety. If I managed to do the task then, the next time something difficult was coming up, Mum would be able to refer back to how scary I had said a previous challenge was, and remind me that I had still managed to do it anyway, and that, afterwards, it had seemed much less scary.

My frustration also helped me to break my silence. I had started to see that other children were being picked over me to do tasks that I knew I could do better. The only time I ever accidentally spoke was towards the end of my SM time and when a friend was doing something wrong. I blurted out 'No, not like that.' I had started to realise that it was holding me back and that I didn't want it to.

Strategies and attitudes that did not help

★ Putting me in a situation where people would try and make me talk. I would feel backed into a corner and anxious and there is no way that they would get anything out of me in that situation.

★ Labelling me as the person who will not speak. This sort of closed the door on the opportunity for me to say something if I did feel brave enough.

While acceptance that I didn't want to talk did help to some degree, labelling me as a person who wouldn't talk did not. In some ways the difference is subtle ... 'Rachel doesn't talk at the moment' versus 'Rachel doesn't talk' but it made a huge difference to the way people treated me. It was important that there was an opportunity for me to speak if I had wanted to (without drawing too much attention to it) but, equally, that I could manage to get by without talking. It was definitely not helpful to label me as 'the girl who didn't talk' because this gave me some sort of undesirable celebrity status.

Whether I am completely over my SM

After I broke my silence at school, I didn't really look back. I was never the first to put my hand up in class to answer a question and I would probably only do so if I was very confident that I had the correct answer. I was given the position of Head Girl in my last year at primary school which involved, to a small degree, representing the school.

I went on to do voluntary work, which involved speaking at meetings with adults present, and gaining leadership certificates. I don't think I particularly enjoy doing presentations but I don't think many people do!

I now have two children and run our village toddler group. I am also on the Parish Council, which involves a degree of public speaking. In many ways, I think the challenge of SM has empowered me because I managed to conquer a major anxiety and every other anxiety that I have seems pretty inconsequential in comparison!

Carl (aged 45)

Age when the SM started

I believe that SM was an innate part of my make-up. As such, I believe SM-like behaviour is perfectly ordinary for many young children who become silent when they feel anxious or scrutinised. I don't therefore see my SM as starting, rather as it never subsiding. My SM became more and more enmeshed with my emotions as I got older.[*]

Earliest memories of being unable to speak fully and freely with everyone

Looking back on my early childhood, it was entirely ordinary behaviour for me to be mute in certain circumstances.[*] As a child, my aunties, uncles and grandparents never heard me speak. My grandparents never heard me before they died. I remember very early on being silent when my mother's friends would look at me and the intentness on my face and say 'He's taking everything in.'

When and how I realised that I had SM

I was perspicacious as a young child and loved learning – particularly maths. I lived very much 'in the moment' and did not concern myself with how others thought about me. As such, I did not realise that I had an issue with speaking, even though it was a firm part of my behaviour, until I was a teenager. If I was mute at school I barely remember, because it didn't matter to me. In the 1970s and 1980s there was much less emphasis on speaking at school.

What caused my SM?

There were issues in my home life, which contributed to my SM, plus inappropriate actions at school made my SM far worse.

In my childhood, my mother had enduring mental health problems. She often could not bear to hear the sound of children. As such, I would be chastised if I made a noise, or 'looked' in a certain way; and my father would threaten me with the belt if I did not obey her.[*] To be clear, I do not blame my mother at all for her mental health issues (it is merely as things were). However I was very affected by her behaviour.[*]

Although it would not happen nowadays in such a way (at least I hope not), my silence invited suspicion amongst teachers – and, without warning, I had to undergo a very invasive examination for signs of sexual abuse at infant school. My parents were not aware and I kept what happened entirely to myself. It caused me to become extremely ashamed of myself for many years and made my SM far worse in hindsight.[*]

As a teenager, my mother and father divorced and my stepfather moved into the house – someone I could not speak to. My mother and stepfather argued very often, very loudly, and were sometimes violent with each other. Particularly at the start of their relationship, I was also often threatened with violence too. I was entirely mute at home for a decade, and it felt inescapable. I lived entirely the opposite double-life to most young people with SM: speaking at school, sixth form, and ultimately university, all the while mute at home.

Any other difficulties as a child

I had childhood depression and am still affected by depression. Anxiety, however, was not something I feel I experienced particularly. There were many situations (eg with strangers, when I was away from my parents) where I could speak. In fact, I was actually bombastic, loud and outgoing, left to my own devices. I do not see SM as an 'anxiety disorder' in my case; rather, I see it as a mixture of conditioning and emotional problems.

Experiences of not being able to speak comfortably

The worst experience was actually my first university graduation ceremony. I had lived a double-life for a very long time, speaking in one situation and not in another. The 'selective' part of my SM by then was, actually, between cities. In London I could generally speak, though there were some exceptions – when people reminded me, in some obscure way, of my parents or family situations. I could not speak to partners in particular. In my home city I was mute.

I spent the graduation ceremony day trying to keep my SM secret. It was something I was deeply ashamed of. I could not tolerate my mother or father knowing I could speak at university; and I could not tolerate my then friends at university knowing I couldn't speak at home. I kept the two groups away from each other, flitting from one to the other to keep them apart. After that day I deliberately lost contact with my friends and lived a 100 per cent mute life until I started my PhD. It was at this stage my own mental health issues became more severe.

Who and what helped and how

I believed that the only way I could break selective mutism was to make myself suffer so much that I could not tolerate it any longer, and I *had* to speak. I started my PhD in another city again, deliberately having isolated myself from everyone, so that I could (one way or another) speak. After abject suffering, I had a nervous breakdown. I was helped just by the existence, rather than in practical terms, of a wonderful psychiatrist who prescribed an SSRI (paroxetine) that had very recently come on the market.

I did then speak to my mother and, in fact, it was she who invented the strategy to help me. I started to whisper the words from a book to her, prompted by her to do so (the book was *Our John Willie* by Catherine Cookson) and, after a day or so, managed to increase my volume.[*] A few days later, I spoke to my stepfather for the first time. A few weeks after that, I joined an amateur dramatic society and appeared on stage in a play (*The Sound of Music*!), just to prove to myself that it was over.

After being so unwell, I continued and completed my PhD. It was a huge emotional, less so academic, achievement.

Strategies and attitudes that did not help

The main strategy or attitude that did not help was inappropriate and invasive scrutiny at school.

SM was unheard of all the way into my twenties (it was still called 'elective mutism' at that stage). My SM pattern was the opposite to the norm, being mute at home, so in many ways it was entirely hidden. As such, no strategy was ever applied to try to help me.

Whether I am completely over my SM

For a number of years after I started speaking to my mother and stepfather, I believed I was over SM. However, I continued to feel the effects of stress, after my experience at university and what I'd had to do to myself to speak again – isolating myself and purposefully making myself unwell. Although not diagnosed, it is clear to me that was I was suffering from PTSD.

Unfortunately, I still have the same triggers and I still become mute – particularly around partners and other relatives. I still have rules (as I always did) about who I can speak to and who I can't. Because there is no tailored therapeutic support out there for adults with SM, it will be something I will have for the rest of my life.

Sarah-Jane (aged 50)

Age when the SM started

From my first memories I cannot remember a time when I didn't have a problem speaking freely and the feelings of the terror that came over me with the very thought of speaking. I don't have any information regarding my language development before this time, but I do remember clearly starting school at around four years old and getting through the whole day without uttering a word other than maybe 'Yes' or 'No' or nodding my head.

Earliest memories of being unable to speak fully and freely with everyone

My memories include: the sense of loneliness and isolation; feeling unwanted; the fear that came over me when I had to speak; the physical sensations of feeling paralysed and frozen. I also strongly remember that I would often end up doing things I didn't want to do and missing out on things I really did want to do.

When and how I realised that I had SM

Approximately five years ago, in my forties, when I came across the term 'selective mutism', while retraining as a neuro-developmental delay practitioner. It was a light-bulb moment during a lecture on a retained Moro reflex (the startle reflex in newborns) and fear–paralysis, involving a description of the physiological effects this can have on a person. I recognised in myself the symptoms and feeling of being on 'red alert' the whole time; my tense muscle tone; difficulty with change and making decisions; low self-esteem; insecurity and dependence; paralysis of the larynx and pharynx.

What caused my SM

Having researched and read around the subject of SM, I believe my SM was a combination of being a highly sensitive child born into a very chaotic family (I was the youngest of five) that misunderstood me and who often responded to my SM with forcefulness, anger and impatience. Consequently, I felt ignored, never heard, unimportant and invisible.(*)

Any other difficulties as a child

Because as a child, from a very early age, the 'goodness-of-fit' between my temperamental style and the patterns of child rearing used by immediate care givers (mainly my neurotic mother and alcoholic grandmother) were unhealthy, I definitely suffered from attachment and trust issues that carried through into adult life. Therefore, although I would not wish SM on any child, I do view my childhood SM as a healthy reaction to an unhappy environment.(*)

Experiences of not being able to speak comfortably

As a child I was abused sexually, both by a member of the family and by an adult outside the family, and never felt able to tell anyone. It didn't cross my mind that I was important and should be protected. Not being able to verbally express how bad and frightened I felt left me unable to report this to anyone. On some level, I hoped that someone would work out what was happening and 'speak' for me.(*)

Who and what helped and how

Firstly, acknowledgement and an understanding that I had suffered from SM and that I was not alone. This was a platform to start working from and included making others around me aware of SM and how it can affect someone's life.

Secondly, having a safe place to start speaking within – in my case, this was with my therapist who I had already been seeing for approximately one year prior to my realisation that I had been an SM sufferer. One main quality of my therapist that helped specifically with SM was developing trust and not fearing that she would judge my silences and difficulty to speak out and possibly reject me.(*)

Specific strategies that helped included EFT (emotional freedom technique) which uses tapping on specific meridian points in the body; and a movement programme developed by the Institute of Neuro-Physiological Psychology (INPP) to overcome the physiological effects of my retained Moro reflex. As a result, I felt able for the first time to take a deep breath, down to my stomach; less constricted by body tension; more able to use eye contact and show my teeth when smiling; and a general diminishing of the terror when speaking.

Thirdly, my personal experiences of recovery have taught me that if my stomach 'churns', I now recognise this as a sign that I want to say something and I am holding back. Once I have recognised this feeling, I am usually able to consciously overcome any anxiety I have about speaking. As I practise this more and more, my speech has become more automatic.[*]

I would also add that a temporary solution in my life was learning a foreign language. I went to Mexico as a teen and felt a real sense of rest, with no expectations to speak their language, for six months. When I did start to speak Spanish, I definitely didn't experience as much anxiety as when I spoke English.

Strategies and attitudes that did not help

Being around anyone who would try and force me to speak or expect me to speak.

Others' assumptions about my silence, such as defiant, rude, spoilt, etc, that would often be followed with some kind of disciplinary measure.[*] This seemed to be because most people struggle to understand why you cannot speak if you have no physical damage that can be 'seen'.

Whether I am completely over my SM

I would say that my significant recovery from SM happened after approximately two years of therapy and one year after realising that SM existed. It was still then a further couple of years until speaking became almost automatic. I shock myself now, as at times I feel like I have verbal diarrhoea and my voice seems louder – something that those around me have also positively commented on.

However, to be absolutely clear, from my experience, I feel one never does totally get rid of early damage (programming) but one can recognise it and can take immediate steps to override it. Sometimes I still freeze. When this happens, I don't panic – I stop and acknowledge that it is just a reminder of my SM, take a breath (including time out) and start again. I still see my therapist as the consequences of suffering SM for decades left me with a lot of 'work' to do, particularly in the areas of relationships and self-esteem.[*]

Interestingly, as I write these words, I can see that my ability to write freely and express myself was also hindered by SM and this has only developed as I now speak freely.[*]

Although regaining my voice has been hard work, it has definitely been worth it because, for me, speaking freely is so very linked to my identity and who I really am – something that I had never been in touch with before.

Vivienne (aged 55)

Age when the SM started

It is hard to pinpoint exactly when my SM started. At three years of age, I can remember hiding behind my carer's back when meeting strangers (especially men). It was well tolerated; it just felt normal and comfortable not to talk and I felt perfectly relaxed because my carer always remained with me. I was not conscious that anything was wrong.[*]

Earliest memories of being unable to speak fully and freely with everyone

On starting school at about four and a half, I suffered badly with separation anxiety. I can remember feeling absolutely terrified – panic-stricken. I did not adapt well to transitions such as playtime; getting ready for PE; or going up on stage to rehearse for the school play.

At the same age, a second difficulty involved my interaction with my mother's new dating partner; I could neither make eye contact nor speak with him, which was perceived as hostility. This was to become the cause of many confrontations and, once he became my stepfather, several beatings.[*] I think it was at this point I came to see myself as a bad child; adults had now become disapproving and angry at behaviours that had once seemed natural and acceptable.[*]

When and how I realised that I had SM

At four and a half, my first experiences of school, alongside my difficulties with my mother's partner, began to ring alarm bells. I felt different and awkward but I did not really know why. It was another 40 years before I came across the term 'selective mutism'.

What caused my SM

My conclusion is that there is generally a strong genetic predisposition to SM; and those affected tend to share a clearly recognisable set of features in common. It is not unusual for SM to traverse generations, passing from parent to child (as in our case).

Any other difficulties as a child

The freeze response proved to be a problem for me, particularly as a young child (below the age of nine), and this was most severe during times of high anxiety. It also caused me to be clumsy which often bothered me more than my inability to talk.

Experiences of not being able to speak comfortably

At the age of six, I was told by my form teacher to go to the head teacher's office where I was asked to read. Initially, I felt a sense of relief because I was not in trouble; and I had always been praised for my good (albeit quiet) reading at my previous school .To my total horror, my throat suddenly felt constricted, as though someone had their hands around my throat. I desperately tried to push out words but they would not come. I eventually managed a single word, but it was the wrong word because I had lost my place on the page. Meanwhile, the head teacher had become exasperated; she accused me of procrastinating because I could not read. This incident left me deeply traumatised. If I had told my parents, they would never have believed me because it made no sense and sounded like a stupid excuse; so I kept it a secret.[*]

My school in Hounslow (in London) was hell – overcrowded and outmoded. There was also a huge influx of Asian refugee children who could not speak English; so the dinner ladies used to manhandle children around, rather than speak to them. I became physically frozen in a way that I had never been before, due to anxiety and not motor-coordination difficulties. There was tight army-like discipline at lunch-time in order to get our hands washed and have us fed and out of the hall within 20 minutes. Within about two weeks of arrival, I had been hit hard from behind by a dinner lady because I had frozen and was therefore moving too slowly; I was yelled at by a teacher because my face had frozen, so she thought that I was smirking. I was also physically picked up and shaken by my form teacher because a boy had stolen my pencil, when she wasn't looking, and she caught me trying to get it back.[*]

In September, when my peer group went up a form, I was kept back. My form teacher told me it was because the head teacher had said that I needed to learn to read. I was deeply upset because I lost my friends, and this led to me being permanently behind at school.

Who and what helped and how

My best experience happened just after my mother remarried. Before I attended the local primary school, I met Mrs W who was the school secretary. She was very positive about the school and told me not to worry, as she would look after me. The first playtime Mrs W introduced me to a group of girls playing together, whom she knew lived nearby, and asked me if I would like to join them (I could now speak to other children, as long as I did not have to initiate). We soon became friends and played together both inside and outside school. Mrs W acted as a mentor, effectively bridging the gap between home and school; and her interventions were always brief and light touch.

My form teacher helped too, by making sure I understood what I had to do and explaining how best to start the set work; this helped reduce my anxiety.

Strategies and attitudes that did not help

One-off or baseline testing was very problematic for both myself and my daughter.

Another unhelpful strategy was being made to repeat school years when I was 12, in a new secondary school – in spite of my exam results placing me more or less in the middle of the year group. My teacher said this was in order for me to gain confidence. Nothing could have been further from the truth. In the absence of knowing that I had SM, I blamed my personality for all my failures; and no matter how hard I tried, I would fail. I pleaded with my mother to persuade the school to let me go up with my peers, but she was fed-up and exasperated with me.

I began to descend into a deep depression and eventually reached the stage where I could not face going to school any more. My parents believed my absence was unwarranted because I was not physically ill. I ended up hiding in my bedroom, and my relationship with my parents reached an all-time low.

Whether I am completely over my SM

No, I am not completely over my SM. I managed to catch up on missed qualifications, gaining 'O' and 'A' levels (end of school public exams), followed by a science degree by my late twenties. However, I believe that I could have gained 'O' levels at school with a minimum of support, if only they had not used my shyness and lack of confidence as a weapon against me. The constant setbacks and failures at school (which were avoidable) have impacted on my confidence as an adult.

I seemed to undergo some degree of spontaneous remission from SM in my twenties. I can now speak in most everyday situations but there are exceptions. These include speaking in groups where there is frequent exchange of conversation; this was especially problematic at university tutorials where there was an expectation that students would be articulate and well able to explore and discuss ideas and concepts. I have always felt unable to join voluntary committees and boards such as school governors.

I find it impossible to answer questions if put on the spot, even if I know the answer, and this made viva voce (oral testing) an ordeal, both at university and for gaining registration in my chosen career. I find job interviews punishing (it took approximately 50 to get my first job). No matter how hard I have tried not to be, I am still taciturn. And, in times of severe anxiety, I still clam up and can lose my ability to speak altogether. I feel strongly that SM is a disability.

Authors' comments

The honest life stories in this chapter illustrate several important points:

★ Maria, Carl and Vivienne demonstrate how the onset of SM is often earlier than the acknowledgement of SM as an issue. All the time their silence was accepted, and they felt no pressure to speak; life felt ordinary and comfortable and they had no sense of anything being 'wrong'.

★ There are good examples of the effects of help from people who know about SM (eg Maria's speech therapist; SMIRA for Katie; Alice Sluckin for Rachel), highlighting the need for good training in SM awareness and management.

★ There are also good examples of the importance of support and acceptance from people who know nothing about SM (eg Carl reading to his mother; Sarah-Jane's therapist; the school secretary for Vivienne).

★ There are tragic descriptions of the effects of late diagnosis, mismanagement and missed opportunities that point to the importance of adult services recognising SM and having the knowledge and skills to manage it effectively, however late (eg Carl, Sarah-Jane and Vivienne).

★ Maria talks about the effect on her of two speech and language therapists who 'quit'. Of course, people change jobs and people's jobs change. But, too often, SLTs are asked to work with children who have SM when they are only in a short-term post. The importance of continuity and good therapist transitions are sometimes overlooked and add to the child's sense of loss or being let down. We believe it is often preferable for the SLT to take on a supportive, advisory role while the children build rapport with people they see on a regular basis (eg a classroom assistant).

★ Katie's examples of mistreatment by her peers at school show that bullying may not always be obvious but is just as painful if it is what some people call 'low level'.

★ The contrast between the level of support given in class to Maria and Katie is stark: Maria's class was informed about her SM and came on board, wanting to help, and sharing in Maria's enjoyment of her achievements. Katie describes the opposite experience. However, Katie made great progress when she had a planned, fresh start at college. Had she been enabled to tell other people at school, she may have been able to break out of her SM earlier, as she had wished.

★ Rachel probably uses the words 'refused' and 'wouldn't' because this is the way she has heard other people speak about her anxious reaction to pressure to talk or open her mouth.

★ Rachel's account shows how parents and teachers who have understood SM can be a great support and help. This illustrates that direct intervention from SLTs or psychologists, and assessment and formal diagnosis, are not essential to recovery.

★ Carl describes the enmeshment of his SM with his emotions; Sarah-Jane describes how she grew up feeling unimportant and invisible; Vivienne came to see herself as a bad child. We believe that not having an explanation of SM affected their self-image.

★ Vivienne's struggle to understand why she couldn't read to her teacher further emphasises the need to explain SM to the people it affects.

★ In Carl's, Sarah-Jane's and Vivienne's early lives they point to a lack of good bonding with their parents, or an 'unhappy environment', playing a significant part in the causes of their SM and lifelong low self-esteem. The positive effects of warm, consistent attachment cannot be underestimated in helping a child get over SM and emerge as a confident young person.

★ Carl's and Sarah-Jane's accounts of inappropriate and invasive physical and sexual contact are disturbing to read. They highlight the importance of ensuring that all children are supported to disclose such events to the people closest to them. It is also important to consider how children who did *not* have SM would have handled these situations; and to reflect on the changes in Safeguarding awareness and legislation over the last 30 years.

★ Sarah-Jane describes well how to recognise her fears and face them – the importance of rational thought to override anxiety and take control. She also describes effective general anxiety-management strategies.

★ The effect of Sarah-Jane's SM on her writing ability is not uncommon. We have seen this in several young people, although it manifests in different ways.

★ There are some examples of unacceptably harsh treatment towards Carl and Vivienne and punishment for Sarah-Jane; thankfully, such reactions seem less common with today's children. However, we also see parents and teachers who have not shown 'tough-enough love'. They have inadvertently made too many allowances and facilitated avoidance, rather than helping their children to face their fears. This can be just as detrimental to the children's progress.

If you would like to read some other helpful life stories, we recommend the stories of Ann and Holly in Benita Rae Smith & Alice Sluckin's book *Tackling Selective Mutism* (2015).

INDEX

Notes:

1. Page numbers may be accompanied by '*b*', '*f*' or '*t*' to denote reference to a box, figure or table.

2. After activating the online resource library, you may use the CTRL + F keys to search for any word or phrase.